RETINOPATHY

of

PREMATURITY

Current Concepts

and

Controversies

ALICE R. McPHERSON, M.D.

Clinical Professor, Department of Ophthalmology
Cullen Eye Institute
Baylor College of Medicine
Houston, Texas

HELEN M. HITTNER, M.D.

Clinical Professor of Ophthalmology and Pediatrics
Cullen Eye Institute and Department of Pediatrics
Baylor College of Medicine
Houston, Texas

FRANK L. KRETZER, PH.D.

Assistant Professor of Ophthalmology and Cell Biology
Cullen Eye Institute
Baylor College of Medicine
Houston, Texas

1986

B.C. DECKER INC • Toronto • Philadelphia

Publisher

B.C. Decker Inc.
3228 South Service Road
Burlington, Ontario L7N 3H8

B.C. Decker Inc.
P.O. Box 30246
Philadelphia, Pennsylvania 19103

Sales and Distribution

United States and Possessions	**The C.V. Mosby Company** 11830 Westline Industrial Drive Saint Louis, Missouri 63146
Canada	**The C.V. Mosby Company, Ltd.** 5240 Finch Avenue East, Unit No. 1 Scarborough, Ontario M1S 4P2
United Kingdom, Europe and the Middle East	**Blackwell Scientific Publications, Ltd.** Osney Mead, Oxford OX2 OEL, England
Australia	**Holt-Saunders Pty. Limited** 9 Waltham Street Artarmon, N.S.W. 2064 Australia
Japan	**Igaku-Shoin Ltd.** Tokyo International P.O. Box 5063 1-28-36 Hongo, Bunkyo-ku, Tokyo 113, Japan
Asia	**Holt-Saunders Asia Limited** 10/F, Inter-Continental Plaza Tsim Sha Tsui East Kowloon, Hong Kong

Retinopathy of Prematurity *Current Concepts and Controversies*   ISBN 0–941158–93–4

Library of Congress catalog card number: 85-073803

10 9 8 7 6 5 4 3 2 1

Publication of this book
was made possible by
The Retina Research Foundation
Houston, Texas

CONTRIBUTORS

JAMES M. ADAMS, M.D.

Associate Professor of Clinical Pediatrics, Baylor College of Medicine; Director, Neonatal Intensive Care Unit, Texas Children's Hospital, Houston, Texas
Intensive Care of the Low-Birth-Weight Infant

ISAAC BEN-SIRA, M.D.

Associate Professor of Ophthalmology, Tel-Aviv University Sackler Medical School; Chairman, Department of Ophthalmology, Beilinson Medical Center, Petach Tikva, Israel
Treatment of Acute Retinopathy of Prematurity with Cryotherapy: The Beilinson Experience

JEROME W. BETTMAN, M.D.

Emeritus Clinical Professor of Ophthalmology, Pacific Medical Center, Stanford University and University of California, San Francisco, California
Medicolegal Aspects of Retinopathy of Prematurity

BARUCH A. BRODY, Ph.D.

Leon Jaworsky Professor of Biomedical Ethics, Baylor College of Medicine, Houston, Texas.
The Vitamin E Study: The Ethics of Experimentation

STEVE CHARLES, M.D.

Clinical Associate Professor, Department of Ophthalmology, University of Tennessee College of Medicine, Memphis, Tennessee
Vitrectomy with Ciliary Body Entry for Retrolental Fibroplasia

DONNA GOAD, M.D.

Research Assistant, Cullen Eye Institute, Baylor College of Medicine, Houston, Texas
Animal Models in Research on Retinopathy of Prematurity

N. WARREN HINDLE, M.D.

Associate Professor of Surgery, Emeritus, Department of Ophthalmology, University of Calgary Faculty of Medicine; Director, Department of Ophthalmology, Alberta Children's Provincial General Hospital, Calgary, Alberta, Canada
Location and Timing of Intervention with Cryotherapy

HELEN MINTZ HITTNER, M.D.

Clinical Professor of Ophthalmology and Pediatrics, Baylor College of Medicine, Houston, Texas
Human Retinal Development: Relationship to the Pathogenesis of Retinopathy of Prematurity
Differential Diagnosis of Retinopathy of Prematurity
Animal Models in Research on Retinopathy of Prematurity
Efficacy of Vitamin E in Retinopathy of Prematurity
Toxicity of Vitamin E in Preterm Infants
Treatment of Acute Retinopathy of Prematurity with Cryotherapy
Treatment of Acute Retinopathy of Prematurity by Scleral Buckling
Treatment of Retrolental Fibroplasia with Open-Sky Vitrectomy

JAMES D. KINGHAM, M.D.

Director, Sarasota Retina Institute, Sarasota, Florida
Classification of Retinopathy of Prematurity

FRANK L. KRETZER, Ph.D.

Assistant Professor of Ophthalmology and Cell Biology, Baylor College of Medicine, Houston, Texas
Human Retinal Development: Relationship to the Pathogenesis of Retinopathy of Prematurity
Differential Diagnosis of Retinopathy of Prematurity
Animal Models in Research on Retinopathy of Prematurity
Efficacy of Vitamin E in Retinopathy of Prematurity
Toxicity of Vitamin E in Preterm Infants
Treatment of Acute Retinopathy of Prematurity with Cryotherapy
Treatment of Acute Retinopathy of Prematurity by Scleral Buckling
Treatment of Retrolental Fibroplasia with Open-Sky Vitrectomy

REKHA S. MEHTA, B.S.

Research Associate, Cullen Eye Institute, Baylor College of Medicine, Houston, Texas
Animal Models in Research on Retinopathy of Prematurity

ALICE R. McPHERSON, M.D.

Clinical Professor, Department of Ophthalmology, Cullen Eye Institute, Baylor College of Medicine, Houston, Texas
Treatment of Acute Retinopathy of Prematurity with Cryotherapy
Treatment of Acute Retinopathy of Prematurity by Scleral Buckling
Treatment of Retrolental Fibroplasia with Open-Sky Vitrectomy

ROBERT A. MOURA, M.D.

Associate Professor, Department of Ophthalmology, Cullen Eye Institute, Baylor College of Medicine, Houston, Texas
Treatment of Retrolental Fibroplasia with Open-Sky Vitrectomy

ILANA NISSENKORN, M.D.

Assistant Professor of Ophthalmology, Tel Aviv University Sackler Medical School; Consultant of Pediatric Ophthalmology, Member of Staff, Beilinson Medical Center Petach Tikva, Israel
Treatment of Acute Retinopathy of Prematurity with Cryotherapy: The Beilinson Experience

JUAN ORELLANA, M.D.

Assistant Professor, Mount Sinai School of Medicine; Assistant Director, Department of Ophthalmology, Director Pediatric Retinal Service, Beth Israel Medical Center, New York, New York
Identification of Retinopathy of Prematurity/Retrolental Fibroplasia
Examination of the Premature Infant

H. HOLLIS OXSPRING, M.D., Ph.D.

Clinical Instructor, Department of Anesthesiology, Baylor College of Medicine; Assistant, Active Staff, Methodist Hospital, Houston, Texas
Anesthetic Considerations in Surgery for Retinopathy of Prematurity

JIM M. PERDUE, B.S., J.D.

Partner, Perdue, Turner & Berry, Houston, Texas
Medicolegal Issues Presented through Retinopathy of Prematurity: The Standard of Care Issue

MAKOTO TAMAI, M.D.

Associate Professor of Ophthalmology, Tohoku University School of Medicine; Vice Director of Ophthalmology, Tohoku University Hospital, Sendai, Japan
Treatment of Acute Retinopathy of Prematurity by Cryotherapy and Photocoagulation

VINCENT WHITEHEAD, M.D., M.B., B.Chir.

Clinical Instructor, Department of Anesthesiology, Baylor College of Medicine; Attending, Active Staff, Methodist Hospital, Houston, Texas
Anesthetic Considerations in Surgery for Retinopathy of Prematurity

PREFACE

Since Terry first described retrolental fibroplasia in 1942, this dread disorder of premature infants has baffled the ophthalmologist, plagued the neonatologist, and blinded thousands of preterm infants. Once oxygen was identified as the offending agent and its use in incubators was curtailed in the 1950s, the incidence of retrolental fibroplasia was reduced markedly. Despite sophisticated monitoring, however, a second epidemic arose in the mid 1970s, coincident with technological advances that made routine the survival of very low birth weight infants. The paradox arose that in order to save the life of the preterm infant weighing less than 1,000 grams, the requisite use of oxygen leads to retinopathy of prematurity, or retrolental fibroplasia.

Our purposes in preparing the present work are threefold: To review the pathogenesis and histopathology in light of the current prevalence of retrolental fibroplasia; to examine the dilemma of vitamin E efficacy versus toxicity; and to survey available surgical modalities including cryotherapy, photocoagulation, vitrectomy, and scleral buckling. The first two sections of the book review fundamental clinical considerations and basic features of the disorder and its diagnosis. A new concept of pathogenesis is set forth in Chapter 4. Medicolegal issues are examined in two separate articles, one by a physician and the other by an attorney.

No single means of prophylaxis or treatment has eliminated or arrested the disorder entirely. Among the newer approaches is the use of vitamin E to protect the retina during the administration of supplemental oxygen; we recognize the controversy surrounding the modality, yet feel that its use as an adjuvant to therapy is sufficiently promising that we examine the role of vitamin E in a separate section of the book entailing four chapters.

The technique and results from five centers are included in the section on surgery. Selection of patients, timing of therapy, surgical procedures, and follow-up care as practiced by several experienced ophthalmologists are detailed so that the reader may compare approaches and results of treatment and apply the experience to his or her own practice.

We would like to express our gratitude to the authors who contributed their expertise to the volume. We would also like to acknowledge a debt of gratitude to the Retina Research Foundation for its support of ongoing research and clinical investigation into the retinopathy of prematurity.

Alice R. McPherson, M.D.
Helen M. Hittner, M.D.
Frank L. Kretzer, Ph.D.

December, 1985

CONTENTS

RETINOPATHY OF PREMATURITY
Current Concepts and Controversies

SURGERY FOR RETINOPATHY OF PREMATURITY AND RETROLENTAL FIBROPLASIA

Identification of Retinopathy of Prematurity/Retrolental Fibroplasia

Juan Orellana, M.D.

W wiliam A. Silverman described in 1980 the events that led to Terry's documentation of retrolental fibroplasia (RLF) in 1941 (Fig. 1–1).[1] Terry's original paper[2] described the initial case seen by a Boston pediatrician, as well as subsequent patients examined by Terry at the Massachusetts Eye and Ear Infirmary. He was unsure if these patients had a persistent vascular structure of the fetal vitreous or a fibroblastic overgrowth of the persistent tunica vasculosa lentis. He thought this tissue developed postnatally, because no anlage existed during embryogenesis. He expected to see these changes in a certain percentage of premature infants.

Overall, 74 of the 100 infants he examined weighed 3.5 pounds or less at birth. Heredity did not seem to play a role; however, he hypothesized that the prematures' nutritional deficiencies, retinal overexposure to light, intraocular inflammation, premature closure of the ductus, an increase or decrease in blood oxygenation, a decreased ambient temperature, and a lack of maternal hormonal support were possibly instrumental in the development of RLF (Table 1–1).[3-8] Several of his published papers dealt with the experimental manipulation of the hyaloid system and tunica vasculosa lentis to produce an animal model for RLF.

Reese and Payne of New York City[9] viewed it as a congenital condition in either premature or full-term babies, comprised of persistent primary vitreous, and vitreous hemorrhage causing secondary changes including a ruptured lens capsule, and glaucoma. There was also an association between RLF and skin hemangiomas, resulting from the angioblastic mesoderm both in the skin and primary vitreous; clinicians had previously noted that hemangiomas occurred more frequently in premature children.[10] Krause[11] studied 18 children in whom he noted retinal atrophy, gliosis, and retinal detachment. His clinical and microscopic findings led him to postulate that the disease represented the sum of various con-

genital defects and was characterized by retinal and cerebral hypoplasia and hyperplasia.

Sporadic cases appeared in the literature over the next several years; however, by 1949 retinopathy of prematurity (ROP)[12] was responsible for 30 percent of blindness seen in preschool children in the United States. In 1948, Owens and Owens of Baltimore ophthalmoscopically observed that normal fundi in premature infants undergo a transformation over several weeks.[13] They noted congested, dilated, tortuous retinal vessels as an early sign (Fig. 1–2). This was followed by peripheral eleva-

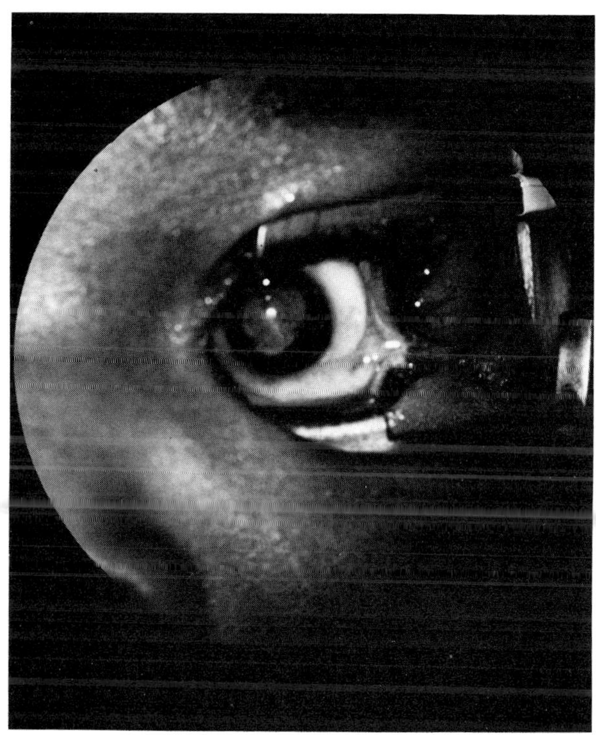

Figure 1–1 Terry's initial case had a white retrolental mass, which he initially diagnosed as a congenital cataract. Subsequently he attempted to produce an animal model of ROP by experimental manipulation of the hyaloid system and tunica vasculosa lentis.

TABLE 1–1 Summary of Major Clinical Ideas Proposed by Terry, 1942-1945

Article	*Findings*
Extreme prematurity and fibroblastic overgrowth of persistent vascular sheath behind each crystalline lens[2]	5 cases noted: the condition might represent a persistent hyperplastic vitreous or an overgrowth of the tunica vasculosa lentis; he believed it developed postnatally in a premature infant
Fibroblastic overgrowth of persistent tunica vasculosa lentis in premature infants[3]	The syndrome was based on the persistence of some part of the tunica vasculosa lentis, growth of connective tissue behind the lens, and persistent fibrillar vitreous; prematurity was important to its development; heredity, drugs, ocular trauma, light toxicity, maternal hormonal insufficiency, nutritional deficiencies, anemia, and erythroblastosis fetalis were considered minor contributors
Retrolental fibroplasia in premature infants[6]	12% of all prematures weighing $\leq 1,307$ g developed RLF; radiation was damaging and did not ameliorate the RLF; glaucoma is a frequent complication; aqueous humor dynamics might leave a lens dependent on the hyaloid system and tunica; both systems were forced to persist; surgical attempts to create new vascular connections between the ciliary body and episclera might be useful
Ocular maldevelopment in extremely premature infants[7]	Terry expected to see 600 cases per year; the basis of the disease was the presence of a functioning hyaloid artery and tunica vasculosa lentis in infants born 3- to 4-weeks premature; increased exposure to light might be a major cause of the disease; he advised that a child be kept in a dark room with a red light; treat the child by preventing glaucoma and posterior synechiae

tions, generalized retinal edema, and finally, vascularized vitreous membranes with organization. The change in blood vessels began 2.5 to 3.5 months postnatally, and by six months four percent had developed RLF. Owens and Owens postulated that this disease had a postnatal etiology, and that a persistence or abnormality of the hyaloid system was not involved.

Kinsey and Zacharias conducted a large encompassing study to determine the relationship of numerous conditions to subsequently developing ROP.[14] Among the factors were maternal age, blood type, delivery of anesthesia, parity, type of delivery, sex of the infant, and anomalies. A relationship existed between ROP, vitamin-E levels, iron levels, and the presence of oxygen. Previously, Unsworth had suggested anemia as an underlying cause of ROP.[15]

Owens and Owens investigated the role of vitamin E, alpha-tocopherol, in the development of ROP.[16] They believed that the infant's depressed vitamin E levels, coupled with experimental evidence of its ability to overcome fibrosis in animals, made its study worthwhile. They administered 150 mg of alpha-tocopheryl acetate by mouth every day—initiated as soon as the infant was able to take it orally—during the ten-month study period, and observed an initial success that could not be repeated at other institutions.

Premature infants were also thought to have low levels of corticotropin (ACTH); since RLF appeared to have a connective tissue component, ACTH was tried. Reese and associates[17] in New York City demonstrated that it was not beneficial.

In other parts of the world, recognition of the disease was slower to evolve. Among the first British reports were those issued by Galloway[18], Martin[19], and Franklin[20] in 1950; however, the incidence remained lower than that seen in the United States. Crosse noted that the early RLF cases were being seen in Birmingham,

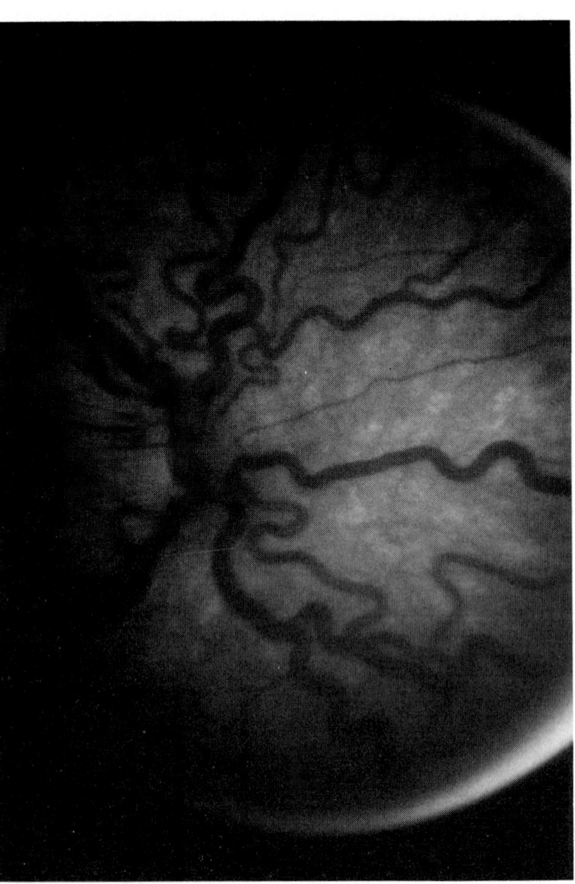

Figure 1–2 Vascular congestion, dilation and tortuosity, as seen here, were thought to be early signs of ROP in the days of direct ophthalmoscopes. As the indirect ophthalmoscope became popular, more infants were examined, and it became evident that the early changes occurred in the periphery.

England between 1946 and 1950, after none had been seen in 1945.[21]

Early cases from France, as well as Sweden, were reported in 1948. Between 1947 and 1951, isolated reports from Switzerland, Italy, Israel, Cuba, Canada, South Africa, and Australia appeared in the literature. Clinicians put forth a plethora of etiologies to explain this disease, and Silverman[22] compiled a summary.

The Role of Oxygen

The question of too much versus too little oxygen as the cause of RLF took some time to resolve. Szewczyk[23] observed changes in vessel caliber and tortuosity in preterm infants when they were taken from an incubator (50% O_2 concentration) to the basinet (22% O_2 concentration). Based on their study of the offspring of hypoxic rats, Ingalls and associates[24] pointed to fetal hypoxia as an etiologic agent. Other investigators also stated that this disease resulted from hypoxia[25,26] or a relative anoxia.[27] Several authors theorized that oxygen was damaging because of its toxic effects, or that the relative early anoxia followed by high levels of continuous oxygen exposure were to blame for RLF. Some failed to see any association between RLF and oxygen administration.[28,29]

Campbell[30] noted that patients who paid for oxygen administration (and thus received less oxygen) had a lower incidence than did the group for which oxygen was given through third-party payment (and thus received more oxygen). Similarly, Ryan in Australia[31], and Goldman and Tobler in Europe[32], noted increased incidence of RLF in infants exposed to higher levels of oxygen while still in incubators. Ryan believed that the prematurity arrested ocular development and that the oxygen then stimulated a superimposed aberrant development.[31] In England, Crosse and Evans[33] pointed out that limited oxygen therapy produced fewer cases of RLF than did liberal administration. Long[34] advised that careful observations be made in the premature infants before definitely implicating oxygen as a cause of RLF.

Patz and associates[35] correlated high oxygen levels with the occurrence of RLF in premature infants. On a random basis, they exposed two groups of infants to oxygen in a "high" or "low" concentration. After one year, 25 percent of those children in the high oxygen group had advanced RLF, whereas no advanced cases were seen in the low oxygen group. A subsequent controlled study reiterated the significant association between RLF and high oxygen exposure.[36] Kinsey's multicentered tri-

al confirmed the correlation between overzealous oxygen therapy and development of the disease.[37] Most important, the concept of high oxygen concentration over a long period, as Ryan[31] previously postulated, was confirmed as detrimental.

Investigators attempted to induce RLF in animals. In 1952, Gyllensten and Hellstrom[38] demonstrated the adverse effects of oxygen on mice showing intraocular hemorrhage, tunica vasculosa lentis hyperplasia, and separation of the neurosensory retina from the pigment layer, as well as vascular, cellular, and fibrous tissue in the retina. Ashton and associates[39] examined kittens and observed vasoconstriction and retinal vessel obliteration under hyperoxic conditions. The obliteration occurred during prolonged hypoxia and paralleled the extent of vessel immaturity, the duration, and concentration of oxygen therapy. Reinstatement of the animal into room air reopened the vessels; however, a network of neovascularization developed. Exposing a more mature feline's retinal vasculature to oxygen did not adversely affect the ocular structures.[40].

Patz and associates[41] demonstrated endothelial nodules in the nerve fiber layer with proliferative neovascularization into the vitreous in mice and rats raised in an oxygen environment. They also pointed out the ocular and systemic effects of oxygen therapy in opossums, kittens, and dogs. Patz suggested that an oxygen analyzer should be placed in premature nurseries, and that oxygen therapy be a specific medical order. These and other laboratory studies provided the early clues that RLF was linked to oxygen therapy.[42-44]

Pathogenesis

The method of oxygen interaction with the retina remains in question. The spindle cells that travel in the nerve fiber layer are derived from the mesenchyme of the hyaloid system. These cells are the precursors of the vascular system as it travels toward the ora serrata.[45] In the human, the spindle cells enter the nerve fiber layer at the disc's edge at 4-months gestation. The nasal ora serrata is reached by inner retinal vasculature[46] at 8 months, and the temporal ora serrata is reached at 9 months. Once vascularization is complete, oxygen will not affect the retina.[39,47] Patz describes two stages of retinal reaction to oxygen: vasoconstriction and secondary vasoproliferation.[48] The concentration of oxygen, duration of exposure, and extent of normal vascularized retina determine the extent to which the retina will undergo vasoconstriction. The return to room air triggers

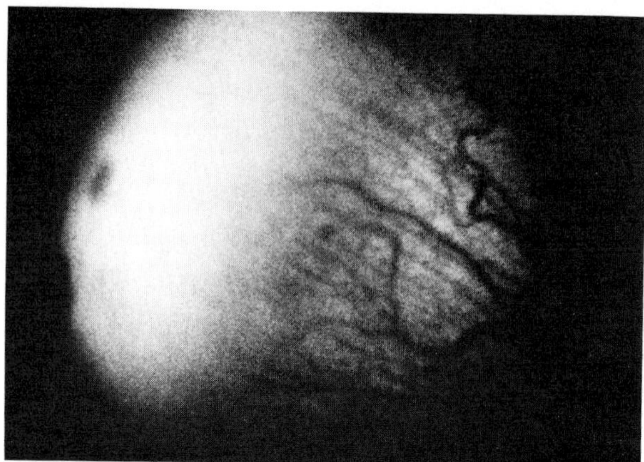

Figure 1–3 Fluorescein angiography using 0.1 cc of 10% fluorescein demonstrates the leakage present at the shunt line due to excessive neovascularization.

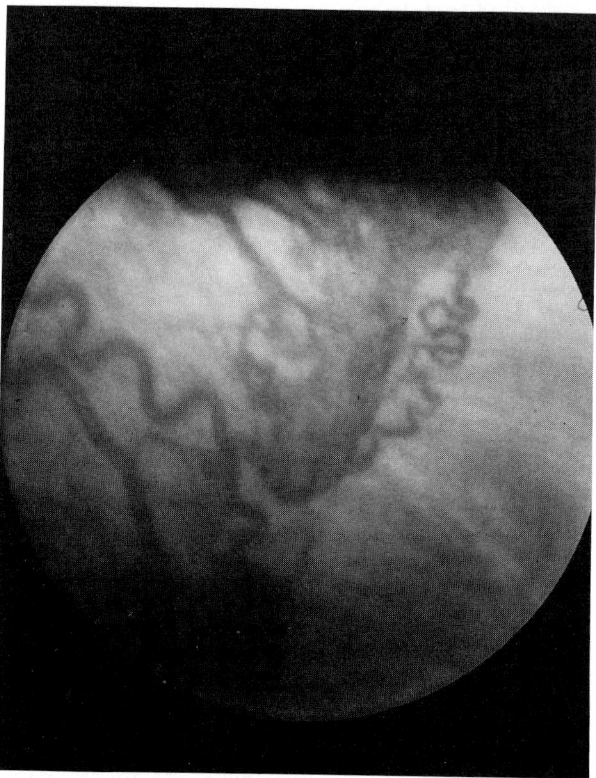

Figure 1–4 Peripheral neovascular vessels are fragile and may produce a vitreous hemorrhage.

the subsequent vasoproliferative stage.[49,50] The new vessels are quite permeable to fluorescein and easily hemorrhage (Fig. 1–3).[51]

Recent studies implicate the spindle cell as the inducer of ROP, because of its interaction with oxygen.[52] This theory is intermingled with the role played by vitamin E, an antioxidant and free-radical scavenger (Chapters 4 and 9).[53-61]

Friedenwald and associates[62] first described proliferating capillary endothelial nodules in the human retina, noting abnormal budding of the capillaries in the nerve fiber layer; moreover, they observed an increased number of what they called "glial cells" in the nerve fiber layer. Serpell[63] noted that these actively proliferating cells were mesenchymal and contained polysaccharide granules (glycogen); they were spindle-shaped precursors of the retinal vascular system. Reese and associates[64] observed neovascularization even when no retinal detachment existed.

Heath, in 1950, studied autopsied eyes of premature children and noted three separate stages: *a* primary retinal disease, *b* vitreous involvement and detachment of the retina, and *c* late repair and atrophy. Histopathological evaluation showed albuminous edema from leaking capillaries and retinal hemorrhages. RLF was "primarily an edematous, hemorrhagic and proliferative process associated with hamartomatous neovascular tissue in the retina."[65] In a subsequent paper[12] Heath called RLF "retinopathy of prematurity" and reiterated his previous findings. He noted endothelial budding and proliferation of superficial neovascular tissue. Angiofibrous changes in the retina resulted in rapid vitreous changes that he believed produced a retinal detachment. The atrophic stage was nonspecific and could be accompanied by glaucoma.

Reese and associates[66] noted that transudation and neovascularization were first seen in the extreme fundus periphery. Proliferating endothelial cells canalized and broke through the internal limiting membrane. The nerve fiber layer in this region became edematous. Newly formed vessels hemorrhaged and this eventually broke into the vitreous (Fig. 1–4). Should a greater portion of the retina become involved, the contracture would produce a retinal detachment. They found no evidence of an inflammatory process, nor that nonattachment of

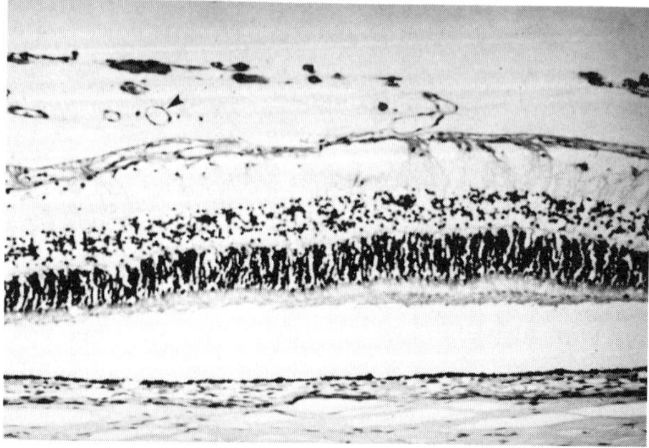

Figure 1–5 Extraretinal neovascularization. There is hemorrhage from these neovascular vessels (arrow). Hematoxylin + Eosin × 120.

the retina played a role in the pathogenesis of the disease, as Wolff[67] previously theorized. In essence, Reese and associates believed it was neovascularization that began in the retina and advanced into the vitreous (Fig. 1–5).

Ashton held that thickening of the nerve fiber layer resulted from endothelial and mesenchymal cells proliferating, thus producing RLF.[68] The earliest histological change was proliferation of vasoformative tissue in the inner layers, with subsequent invasion into the vitreous through the internal limiting membrane and hyaloid face. Ward histologically examined premature infant eyes to find early signs of RLF, or changes that might predispose an infant to develop it.[69] He noted that 13 percent of infants had increased vasoformative tissue in the nerve fiber layer; however, no other changes of RLF accompanied these findings.

Foos catalogued a progression of the disease, starting with a thickening of the vanguard region into a ridge in which vessels lay posterior to the advancing vanguard.[70] He noted spindle cells in the nerve fiber layer and the rearguard composed of endothelial cells.

The extraretinal aspect consisted of the passing of neovascular capillaries in the rearguard into the vitreous (Fig. 1–6). These vessels contained endothelial cells and pericytes. With additional development, the extraretinal tissue also contained endothelial cell nodules. Kushner and associates[71] studied the ridge region and documented the intraretinal ridge as a "circumferentially oriented arterial-venous shunt" in the eye; they also noted capillary obliteration around arteries and veins.

RLF can also occur in full-term infants, either in those briefly exposed[72] or not exposed to oxygen.[73] Tissue hypoxia, or the reversal of a congenital condition that interferes with the oxygen-carrying capacity of the blood, will end in a picture consistent with RLF.[73-75]

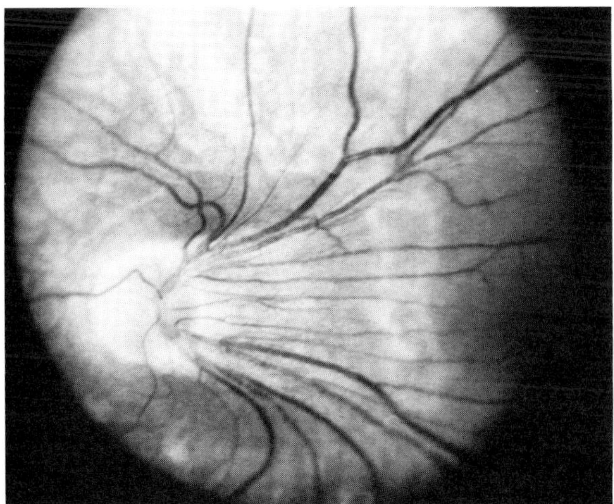

Figure 1–7 Mild dragging of the retina and retinal vessels. Visual acuity is 20/40 in this patient, even with temporal displacement of the macula.

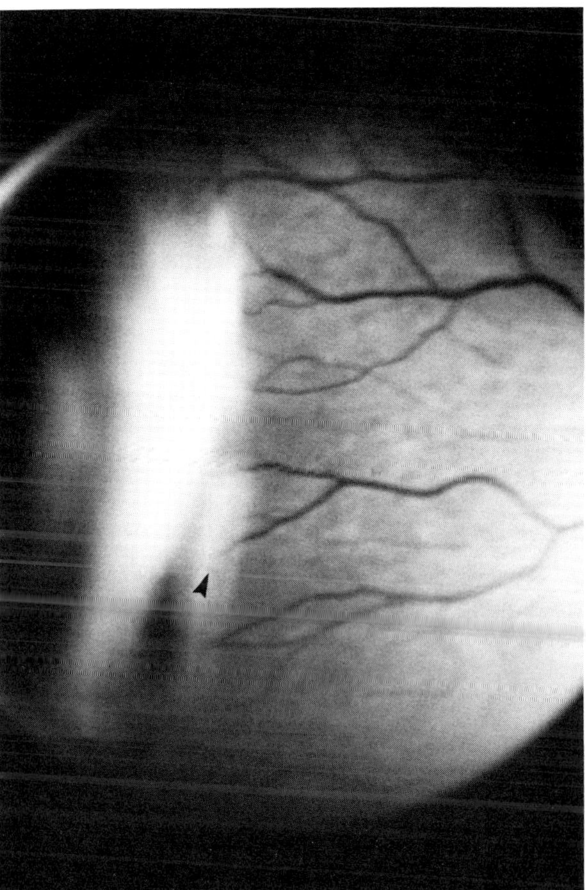

Figure 1–8 A vitreous membrane over the retina (arrow). This is the only indication of prior active disease.

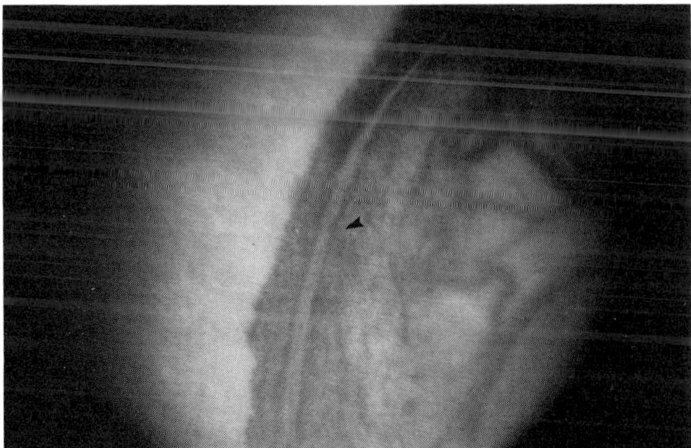

Figure 1–6 Excessive intraretinal and extraretinal neovascularization. The extraretinal vessels are originating from the rearguard retina and passing into the vitreous (arrow).

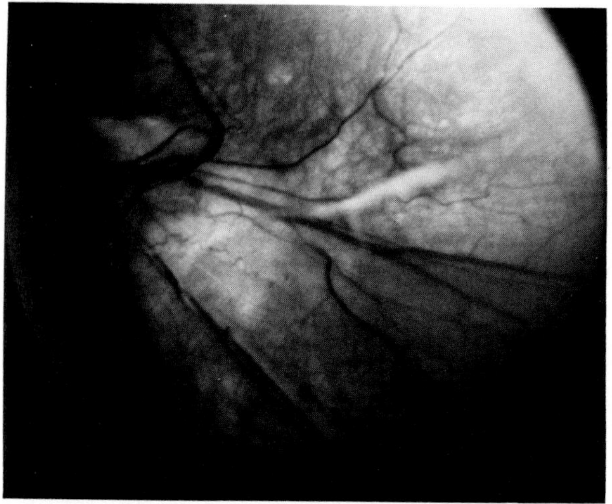

Figure 1–9 Dragging of the disc, retina and retinal vessels. A vitreous membrane lies over the retina. Although the retina is dragged inferio-temporal, the macula lies just above the membrane.

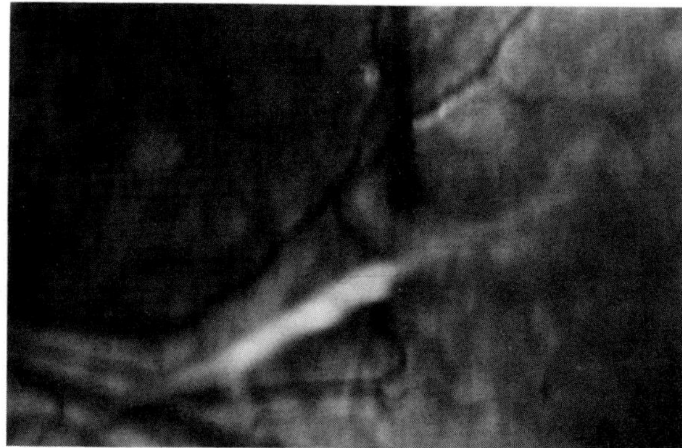

Figure 1–10 When asked to fixate, the patient depicted in Figure 1–9 is able to do so. This photograph was taken when the patient was asked to fixate at a target inside the fundus camera.

However, hyperoxemia does not always produce a cicatricial end product.[76] Of 20 infants who had sustained aortic PO_2 values greater than 150 mm for 10 to 43 hours, only one child had cicatricial disease after 5 months.

Classification and Incidence

Cicatricial disease can vary from mild to severe. Spontaneous resolution of active ROP can occur at any stage; a majority of Stages 1 and 2 resolve without sequelae or intervention.[13,77] A smaller percentage of cases (Stages 3 and 4) resolve on their own; however, clues will be evident that suggest a prior active state. Reese and associates[78] set forth the original classification of RLF that has, for the most part, remained unchanged. In essence, Grade I is characterized by myopia,[79] retinal pigmentation, equatorial retinal folds, and vitreous membranes (Fig. 1–7).[80] Asymmetric myopia can be present, and adequate visual function seems to be the rule in these cases.[79] Features of Grade II include a dragged macular region,[80,81] peripheral patches of neovascularization, and elevated blood vessels that can hemorrhage in later years (Figs. 1–8 to 1–10). A higher incidence of lattice degeneration (15%) is present in these patients, versus the general population (6 to 7%). Temporal vitreoretinal traction, producing breaks, can also be present. Falciform retinal folds are seen in Grade III, primarily in the temporal quadrants (Fig. 1–11). These folds can traverse the macula and limit visual function. Retinal detachment is present in Grade IV; it can be serous or tractional. Leukocoria with an organized retrolental mass is seen in Grade V disease (Fig. 1–12).

The topic of oxygen concentration went through a stage of initial curtailment, reducing the numbers of RLF cases.[35,36] This, however, was followed by the awareness that curtailment of oxygen would increase the perinatal mortality.[82]

Kalina and Karr[83] noted the incidence of ROP/RLF in surviving neonates from 1960 through 1980. From 1960 through 1967, there was a 14 percent incidence of cicatricial RLF, and from 1968 through 1980, 20 percent of 140 infants developed cicatrical disease.

Davidorff[84] reported no incidence in 1971, which blossomed into an incidence of 34 percent in 1979. Phelps[85] calculated, based on birth-weight-specific published survival figures and ROP incidence data, that 546 children would be blinded by RLF in 1979. Harris[86] noted that the incidence in Canada was 18 cases per year from 1970 to 1974, and the disease still represented a significant cause of blindness in Canada.

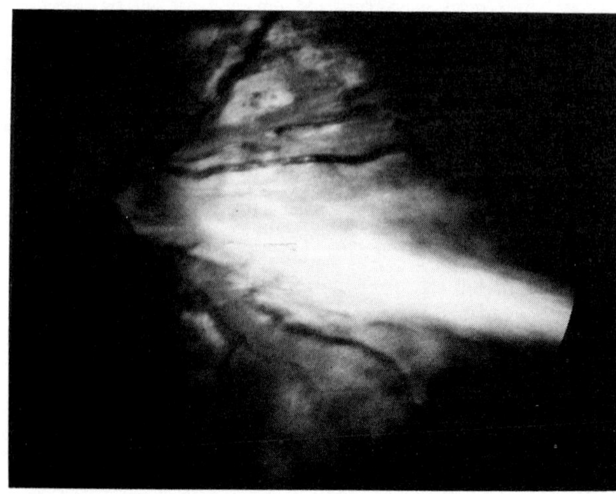

Figure 1–11 A falciform fold traverses the macula, severely limiting visual acuity.

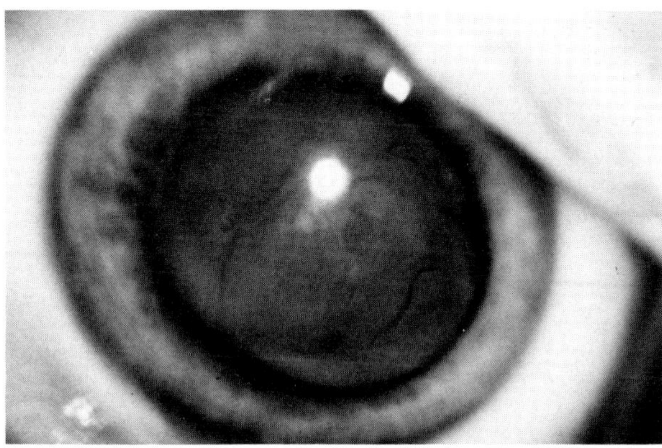

Figure 1–12   A retrolental cicatricial mass. Surgery in these cases is currently being done; however, the visual prognosis is guarded. Early treatment with vitamin E may serve to reduce the number of these cases. Earlier surgical intervention may have prevented this previously untreated result.

Several factors might be responsible for the increase in new cases of RLF. Improved respiratory and nutritional support in specialized neonatal centers, as well as an improved physiological understanding of premature infants, have increased the infants' survival rate. In 1978, the survival rate for infants weighing between 1 and 1.5 kg was 70 percent, but for those less than 1 kg, it was 26 percent.[87] In 1979, it was 50 percent for those weighing between 750 g and 1 kg.[88] As in earlier years, those children under 1.5 kg are at greater risk of developing RLF and more of these neonates are surviving. Studies assessing factors can be used to predict which neonate (less than 1.5 g) will develop acute disease.[89]

The story of ROP is still unfolding. The notion of establishing a uniform classification for acute ROP has only recently come to fruition as the International Classification (see Chapter 3). Prior to this, several authors proposed classifications.[75, 90–96]

REFERENCES

1. Silverman WA. Retrolental Fibroplasia. A Modern Parable. New York: Grune and Stratton, 1980, 1–7.
2. Terry TL. Extreme prematurity and fibroplastic overgrowth of persistent vascular sheath behind each crystalline lens. I. Preliminary report. Am J Ophthalmol 1942; 25:203–204.
3. Terry TL. Fibroplastic overgrowth of persistent tunica vasculosa lentis in infants born prematurely. III. Studies in development and regression of hyaloid artery and tunica vasculosa lentis. Am J Ophthalmol 1942; 25:1409–1423.
4. Terry TL. Fibroplastic overgrowth of persistent tunica vasculosa lentis in premature infants. II. Report of cases—clinical aspects. Arch Ophthalmol 1943; 29:36–53.
5. Terry TL. Fibroplastic overgrowth of persistent tunica vasculosa lentis in premature infants. IV. Etiologic factors. Arch Ophthalmol 1943; 29:54–68.
6. Terry TL. Retrolental fibroplasia in premature infants. V. Further studies on fibroblastic overgrowth of persistent tunica vasculosa lentis. Arch Ophthalmol 1945; 33:203–208. Trans Am Ophthalmol Soc 1944; 42:383–396.
7. Terry TL. Ocular maldevelopment in extremely premature infants: retrolental fibroplasia; general considerations. JAMA 1945; 128:582–585.
8. Terry TL. Retrolental fibroplasia. In: Levine SZ, et al, eds. Advances in pediatrics, Vol 3. New York: Interscience Publishers, Inc., 1948.
9. Reese AB, Payne J. Persistence and hyperplasia of the primary vitreous. Tunica vasculosa lentis or retrolental fibroplasia. Am J Ophthalmol 1946; 29:1–24.
10. Howard H. A case showing multiple congenital abnormalities of the eye, the origin of the vitreous indicated by one of them. Trans Am Ophthalmol Soc 1917; 15:244–301.
11. Krause AC. Congenital encephalo-ophthalmic dysplasia. Arch Ophthalmol 1946; 36:387–444.
12. Heath P. Pathology of retinopathy of prematurity: retrolental fibroplasia. Am J Ophthalmol 1951; 43:1249–1259.
13. Owens WC, Owens EW. Retrolental fibroplasia in premature infants. Trans Am Acad Ophthalmol Otolaryngol 1948; 53:18–41.
14. Kinsey VE, Zacharias L. Retrolental fibroplasia. JAMA 1949; 139:572–578.
15. Unsworth AC. Retrolental fibroplasia. A preliminary report. Arch Ophthalmol 1948; 40:341–346.
16. Owens WC, Owens EU. Retrolental fibroplasia in premature Infants. II. Studies on the prophylaxis of the disease: the use of alpha tocopheryl acetate. Am J Ophthalmol 1949; 32:1631–1637.
17. Reese AB, Blodi FC, Locke JC, Silverman WA, Day RL. Results of use of corticotropin (ACTH) in treatment of retrolental fibroplasia. Arch Ophthalmol 1952; 47:551–555.
18. Galloway NPR. Fibrosis of the posterior vascular sheath of the lens. Proc Roy Soc Med 1948; 4:724.
19. Martin, JK. Retrolental fibroplasia occurring in twins. Proc Roy Soc Med 1950; 43:235.
20. Franklin AW. Retrolental fibroplasia in a premature baby. Proc Roy Soc Med 1950; 43:235–236.
21. Crosse VM. Retrolental fibroplasia. Proc Roy Soc Med 1950; 43:232–236.
22. Silverman WA. Retrolental Fibroplasia. A Modern Parable. New York: Grune and Stratton, 1980; 165–172.
23. Szewczyk TS. Retrolental fibroplasia; etiology and prophylaxis. A preliminary report. Am J Ophthalmol 1951; 34:149–165.
24. Ingalls TH, Tedeschi CG, Halpern MM. Congenital malformations of the eye induced in mice by maternal anoxia: with particular reference to the problem of retrolental fibroplasia in man. Am J Ophthalmol 1952; 35:311–329.
25. Jefferson E. Retrolental fibroplasia. Arch Dis Child 1952; 27:329–336.
26. Klien BA. Histopathologic aspects of retrolental fibroplasia. Arch Ophthalmol 1949; 41:553–561.
27. Szewczyk TS. Retrolental fibroplasia; etiology and prophylaxis. Am J Ophthalmol 1952; 35:301–310.
28. Zacharias L. Retrolental fibroplasia. Survey. Am J Ophthalmol 1952; 35:1427–1454.
29. Exlive AL Jr, Harrington MR. Retrolental fibroplasia: clinical statistics from the Premature Center of Charity Hospital of Louisiana at New Orleans. J Pediatr 1951; 38:1–7.
30. Campbell K. Intensive oxygen therapy as a possible cause of retrolental fibroplasia: a clinical approach. Med J Aust 1951; 2:48–50.
31. Ryan H. Retrolental fibroplasia. A clinicopathologic study. Am J Ophthalmol 1952; 35:329–342.
32. Goldman H von, Tobler W. Etiology of retrolental fibroplasia. Schweiz Med Wochenschr 1952; 82:381–385.
33. Crosse VM, Evans PJ. Prevention of retrolental fibroplasia. Arch Ophthalmol 1952; 48:83–87.
34. Long HD. Retrolental fibroplasia. Am J Ophthalmol 1952; 35:431.
35. Patz A, Hoeck LE, DeLaCruz E. Studies on the effect of high oxygen administration in retrolental fibroplasia. Nursery observations. Am J Ophthalmol 1952; 27:1248–1253.
36. Lanman JT, Guy LP, Dancis J. Retrolental fibroplasia and oxy-

gen therapy. JAMA 1954; 155:223–226.

37. Kinsey VE. Retrolental fibroplasia: Cooperative study of retrolental fibroplasia and the use of oxygen. Arch Ophthalmol 1956; 56:481–543.

38. Gyllensten LJ, Hellstrom BE. Retrolental fibroplasia: animal experiments—the effect of intermittently administered oxygen on the postnatal development of the eyes of full-term mice. A preliminary report. Acta Paediatr Scand 1952; 41:577–582.

39. Ashton N, Ward B, Serpell G. Role of oxygen in the genesis of retrolental fibroplasia; preliminary report. Br J Ophthalmol 1953; 37:513–520.

40. Ashton N, Cook C. Direct observation of the effect of oxygen on developing vessels. Preliminary report. Br J Ophthalmol 1954; 38:433–440.

41. Patz A, Eastham A, Higginbotham DH, Kleh T. Oxygen studies in retrolental fibroplasia. II. The production of microscopic changes of retrolental fibroplasia in experimental animals. Am J Ophthalmol 1953; 36:1511–1522.

42. Gyllensten LJ, Hellstrom BE. Experimental approach to the pathogenesis of retrolental fibroplasia. I. Changes of the eye induced by exposure of newborn mice to concentrated oxygen. Acta Paediatr Scand 1954; 43, Suppl 100:131–148.

43. Gerschman R, Nadig PW, Snell AC Jr, Nye SW. Effect of high oxygen concentrations on eyes of newborn mice. Am J Physiol 1954; 179:115–118.

44. Michaelson IC, Herz N, Lewkowitz E, Kertesz D. Effect of increased oxygen on the development of the retinal vessels. An experimental study. Br J Ophthalmol 1954; 38:577–587.

45. Kretzer FL, Hittner HM, Johnson AT, Mehta RS, Godio LB. Vitamin E and retrolental fibroplasia: ultrastructural support of clinical efficacy. Ann NY Acad Sci 1982; 393:145–166.

46. Cogan DG. Development and senescence of the human retinal vasculature. Trans Ophthalmol Soc UK 1963; 83:465–489.

47. Patz A. The role of oxygen in retrolental fibroplasia. E Mead Johnson Award Address. Pediatrics 1957; 19:504–524.

48. Patz A. Retrolental fibroplasia. In: Ryan S, Smith M, eds. Selected topics on the eye in systemic disease. New York: Grune and Stratton, 1974;

49. Ashton N. Oxygen and the growth and development of retinal vessels: in vivo and in vitro studies. Am J Ophthalmol 1966; 62:412–435.

50. Patz A. Oxygen studies in retrolental fibroplasia. IV. Clinical and experimental observations. The First Edward L. Holmes Lecture. Am J Ophthalmol 1954; 38:291–308.

51. Flynn JT. Acute proliferative retrolental fibroplasia: evolution of the lesion. Graefes Arch Clin Exp Ophthalmol 1975; 195:101–111.

52. Kretzer FL, Mehta RS, Johnson AT, Hunter DG, Hittner HM. Vitamin E protects against retinopathy of prematurity through action on spindle cells. Nature 1984; 309:793–795.

53. Phelps DL, Rosenbaum AL. The role of tocopheryl in oxygen induced retinopathy: kitten model. Pediatrics 1977; 59:998–1005.

54. Johnson L, Schaffer D, Boggs TR. The premature infant, vitamin E deficiency and retrolental fibroplasia. Am J Clin Nutr 1974; 27:1158–1173.

55. Johnson L, Schaffer D, Quinn G, Goldstein D, Mathis MJ, Otis C, Boggs TR Jr. Vitamin E supplementation and the retinopathy of prematurity. Ann NY Acad Sci 1982; 393:473–495.

56. Hittner HM, Godio LB, Rudolph AJ, et al. Retrolental fibroplasia: efficacy of vitamin E in a double-blind clinical study of preterm infants. N Engl J Med 1981; 305:1365–1371.

57. Millner RA, Watts JL, Paes B, et al. RLF in 1500-gram neonates: part of a randomized clinical trial of the effectiveness of vitamin E. Retinopathy of prematurity conference syllabus, Washington, DC, December 4–6, 1981; 2:703–716.

58. Puklin JE, Simon RM, Ehrenkranz RA. Influence on retrolental fibroplasia of IM vitamin E during respiratory distress syndrome. Ophthalmology 1982; 89:96–103.

59. Finer NN, Schindler RF, Grant GD, et al. Effect of intramuscular vitamin E on the frequency and severity of retrolental fibroplasia: a controlled trial. Lancet 1982; 1:1087–1091.

60. Finer NN, Schindler RF, Peters KL, Grant GD. Vitamin E and retrolental fibroplasia. Improved visual outcome with early vitamin E. Ophthalmology 1983; 90:428–435.

61. Phelps DL. Vitamin E and retrolental fibroplasia in 1982. Pediatrics 1982; 70:420–425.

62. Friedenwald J, Owens WC, Owens EU. Retrolental fibroplasia in premature infants. III. The pathology of the disease. Trans Am Ophthalmol Soc 1951; 49:207–234.

63. Serpell G. Polysaccharide granules in association with developing retinal vessels and with retrolental fibroplasia. Br J Ophthalmol 1950; 44:245–274.

64. Reese AB, Blodi F. Retrolental fibroplasia: Fifth Francis I. Proctor Lecture. Am J Ophthalmol 1951; 34:1–24.

65. Heath P. Retrolental fibroplasia as a syndrome. Pathogenesis and classifications. Arch Ophthalmol 1950; 44:245–274.

66. Reese AB, Blodi FC, Locke JC. The pathology of early retrolental fibroplasia, with an analysis of the histologic findings in the eyes of newborn and stillborn infants. Am J Ophthalmol 1952; 35:1407–1426.

67. Wolff E. Pathologic aspects of retrolental fibroplasia. Am J Ophthalmol 1950; 33:1768–1774.

68. Ashton N. Pathological basis of retrolental fibroplasia. Br J Ophthalmol 1954; 38:385–396.

69. Ward BA. Ocular histology in premature infants with reference to retrolental fibroplasia. Br J Ophthalmol 1954; 38:445–459.

70. Foos RY. Pathological basis of retrolental fibroplasia. Graefes Arch Clin Ophthalmol 1975; 195:87–100.

71. Kushner BJ, Essner D, Cohen IJ, Flynn JT. Retrolental fibroplasia. II. Pathologic correlation. Arch Ophthalmol 1977; 95:29–38.

72. Kraushar MF, Harper RG, Concepcion GS. Retrolental fibroplasia in a full-term infant. Am J Ophthalmol 1975; 80:106–108.

73. Schulman J, Jampol LM, Schwartz H. Peripheral proliferative retinopathy without oxygen therapy in a full-term infant. Am J Ophthalmol 1980; 90:509–514.

74. Naiman J, Green WR, Patz A. Retrolental fibroplasia in hypoxic newborn. Am J Ophthalmol 1979; 88:55–58.

75. Kalina RE, Hodson WA, Morgan BC. Retrolental fibroplasia in a cyanotic infant. Pediatrics 1972; 50:765–768.

76. Aranda JV, Sweet AY. Sustained hyperoxemia without cicatricial retrolental fibroplasia. Pediatrics 1974; 54:434–437.

77. Kingham J. Acute retrolental fibroplasia. Arch Ophthalmol 1977; 95:39–47.

78. Reese AB, King M, Owens WC. A classification of retrolental fibroplasia. Am J Ophthalmol 1953; 36:1333–1335.

79. Tasman W. Late complications of retrolental fibroplasia. Ophthalmology 1979; 86:1724–1740.

80. Faris B, Tolentino FI, Freeman HM, Brockhurst RJ, Schepens CL. Retrolental fibroplasia in the cicatricial stage. Arch Ophthalmol 1971; 85:661–668.

81. O'Grady GE, Flynn JT, Herrara JA. The clinical course of retrolental fibroplasia in premature infants. South Med J 1972; 65:655–658.

82. Avery ME, Oppenheimer EH. Recent increase in mortality from hyaline membrane disease. J Pediatr 1960; 57:553–559.

83. Kalina RE, Karr DJ. Retrolental fibroplasia: experience over two decades in one institution. Ophthalmology 1982; 89:91–95.

84. Davidorff FH, Weiss ET. Retrolental fibroplasia: a new look at an old problem. Ohio State Med J 1982; 78:662–664.

85. Phelps D. Retinopathy of prematurity: an estimate of vision loss in the United States—1979. Pediatrics 1981; 67:924–926.

86. Harris GS. Retinopathy of prematurity and retinal detachment. Can J Ophthalmol 1976; 11:21–25.

87. Hack M, Fanaroff AA, Merkatz IR. The low-birth-weight-infant—evolution of a changing outlook. N Engl J Med 1979; 301:1162–1165.

88. Kumar S, Anday E, Sacks L, et al. Survival of the extremely low-birth-weight infant (LBW)—current limits of successful support. Pediatr Res 1980; 14:602.

89. Manroe B, Wright W, Browne R. Risk factors for retinopathy of prematurity. Pediatr Res 1979; 13:500.

90. McCormick A. The retinopathy of prematurity in the newborn. Curr Probl Pediatr 1977; 7:1–28.

91. Uemura Y. Current status of retrolental fibroplasia. Jpn J Ophthalmol 1974; 21:366–378.
92. Cantalino SJ, Curran JS, Van Cader TC, Edward WC. Acute retrolental fibroplasia: classification and objective evaluation of incidence, natural history, and resolution by fundus photography and intravenous fluorescein angiography. Perspect Ophthalmol 1978; 2:175–187.
93. Payne JW, Patz A. Current status of retrolental fibroplasia. The retinopathy of prematurity. Ann Clin Res 1979; 11:205–221.
94. Schaffer DB, Johnson L, Quinn GE, Boggs TR. A classification of retrolental fibroplasia to evaluate vitamin E therapy. Ophthalmology 1979; 86:1749–1760.
95. Hindle NW. International classification of retrolental fibroplasia: a proposal. Can J Ophthalmol 1982; 17:107–109.
96. Committee for the classification of retinopathy of prematurity: an international classification of retinopathy of prematurity. Arch Ophthalmol 1984; 102:1130–1134.

Juan Orellana, M.D.

The examination of the premature infant in the nursery is the first step in screening for retinopathy of prematurity.

PATIENT HISTORY

A detailed history should be obtained. Important data regarding birth weight and gestational age should be recorded. Questions regarding pregnancy history should focus on maternal exposure to infectious agents, breech presentation, maternal disease, trauma during pregnancy, type of delivery (caesarean section, spontaneous vaginal) and medications taken during pregnancy. The amount and duration of oxygen exposure are important. The history should note the presence or absence of anemia, intraventricular hemorrhage, septicemia, respiratory distress syndrome, patent ductus arteriosus or other abnormality, and amount of blood transfused. All these can contribute to the development of ROP/RLF. It should be noted whether vitamin E has been administered continuously and how soon after birth it was initiated.

OCULAR EXAMINATION

In the nursery, a nurse or nurse's aide may help gently restrain the infant while the ophthalmologist works. In the office, the older infant may be wrapped in a sheet and restrained by either office personnel or the mother (Fig. 2–1). Rarely, if ever, is medication needed to sedate the child.

EXTERNAL APPEARANCE

External examination should note any lid abnormalities. Prenatally, lid differentiation begins nasally and ends temporally, when the lids separate at the end of the sixth month. In very premature infants, the lids may not have separated. The cornea can be examined for clarity and size by using a 20- or a 14–D indirect lens as a magnifier. Persistent tunica vasculosa lentis, pupillary remnants, as well as posterior synechiae, should be noted (Fig. 2–2). The child's pupillary reactions to light, direct and consensual, should be recorded.

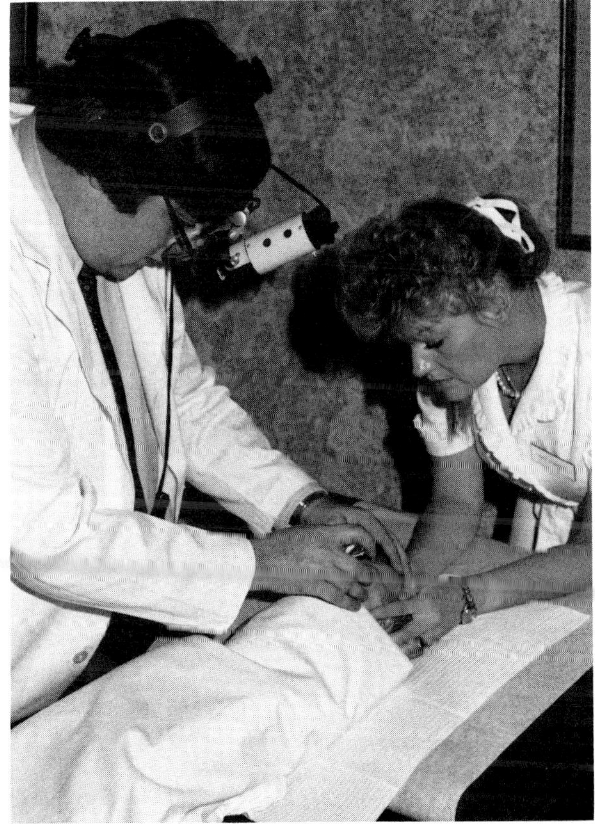

Figure 2–1 Wrapping the child in a sheet effectively limits excessive movement of the limbs. The technician or mother gently restrains the child's head.

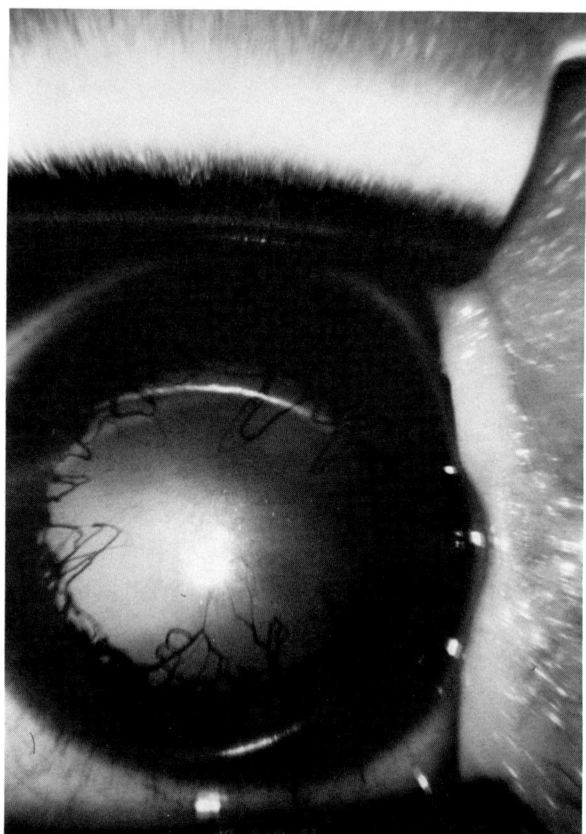

Figure 2–2 A persistent tunica vasculosa lentis can be present in premature infants; however, it should not be recorded as neovascularization. Pediatricians should be aware of these vessels, because some face masks can fit poorly, and undue pressure over the eyes will result in a massive hyphema and vitreous hemorrhage.

ANTERIOR SEGMENT

The anterior chamber should be examined for clarity and depth. Angle evaluation can be useful in the infants: children with RLF can develop secondary glaucoma.

Premature infants can exhibit transient cataracts that are reversible.[2] The ophthalmologist will be able to follow the lens changes as they gradually subside. No treatment is necessary for this type of cataract.

POSTERIOR SEGMENT

Visualization of both the posterior pole and retina periphery is indispensible if the eyes are to be adequately evaluated. Gonioscopy, utilizing a Koeppe or Layden lens after topical corneal anesthesia, yields valuable information regarding the posterior pole (Fig. 2–3). Photography can also be performed through these lenses with a handheld camera. Mydriacyl 1 percent (tropicamide) and Neo-Synephrine 2.5 percent (phenylephrine hydrochloride), instilled once or twice in both eyes, combined with punctal occlusion to decrease systemic absorption, provide adequate dilation over 30 minutes. Cyclogyl (cyclopentolate hydrochloride) is avoided because of its occasional side effects.[3] Neo-Synephrine 10 percent is too concentrated and can be very toxic to these infants[4]; systemic absorption of phenylephrine hydrochloride at a concentration of 10 percent causes a wide range of toxic reactions.[5]

Oculocardiac reactions, identified as alterations in cardiac rhythm or rate, have been reported to occur in

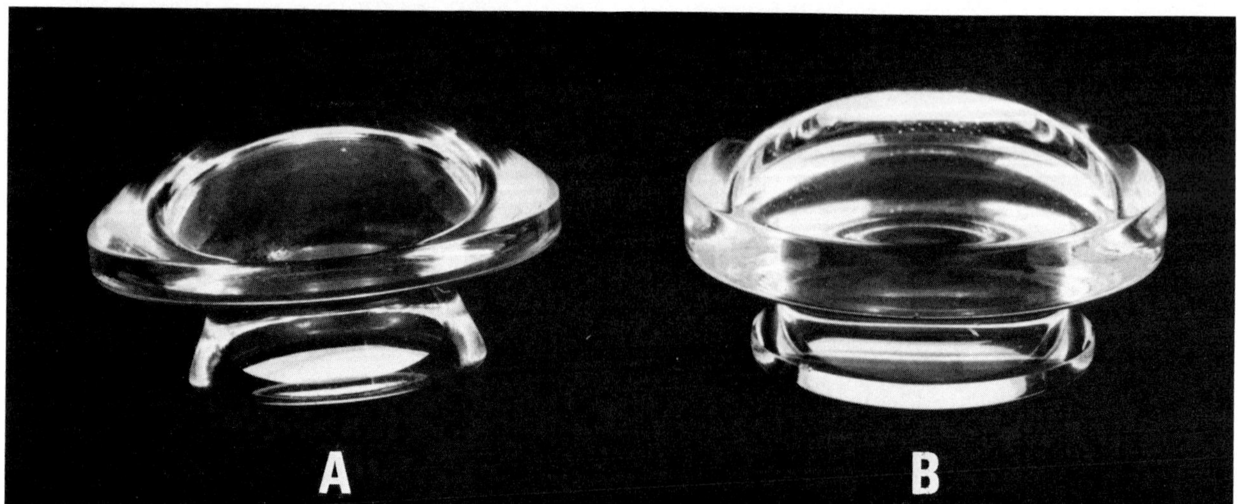

Figure 2–3 A Koeppe lens A and a Layden lens B may be used to examine the child in the nursery or office. The Layden lens can be used without a speculum and affords easy examination of the ora serrata, including photography.

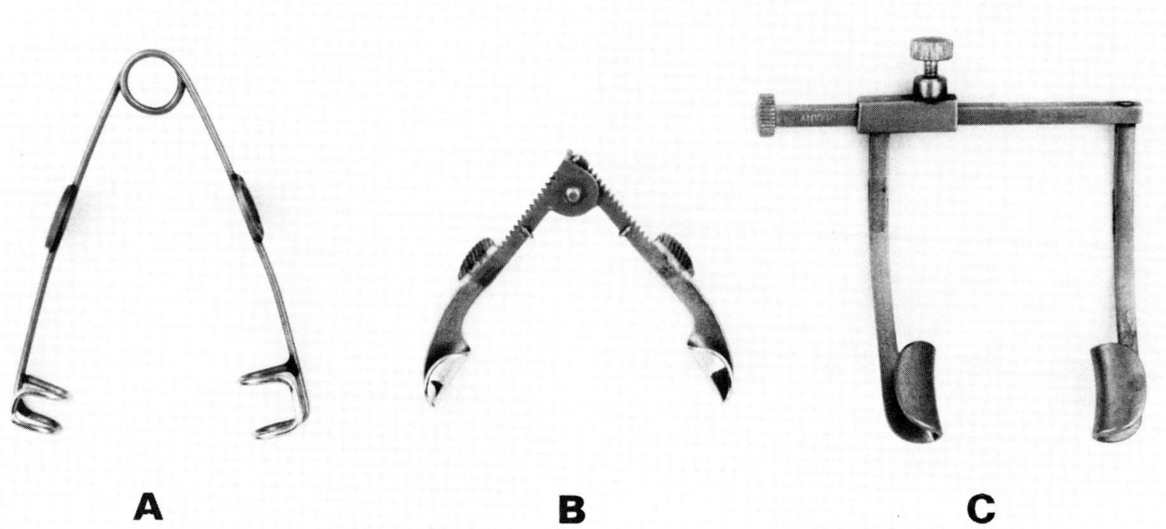

Figure 2–4   The Alfonso A, Sauer B, or Cook C speculums can be used in the nursery or office. The Alfonso and Sauer speculums are easier and quicker to use.

premature infants from stimuli that might be associated with examination, such as traction on extraocular or eyelid muscles, pressure on the globe, intraorbital injection (retrobulbar block), scleral depression and use of a lid speculum.[6]

If a speculum is needed, an Alfonso or Sauer instrument can be used after topical anesthesia has been applied (Fig. 2–4). Examination of the temporal periphery is done by rotating the head, producing an abduction of the eye to be examined.

Attention is paid to the optic nerve first, i.e., documenting its size, shape and color. Congenital, optic-nerve anomalies, should be noted. The presence of persistent hyaloid remnants should be recorded. In the posterior pole, vascular tortuosity, congestion, and dilatation should be documented (Fig. 2–5). A vitreous

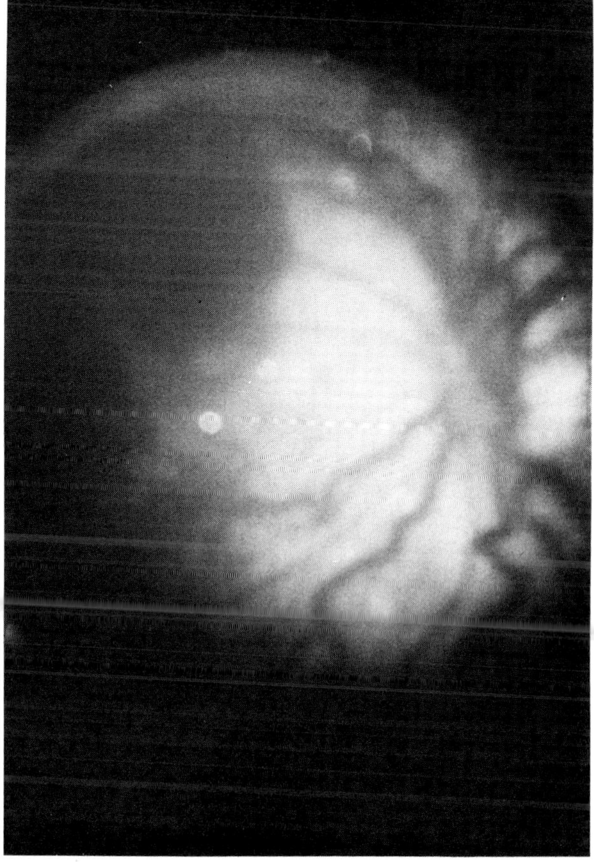

Figure 2–6   A vitreous hemorrhage originates from the extensive neovascularization present. In eyes where the shunt line is very posterior, the hemorrhage will obscure part of the posterior pole. There will be a definitive vitreous haze throughout.

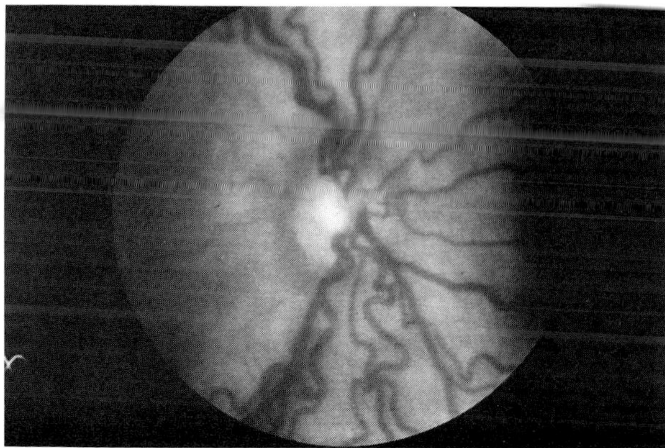

Figure 2–5   Dilated, congested, and tortuous vessels are present in the posterior pole once the low-resistance shunt has been established.

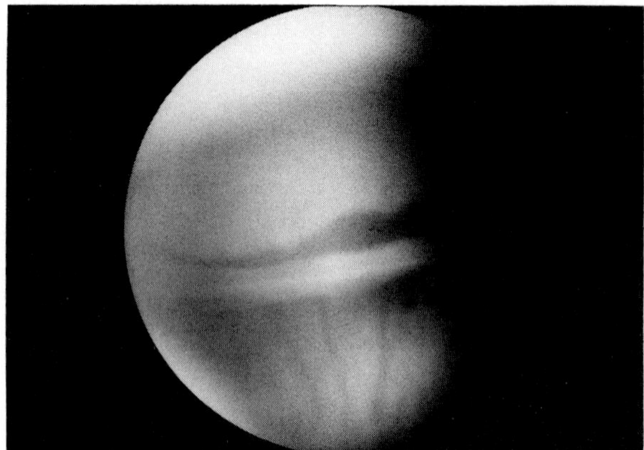

Figure 2–7   The arteriovenous shunt line begins as a thickening between the avascular vanguard (above) and vascularized rearguard (below). It is important to realize that the grayish vanguard is not a retinal detachment.

hemorrhage can overlie the posterior pole, limiting the view of the fundus details (Fig. 2–6). This is distinct from the retinal hemorrhages in the posterior pole, related to vaginal delivery. These hemorrhages are not associated with neovascularization and are not to be confused with ROP.

The ophthalmologist should follow the vessels peripherally and note the extent of vascularized retina (rearguard retina). The avascular retina anterior to the rearguard is the vanguard retina. The junction between the rearguard and vanguard retina is the arteriovenous shunt line, or ridge; it can vary from a demarcation line to a highly elevated ridge (Figs. 2–7 to 2–9). Note the neovascular membranes, the presence or absence of capillary tufts, and both the position and width of the shunt line. These should be carefully recorded, since they are important prognostic signs. The combination of a wide ridge located posterior to the equator has a poorer prognosis than a narrow, anterior ridge. Additional, poor prognostic signs are iris neovascularization (Fig. 2–10), not to be confused with a persistent tunica vasculosa lentis; pupillary synechiae; and extensive vitreous hemorrhage. A small vitreous hemorrhage does not appear to significantly affect the prognosis.

Peripheral traction detachments can involve the shunt line and can either remain stable, resolve, or extend into the posterior pole. Documentation by drawings will assist the ophthalmologist in determining the

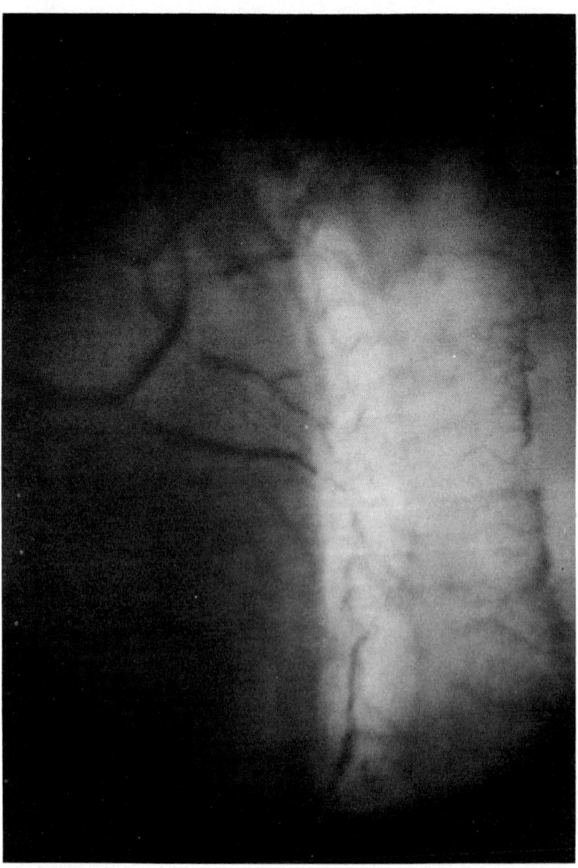

Figure 2–8   As the active disease progresses, there is elevation, thickening, and contraction of the arteriovenous shunt line or ridge. An early peripheral detachment is present.

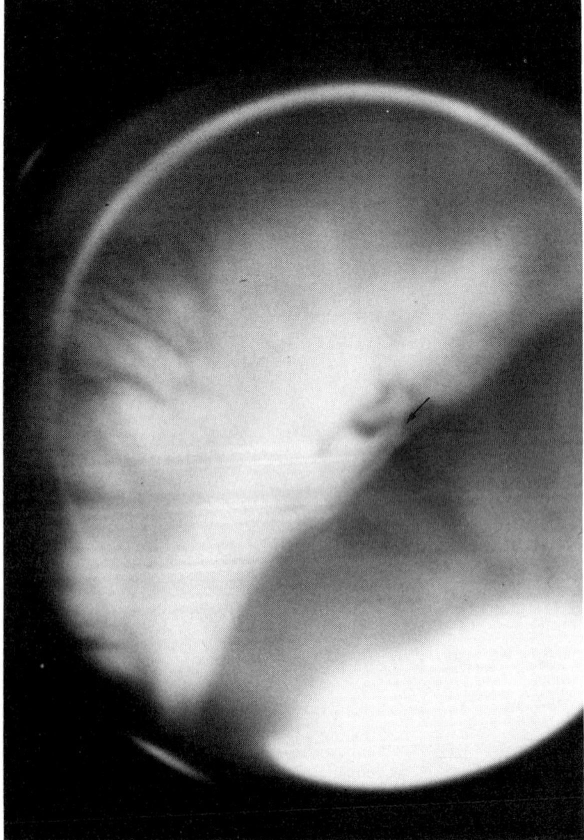

Figure 2–9   Marked ridge elevation will occur in some patients. This ridge is thickened and elevated. A rim of thickened vitreous (arrow) is present, which turns in the ridge as it contracts.

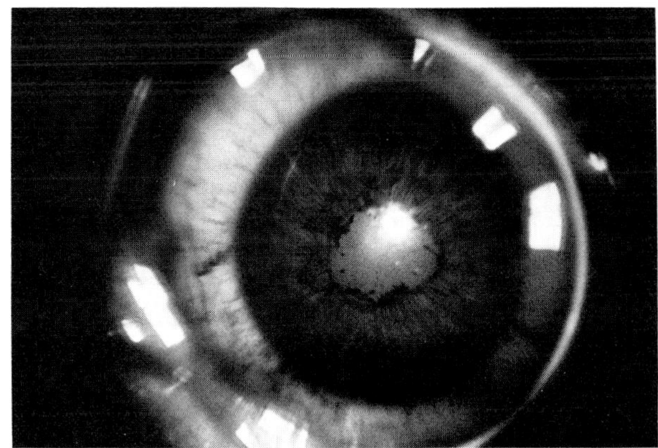

Figure 2–10 Iris neovascularization and pupillary synechiae are prognostic signs of a poor outcome, whether or not treatment is instituted.

course these detachments are taking. The active stage of the disease is frequently accompanied by serous exudation, adding a serous component to an initial traction detachment. In other cases, the detachment is mostly serous, with a minimal, tractional component.

After assessing all the data gathered, the stages of the diseases are noted by using the International Classification[7,8] for active ROP and the Reese system for classification of cicatricial RLF.[9]

It is important to note when disease regression is taking place. Observe the vascular dilation and tortuosity, a result of the low-resistance shunt present at the arteriovenous ridge. When the ridge begins to flatten, the resistance will be altered, and the dilation and tortuosity will be reversed, producing a normalized vasculature. Vessels observed traversing the ridge and beginning vascularization of the vanguard retina indicates that the ROP is resolving.

If the ophthalmologist can examine the baby only once in the nursery, this should be done 7 weeks after birth.[10] This will yield the maximum ROP detection, while later examinations might be too late for treatment to be of help. Continued follow-up examinations are crucial. Extensive changes can occur in a matter of days. Examinations done infrequently will overlook a great deal of pathology and deny the infant the chance for earlier surgical intervention.

REFERENCES

1. Hittner HM, Rhodes LM, McPherson AR. Anterior segment abnormalities in cicatricial retinopathy of prematurity. Ophthalmology 1979; 86:803–816.
2. Alden ER, Kalina RE, Hodson WA. Transient cataracts in low-birth-weight infants. J Pediatr 1973; 82:314–318.
3. Bauer CR, Trottier MCT, Stern L. Systemic cyclopentolate (Cyclogyl) toxicity in the newborn infant. J Pediatr 1973; 82:501–505.
4. Borromeo-McGrail V, Bordiuk JM, Keitel H. Systemic hypertension following ocular administration of 10 percent phenylephrine in the neonate. Pediatrics 1973, 51:1032–1036.
5. Fraunfelder FT, Scafidi AF. Possible adverse effects from topical ocular 10 percent phenylephrine. Am J Ophthalmol 1978; 85:447–453.
6. Clark WN, Hodges E, Noel LP, Roberts D, Coneys M. The oculocardiac reflex during ophthalmoscopy in premature infants. Am J Ophthalmol 1985; 99:649–651.
7. Hindle NW. International classification of retrolental fibroplasia: a proposal. Can J Ophthalmol 1982; 17:107–109.
8. Committee for the classification of retinopathy of prematurity: an international classification of retinopathy of prematurity. Arch Ophthalmol 1984; 102:1130–1134.
9. Reese AB, King MJ, Owens WC. A classification of retrolental fibroplasia. Am J Ophthalmol 1952; 35:1333–1335.
10. Palmer EA. Optimal timing of examination for acute retrolental fibroplasia. Ophthalmology 1981; 88:662–668.

Classification of Retinopathy of Prematurity

3

James D. Kingham, M.D.

HISTORY OF RETINOPATHY OF PREMATURITY

Terry[1] first reported retrolental fibroplasia (RLF) in 1942 in a premature infant. In the decade immediately after his initial description, RLF assumed almost epidemic proportions and became a common cause of blindness in preschool children. In 1951, Parker Heath, in describing the pathology of RLF, first used the term "retinopathy of prematurity" (ROP).[2] At about that time, Kate Campbell in Australia associated intensive oxygen therapy with the development of RLF.[3] This theory was then proven clinically and in the laboratory by Patz and coworkers.[4,5]

In using the direct ophthalmoscope, the diagnostic tool available then, Reese and associates devised a clinical classification of RLF.[6] This classification was divided into active and cicatricial groups. The active stages were:

1. Dilation and tortuosity of retinal vessels
2. Stage 1 plus neovascularization and some peripheral retinal clouding; spontaneous regression can occur
3. Stage 2 plus retinal detachment in the periphery of the fundus; spontaneous regression unlikely
4. Hemispheric or circumferential retinal detachment
5. Complete retinal detachment

With the discovery of oxygen toxicity to immature retinal vessels, the use of oxygen was dramatically curtailed, with a concomitant increase in infant mortality from respiratory distress and morbidity associated with cerebral palsy.[7,8] In the mid and late 1960s, neonatology emerged as a subspecialty of pediatrics. Life-support systems were developed and maintained for low-birth-weight premature infants who had a variety of systemic diseases. The survival rate of infants who weigh less than 1 kg has changed from 8 percent to 35 percent in 1980.[9] Accordingly, there has been an increase in the incidence of ROP in the United States since 1965.[10]

In 1971, the Committee on Fetus and Newborn of the American Academy of Pediatrics recommended that a person experienced in recognizing RLF should examine the eyes of all infants born at less than 36-weeks gestation or weighing less than 2,000 grams.[11] Unfortunately, few physicians were experienced in recognizing RLF; even more unfortunately, in using the technique of indirect ophthalmoscopy, it was learned that Reese's classification and stages of RLF bore little or no resemblance to what was seen in the perinatal intensive care nursery. Kingham in 1977, with the use of the indirect ophthalmoscope,[12] revised the acute RLF classification system to more accurately parallel the findings seen in the nursery. He graded the acute stages of RLF as follows:

Grade I	Abnormal peripheral aborization
Grade II	Demarcation line
Grade III	Intraretinal ridge with extrarctinal neovascularization
Grade IV	Partial retinal detachment
Grade V	Total retinal detachment

As a result of refinement in neonatology, the 1970s saw a worldwide explosion of new cases of RLF or ROP. Interest in RLF was especially keen in Japan, and the Japanese recognized two types[13] of RLF:

Type I	Roughly classified along conventional lines, as in the Kingham classification
Type II	A rare but fulminant type of retinopathy found in very small, very sick premature infants whose clinical

course was rapidly progressive with extremely poor prognosis for vision.[14-17]

This "rush disease" was characterized by engorgement of the posterior vessels whose most peripheral development was still in the posterior pole, and it was accompanied by a broad expanse of anterior, nonvascularized retina.

Fundus examination of 3,400 premature infants led David Schaffer and his colleagues to further refine the Kingham classification, with the important observation that vascular dilation and tortuosity in the posterior pole constituted an additional parameter in the manifestation and severity of the disease.[18,19] They found that with increasing posterior polar vascular dilation and tortuosity, there was often engorgement of iris vessels and increased resistance to pharmacological dilation. When retinopathic changes of ROP were found with associated posterior vascular dilation and tortuosity, the condition was termed "plus disease," and they believed this should be regarded as a distinct clinical entity.

An attempt at surgical treatment of RLF[20-25] made the ophthalmic community painfully aware of the need for a standardized classification system, so that indications and timings for treatment could be standardized from center to center and from country to country. At that point, results could be accurately compared. At the urging of Warren Hindle, a pediatric ophthalmologist at the Univerity of Alberta, a symposium was held in Calgary in September of 1982.[26] There, 22 ophthalmologists and one ocular pathologist from 11 countries met and agreed upon a classification of ROP. A computer-friendly flow sheet was designed to record the findings in the nursery. The symposium participants then returned to their respective countries and used the new classification system and flow sheets, before meeting again in Baltimore one year later to compare results and to refine the new classification. The result was an "International Classification of Retinopathy of Prematurity."[27] This new classification is unique in that it not only stages ROP as to quality and severity, but it describes the anteroposterior or radial location of the abnormal findings, as well as the circumferential extent of the disease.

CLASSIFYING RETINOPATHY OF PREMATURITY

The overall disease is called retinopathy of prematurity (ROP). Terry's term, "retrolental fibroplasia" (RLF), is inappropriate for the acute phases, because most of

the ROP changes seen acutely resolve spontaneously to normal or near normal, and neither cicatrix nor fibroplasia is seen clinically. RLF is a more suitable term both histologically and clinically, for the cicatricial residuum in the late, severe forms of the disease.

The Normal Premature Retina

The human fetus has no retinal blood supply until the fourth month of gestation.[28] Then retinal vessel growth proceeds centrifugally and is complete on the nasal side at about 8 months, and on the temporal side at about 9 months, or just shortly before birth. Premature infants show incomplete vascularization, especially on the temporal side; this incompleteness is proportional to their prematurity. In the normal infant, without ROP, the vessel size decreases as it approaches the retinal periphery. The branching angles of the fourth- or fifth-order vessels are 20 to 40 degrees, or the angle can be as high as 60 to 70 degrees. Arteries and veins are definable almost out to the limits of their resolution. There is no peripheral engorgement or enlargement of vessels. The peripheral retina and the nonvascular retina anterior to the limits of vascularization have a silver-gray, opaque, wet, glistening, and silky appearance. This is probably a manifestation of the paucity or absence of vascularization in the peripheral retina, combined with an oblique viewing angle. The transition between vascular retina and nonvascular retina is gradual.

STAGING THE DISEASE

Stage 1 ROP: Demarcation Line

The sine qua non of Stage 1 ROP is a demarcation line separating the posterior vascularized retina from the anterior nonvascularized retina (Fig. 3–1). It is a thin, distinct, relatively flat, circumferentially-oriented, intraretinal line. It can be white, or it can have a yellowish tint. There are usually abnormal terminal arborizations of small vessels immediately posterior to the demarcation line, characterized by small-vessel dilation and acutely-branching small vessels, sometimes in tufts like the bristles of a broom. Although abnormal vessel configuration can precede the appearance of the line, a line must be present to clearly diagnose Stage 1 ROP.

Stage 2 ROP: Intraretinal Ridge

The demarcation line has increased in volume to occupy both height and width, but this proliferative tissue remains intraretinal (Fig. 3–2). The color of the ridge can be white to cream. Posterior to the ridge, vessels can leave the plane of the retina to enter it; this phenomenon should not be confused with localized retinal detachment. Small tufts of new vessels can be seen lying on the retina's surface, posterior to the ridge, but these are not the extraretinal fibrovascular proliferation (EFP) necessary for Stage 3 disease. In Stage 1 and Stage 2 disease, vessels in the posterior pole are usually not dilated or tortuous (Fig. 3–3).

cularization accompanied by fibrous proliferation emerges through the internal limiting membrane into the vitreous. The neovascularization can arise as small tufts along the posterior edge or crest of the ridge (Fig. 3–4). As proliferation becomes more extensive, these tufts can coalesce and present a ragged appearance (Fig. 3–5). Immediately posterior to the ridge, but not always appearing to be connected with it, can be seen coalesced formations resembling sausages, running parallel to the ridge.[19] The retinal vessels entering the ridge are dilated and engorged (Fig. 3–6). The presence of hemorrhage on or adjacent to the ridge is not uncommon in this stage of disease.

Stage 3 ROP: Ridge Plus Extraretinal Fibrovascular Proliferation (EFP)

The intraretinal ridge continues to increase in volume with increased height and width. From this ridge, neovas-

Stage 4 ROP: Retinal Detachment

Unequivocal retinal detachment occurs posterior to the ridge. It usually starts peripherally and can be in one quadrant or two or more quadrants (Fig. 3–7). As the

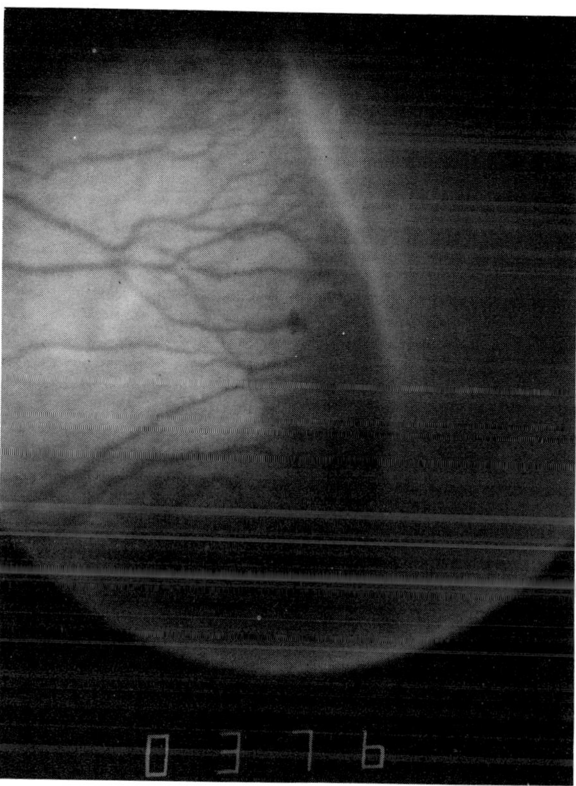

Figure 3-1 Stage 1 ROP. A distinct equatorially oriented intraretinal demarcation line separates the posterior vascularized retina from the anterior zone of the nonvascularized retina. The vessels approaching the line exhibit some engorgement, and they arborize abnormally with multiple terminal branches with hyperacute branching angles.

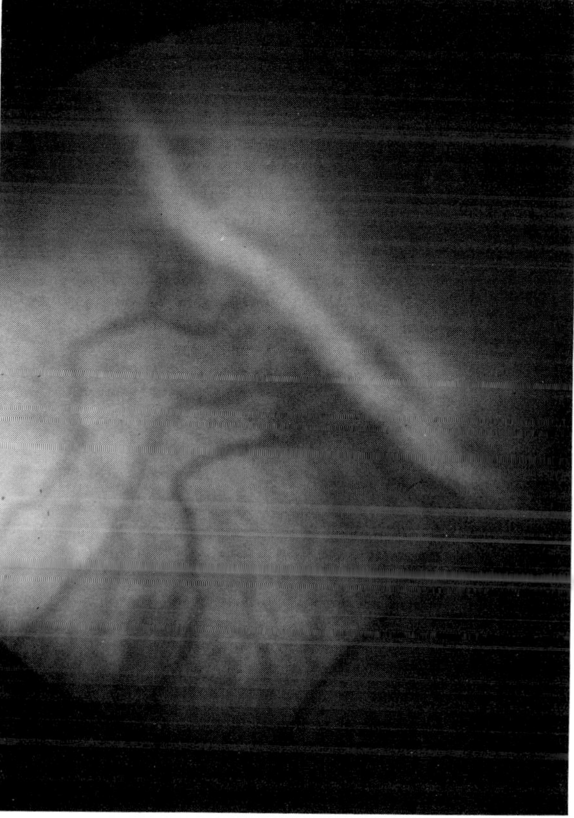

Figure 3-2 Stage 2 ROP. The demarcation line has increased in height and width, and therefore volume, to form a ridge that remains intraretinal. Note the engorgement of the vessels approaching the ridge.

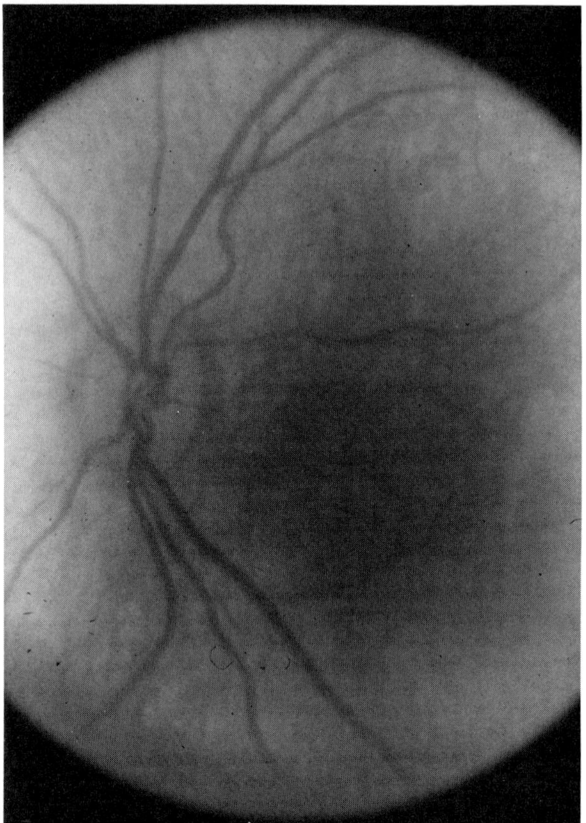

Figure 3-3 Posterior pole of the infant with Stage 2 ROP. Venules are not abnormally dilated, and arterioles are not tortuous.

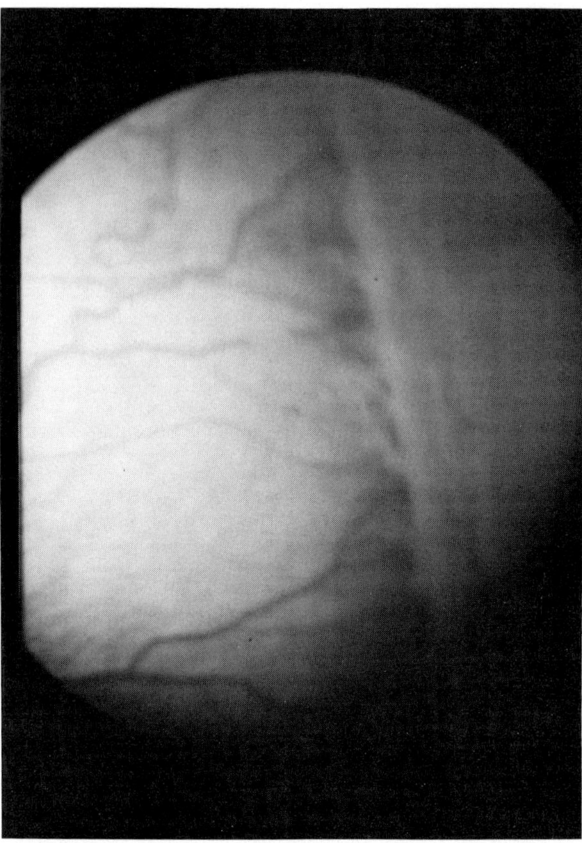

Figure 3-4 Stage 3 ROP. Neovascular tufts along the posterior border of the ridge have extended into the vitreous.

retinal detachment progresses, it is observed posteriorly. Anterior to the ridge, the opaque retina might be difficult to distinguish from shallow retinal detachment. The detachment can be exudative, caused by the serous effusion from the incompetent neovascularization from the fibrovascular ridge, or there can be some tractional component, secondary to early cicatrization occurring within the EFP. Both exudative and tractional forms can be present simultaneously, indicating components of acute ROP and cicatricial ROP. In advanced, acute disease, the retinal detachment can extend all the way to the optic disc with a convex, bullous appearance to the detachment,[21] indicative of the disease's exudative component (Fig. 3–8).

Usually with increasing severity of the disease, changes in the caliber of established vasculature will be

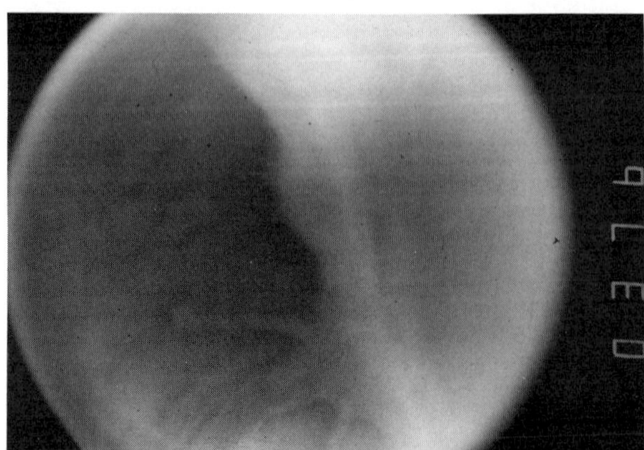

Figure 3-5 Stage 3 ROP. Extraretinal neovascularization has coalesced into an extensive arteriovenous shunt.

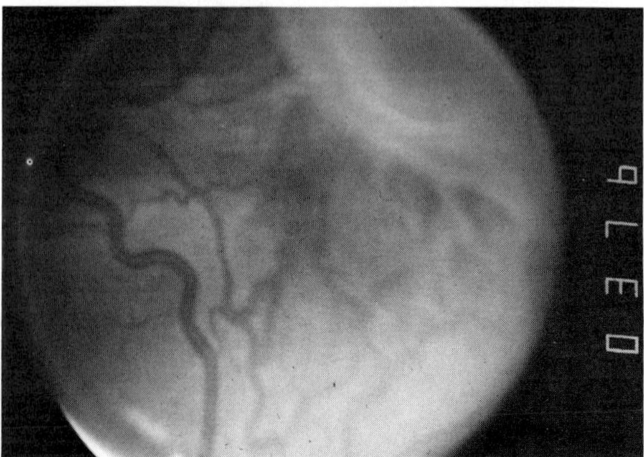

Figure 3-6 Stage 3 ROP. Same patient as Figure 3-5. Note the vessel dilation and tortuosity approaching the peripheral shunt.

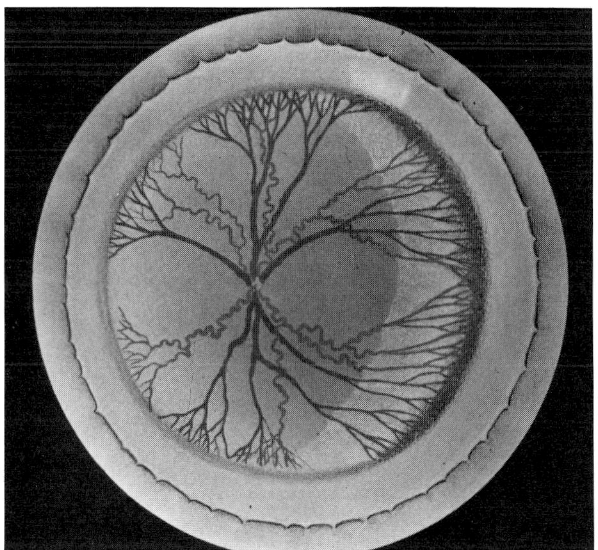

Figure 3-7 Stage 4 ROP. Extraretinal fibrovascular proliferation (EFP) with subretinal fluid in temporal periphery. Vessels are dilated and tortuous posteriorly as well as peripherally.

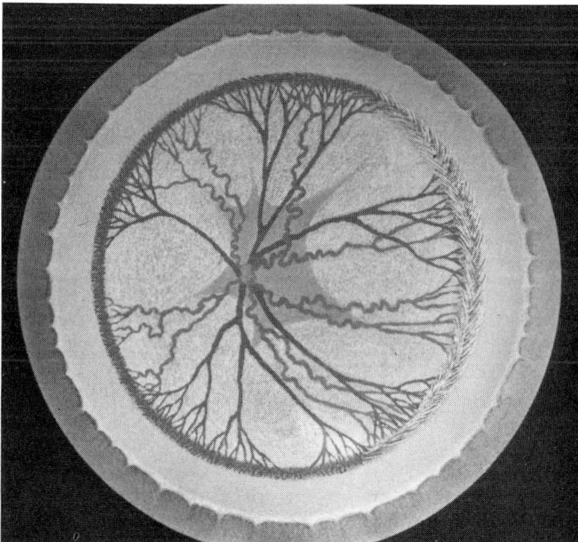

Figure 3-8 Stage 4 ROP. Total retinal detachment. Bulbous appearance indicates exudative subretinal fluid rather than tractional retinal detachment.

observed immediately posterior to the events at the vascular-avascular border. The vessels leading to and from the ridge structures cannot always be identified as arterioles or venules. However, when the veins are definitely dilated and the arteries tortuous in the posterior pole, the designation "plus disease" is added to this stage (Fig. 3–9). In addition, hemorrhage can occur intraretinally or preretinally in proximity to the EFP.

Iris vessel dilation, incomplete pharmacological pupillary dilation, and increasing vitreous haze can also be observed. Posterior polar venous dilation, arterial tortuosity, and lush overgrowth of neovascularization within Zone I or posterior Zone II indicate the unusual variation called "rush disease" (Fig. 3–10). Its progression can be such that the usual staging is altered or so rapid that successive stages are not observed, and extensive serous detachment and fibrovascular cicatrization occur following the appearance of "rush disease."

LOCALIZATION OF THE DISEASE

The disease in its various stages can be identified according to its anteroposterior location within the retina. The retina from optic disc to ora serrata is divided into three zones, with the optic disc as the approximate center (Fig. 3–11).

Zone I   A circle in the posterior pole, the radius of which extends from the center of the optic disc to twice the distance from the optic disc to the center of the macula;

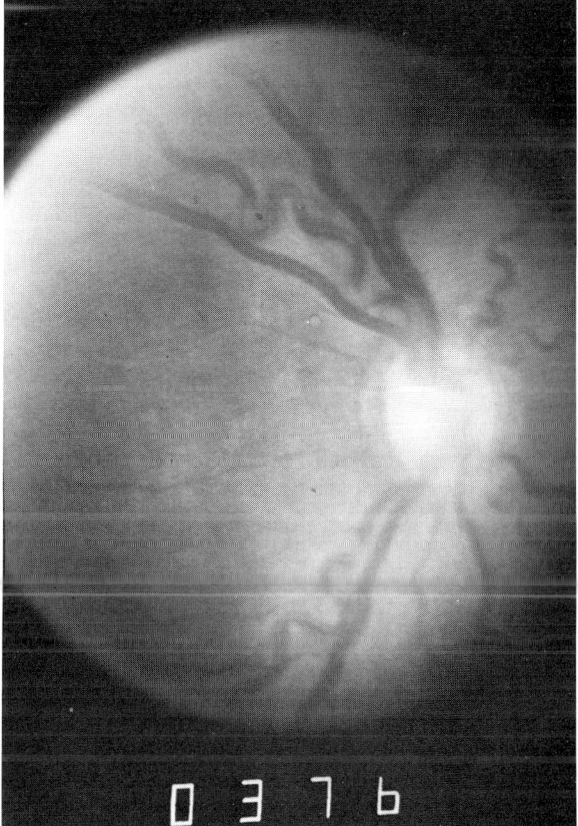

Figure 3-9 "Plus disease." Posterior pole vessels are dilated and tortuous, indicating high-flow shunt in periphery. Prognosis for such eyes is generally poorer than for eyes without this shunt.

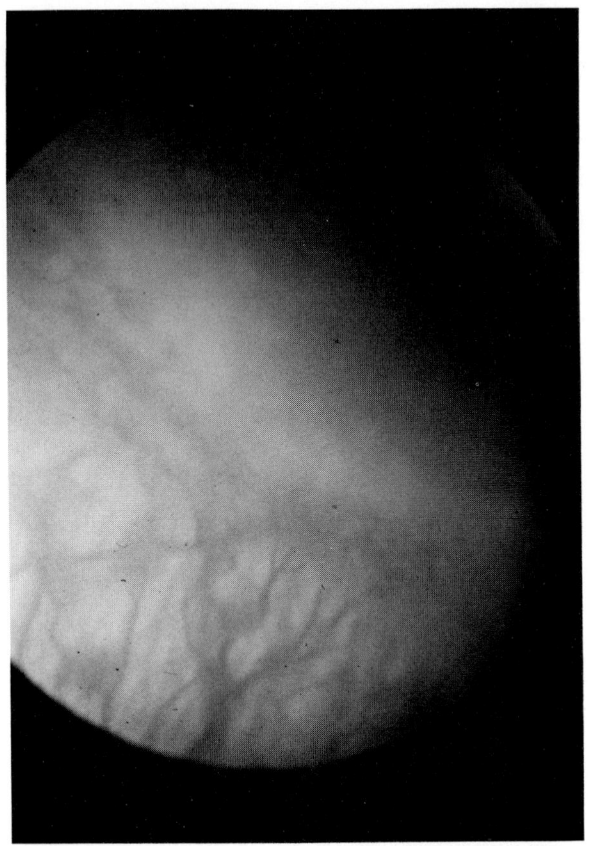

Figure 3-10 "Rush disease." An unusual form of ROP shows vascular-avascular border located in Zone I or posterior Zone II. There is profuse abnormal vascularization up to the avascular retina. Later, a lush neovascular overgrowth will emerge, and the retina will become totally detached.

Zone II   A circle that extends from the outer edge of Zone I to a point tangential to the ora serrata nasally and around to an area near the temporal anterior equator;

Zone III   The residual crescent of retina outside Zone II to the ora serrata; accordingly, there is more Zone III temporally than nasally, and this is the last area vascularized in the premature eye.

EXTENT OF THE DISEASE

The amount of the disease in its various stages and anteroposterior location can also be quantitated in a schematic according to its circumferential extent, on the basis of the clock. Each clock hour is called a sector. As the observer looks at each eye, the temporal horizontal meridian is nine o'clock for the right eye and three o'clock for the left eye (Fig. 3–11).

RECORDING THE OBSERVATIONS

With the disease staged, localized anteroposteriorly, and quantitated circumferentially with the associated ocular findings, a reproducible quantitation of disease at any given time is available. These observations are officially recorded on the computer-compatible flow sheet at each examination (Fig. 3–12).

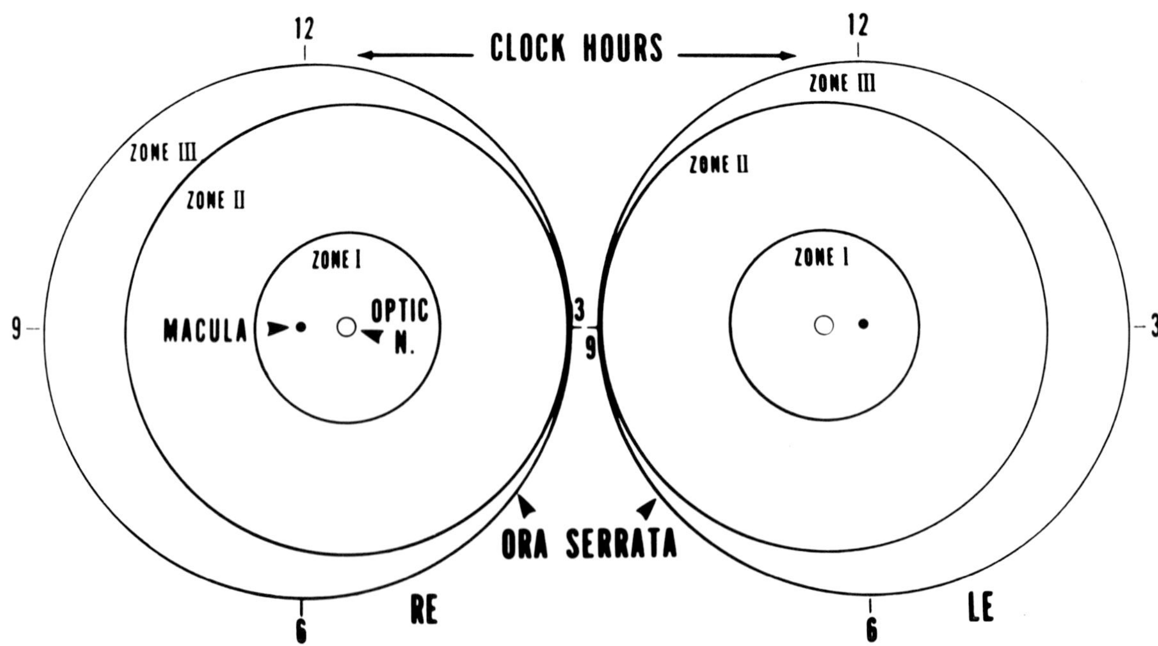

Figure 3-11 Location schematic identifies three zones in relation to the optic nerve and ora serrata.

Anatomical landmarks other than the disc and the ora serrata are difficult to discern in the premature eye; thus, the boundary between zones is arbitrary and can only be approximated. When doubt exists, disease should be located in the more posterior zone. Serial observation is necessary to determine whether the disease is in its progressing or regressing phase. Generally the more posterior the disease and the more extensive the EFP, the more serious the prognosis for the eye.

International Classification of ROP

Retinopathy of Prematurity (ROP) Ophthalmic Examination Record

Biographical Data

Name _______________________________________   Hospital # ___ ___ ___ ___ ___ ___ ___

Birth date
(Mo/D/Yr)   ___ ___ / ___ ___ / ___ ___   Sex (M=1, F=2) ___

Birth weight (grams) ___ ___ ___ ___   Gestational age (weeks) ___ ___

Multiple births (single=1, twin=2, triplet=3) ___

Examination

Date of Exam ___ ___ / ___ ___ / ___ ___   Examiner's Initials or # ___ ___ ___

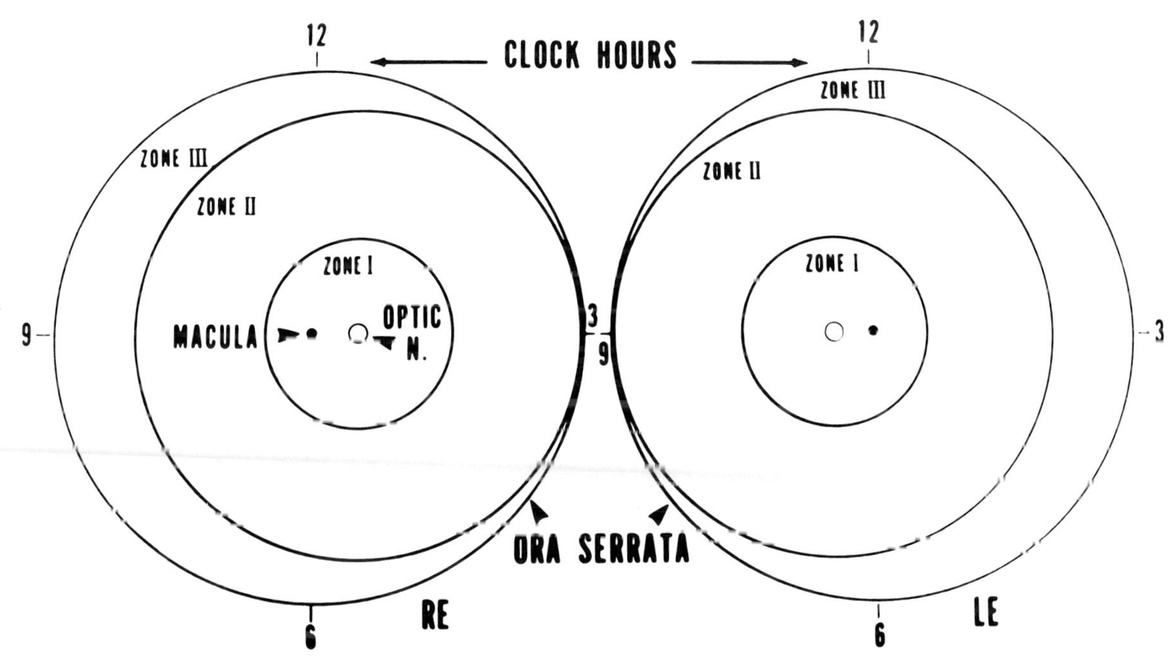

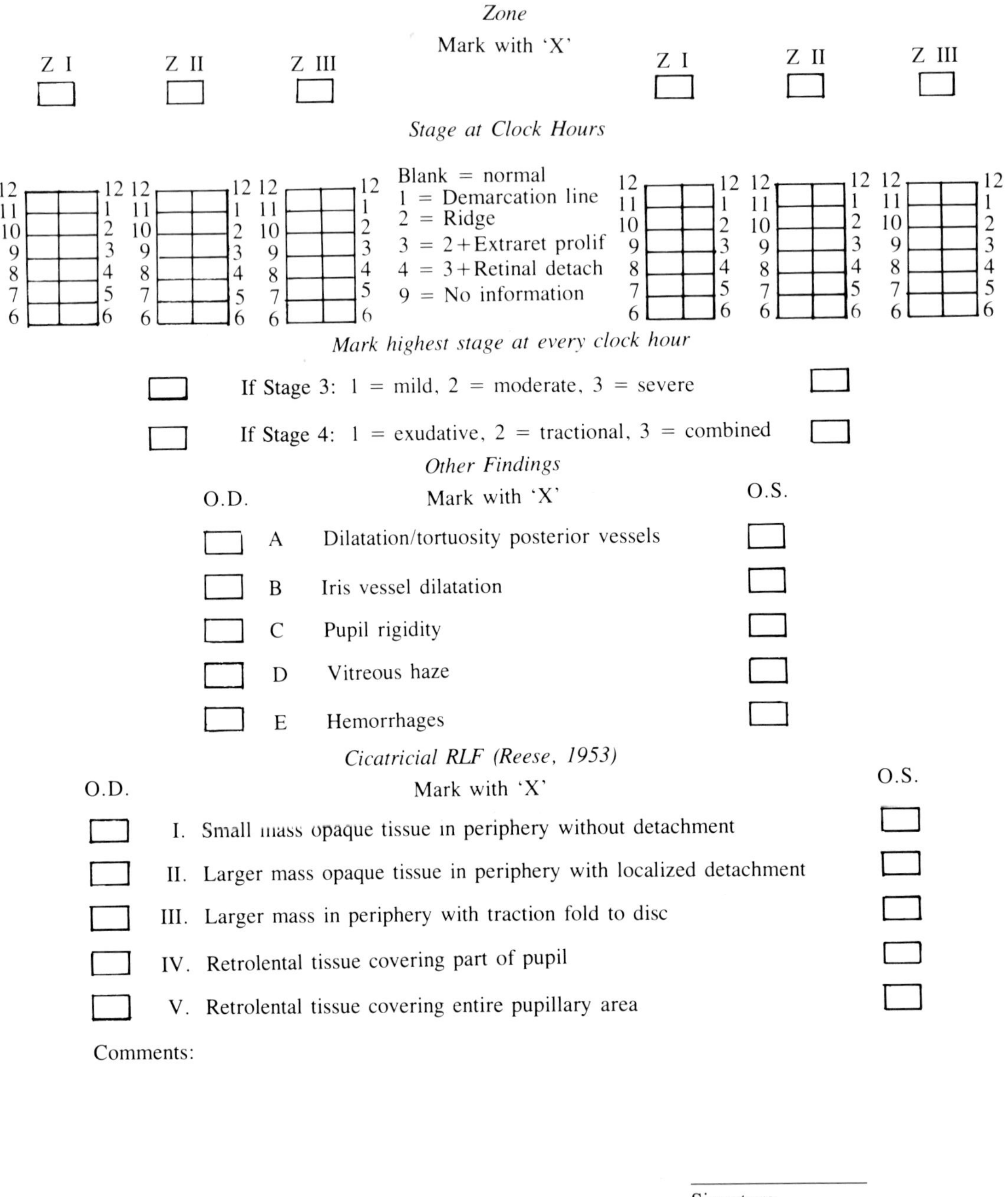

Figure 3-12 Examination record to be used in serial exams collates biographical data and identifies stage, anteroposterior location, and circumferential extent of ROP in a computer family form.

REFERENCES

1. Terry TL. Extreme prematurity and fibroblastic growth of persistent vascular sheath behind each crystalline lens. I. Preliminary report. Am J Ophthalmol 1942; 25:203-204.

2. Heath P. Pathology of the retinopathy of prematurity: retrolental fibroplasia. Am J Ophthalmol 1951; 34:1249-1268.

3. Campbell K. Intensive oxygen therapy as a possible cause of retrolental fibroplasia. A clinical approach. Med J Aust 1951; 2:48-50.

4. Patz A, Hoeck LE, DeLaCruz E. Studies on the effect of high oxygen administration in retrolental fibroplasia. I. Nursery observations. Am J Ophthalmol 1952; 35:1248-1253.

5. Patz A, Eastham A, Higgenbotham DH, et al. Oxygen studies in retrolental fibroplasia: II. The production of the microscopic changes of retrolental fibroplasia in experimental animals. Am J Ophthalmol 1953; 36:1511-1522.

6. Reese AB, King MJ, Owens WC. A classification of retrolental fibroplasia. Am J Ophthalmol 1953; 36:1333-1335.

7. Avery ME, Oppenheimer EH. Recent increase in mortality from hyaline membrane disease. J Pediatr 1960; 57:533.

8. McDonald AD. Cerebral palsy in children of very low birth

weight. Arch Dis Child 1963; 38:579.

9. Phelps DL. Vision loss due to retinopathy of prematurity. Lancet 1981; 1:606.

10. Patz A. Retrolental fibroplasia (retinopathy of prematurity). Am J Ophthalmol 1982; 94:552-554.

11. Graven SN. Oxygen therapy in the newborn infant: a statement of the Committee on Fetus and Newborn by the American Academy of Pediatrics. Wis Med J 1971; 70:224.

12. Kingham JD. Acute retrolental fibroplasia. Arch Ophthalmol 1977; 95:39-47.

13. Majima A. Studies on retinopathy of prematurity. I. Statistical analysis of factors related to occurrence and progression in active phase. Jpn J Ophthalmol 1977; 21:404-420.

14. Oshima K, Nishimura Y, Kano M, et al. Photocoagulation treatment on rapidly progressive cases of retinopathy of prematurity. Jpn J Clin Ophthalmol 1974; 28:217-223.

15. Morizane H. Initial sign and clinical course of the most severe form of acute proliferative retrolental fibroplasia (type II). Acta Soc Ophthalmol Jpn 1976; 80:54-61.

16. Soejima N, Takagi I, Takashima Y. Clinical studies on retinopathy of prematurity, severe and rapidly progressive type. Folia Ophthalmol Jpn 1976; 27:155-161.

17. Uemura Y. Current status of retrolental fibroplasia. Report of the joint committee for the study of retrolental fibroplasia in Japan. Jpn J Ophthalmol 1977; 21:366-378.

18. Schaffer D, Johnson L, Quinn G, et al. A classification of retrolental fibroplasia to evaluate vitamin E therapy. Ophthalmology 1979; 86:1749-1760.

19. Quinn GE, Schaffer DB, Johnson L. A revised classification of retinopathy of prematurity. Am J Ophthalmol 1982; 94:744-749.

20. Nagata M. Treatment of acute proliferative retrolental fibroplasia with xenon-arc photocoagulation: its indications and limitations. Jpn J Ophthalmol 1977; 21:436-459.

21. Kingham JD. Acute retrolental fibroplasia. II. Treatment by cryosurgery. Arch Ophthalmol 1978; 96:2049-2053.

22. Koerner FH. Retinopathy of prematurity. Natural course and management. Metabol Ophthalmol 1978; 2:325-329.

23. Ben-Sira I, Nissenkorn E, Grunwald E, et al. Treatment of acute retrolental fibroplasia by cryopexy. Br J Ophthalmol 1962; 64:758-762.

24. Hindle NW. Cryotherapy for retinopathy of prematurity to prevent retrolental fibroplasia. Can J Ophthalmol 1982; 17:207-212.

25. McPherson AR, Hittner HM, Lemos R. Retinal detachment in young premature infants with acute retrolental fibroplasia. Ophthalmology 1982; 89:160-169.

26. Hindle NW. International classification of retrolental fibroplasia: a proposal. Can J Ophthalmol 1982; 17:107–109.

27. Committee for the classification of retinopathy of prematurity. An international classification of retinopathy of prematurity. Arch Ophthalmol 1984; 102:1130–1134.

28. Cogan DG. Development and senescence of the human retinal vasculature. Trans Ophthalmol Soc UK 1963; 83:465-489.

Human Retinal Development: Relationship to the Pathogenesis of Retinopathy of Prematurity

4

Frank L. Kretzer, Ph.D.
Helen M. Hittner, M.D.

The classic pathogenesis of retinopathy of prematurity (ROP)[1-3] has been suggested to involve the following events: oxygen administration to the preterm infant triggers vasoconstriction, vaso-obliteration, and endothelial cell necrosis of nascently formed, inner retinal vessels; when the infant is returned to ambient air, the patency of these vessels is not restored, and there is increased hypoxia within the inner retinal layers, which induces retinal and vitreal neovascularization.

In contrast, the highlights of the spindle cell pathogenesis of ROP[4-9] are summarized in Table 4–1. This pathogenesis proposes that the inducers of the retinal and vitreal neovascularization are spindle cells in the hyperoxygenated avascular vanguard retina. A cluster of oxidative insults to spindle cells, which are precursors of the inner retinal vasculature, causes biochemical alterations, halts normal vasoformation, and triggers gap junction formation. There is subsequent proliferation of the cytoplasmic volume of the rough endoplasmic reticulum within spindle cells, such that these endothelial cell precursors are transformed into sites of synthesis and secretion of angiogenic factors. While the infant is still on continuous oxygen administration, and in the absence of inner retinal hypoxia, ROP may develop clinically. If factors trigger early down modulation of gap junctions, spontaneous regression ensues, ROP Stages 1 or 2 are observed clinically, and spindle cell stacking within the nerve fiber layer does not occur. If spindle cells remain gap junction linked, neovascularization from nascent vessels continues, with migration of significant numbers of myofibroblasts into the vitreous body, and ROP Stage 3 is observed clinically. When these myofibroblast sheets contract, retinal separation develops, and ROP Stage 4 is observed clinically. The vitreous invasion of myofibroblasts occurs just prior to spindle cell maturation. Maturation involves a down modulation of gap junctions, a decrease in the cytoplasmic volume of the rough endoplasmic reticulum, a cessation of synthesis and secretion of angiogenic factors, and a stacking of spindle cells within the nerve fiber layer.

TABLE 4–1   Highlights of the Spindle Cell Pathogenesis of ROP

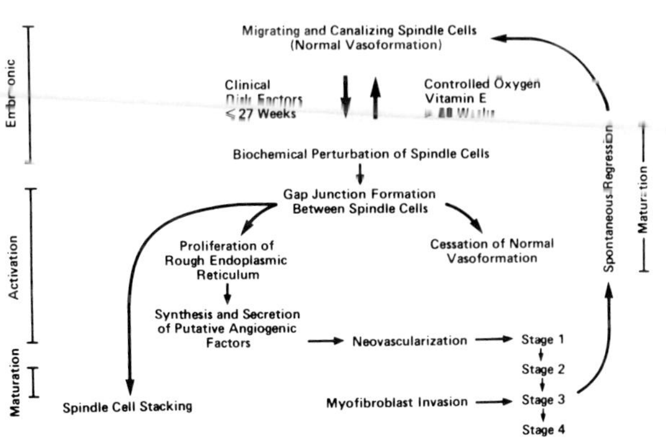

THE DATA BASE

The role of spindle cells in the induction of ROP, as modulated by gestational age and vitamin E supplementation, is based upon a data base of 97 pairs of whole-eye donations obtained within 1 to 5 hours post mortem (Tables 4–2 to 4–8). Seventy-three pairs of eyes were from live-born, anomaly-free, preterm infants who weighed 1,500 grams or less at birth, were in respiratory distress, and received continuous oxygen administration until death. Of these infants, 22 controls achieved mean plasma vitamin E levels of 0.3 to 0.6 mg per deciliter (Tables 4–2 and 4–3) with oral supplementation (5 mg per kilogram per day) of dl-alpha-tocopherol.[10] Fifty-one treatments achieved mean plasma vitamin E levels of 1.2 to 3.3 mg per deciliter (Tables 4–4 to 4–7), with oral

TABLE 4-2 Control Embryonic Infants Surviving < 4 Days

Infant	Gestational Age (wk)	Birth Weight (g)	Spindle Cell Volume of Nerve Fiber Layer (%)	Average Gap Junction Area (%)	RER (%)*	Photoreceptor Maturation Studied	Search for Endothelial Necrosis Performed	Life (hr)
Control Embryonic (N=14)								
(1) 82-6	20	300	4.5	5.3		+		3.0
(2) 82-81	23	450	7.9	2.4	4.6			3.0
(3) 82-54	23	500	9.3	2.4		+		1.0
(4) 82-53	24	540	6.3	3.1				2.0
(5) 82-59	24	560	12.6	5.8	8.2			1.0
(6) 82-16	25	640	10.8	4.0			+	2.0
(7) 82-101	25	650	11.8	4.5				8.0
(8) 82-112	25	700	4.8	7.7	12.3	+		0.3
(9) 82-116	25	780	11.0	15.7				2.0
(10) 82-21	26	810	7.0	3.4				1.0
(11) 82-22	27	770	13.4	5.8				17.0
(12) 82-115	27	910	5.6	3.4	6.4	+		2.0
(13) 82-108	28	950	5.5	1.8			+	36.0
(14) 82-70	28	990	8.6	8.8	9.8	+		8.0
			8.5	5.0				

* Percentage volume of the spindle cell cytoplasm occupied by rough endoplasmic reticulum (RER)

TABLE 4-3 Control Activation and Control Maturation Infants Surviving > 4 Days

Infant	Gestational Age (wk)	Birth Weight (g)	Spindle Cell Volume of Nerve Fiber Layer (%)	Average Gap Junction Area (%)	RER (%)#	Search for Endothelial Necrosis Performed	Life (days)
Control Activation (N = 6)							
(15) 82-14	24	520	8.7	30.3	40.0		4.25
(16) 81-96	25	700	19.7	67.1	32.0	+	56.00
(17) 82-122	26	710	12.8	56.3			39.00
(18) 82-49	27	880	12.5	28.3	37.0		4.25
(19) 82-133	27	900	10.6	40.7	35.0	+	23.00
(20) 81-67	28	1,060	5.1	43.8		+	5.00
			11.6*	44.4†			
Control Maturation (N=2)							
(21) 79-126¶	26	625	53.9	11.9	3.2	+	70.00
(22) 81-16¶	27	900	31.6	2.5	10.1	+	84.00
			42.8‡	7.2§			

* Comparable (p = 0.09) to control-embryonic levels
† Significantly different (p < 0.0000) from control-embryonic levels
‡ Significantly different (p < 0.0000) from the average spindle-cell volume of the entire data base (excluding infant 55)
§ Comparable (p = 0.5) to control-embryonic levels
¶ ROP Stage 3
# Percentage volume of the spindle cell cytoplasm by rough endoplasmic reticulum (RER)

TABLE 4–4 Treatment-Embryonic Infants Surviving <4 Days

Infant	Gestational Age (wk)	Birth Weight (g)	Spindle Cell Volume of Nerve Fiber Layer (%)	Average Gap Junction Area (%)	RER (%)‡	Photoreceptor Maturation Studied	Search for Endothelial Necrosis Performed	Life (hr)
Treatment Embryonic (N = 13)								
(23) 82–46	24	740	13.6	2.4	10.2	+		8.0
(24) 82–15	25	660	12.6	3.5			+	84.0
(25) 82–60	25	770	12.6	6.2		+		6.0
(26) 82–58	26	790	10.1	3.7				36.0
(27) 82–38	26	860	12.1	4.9		+	+	9.0
(28) 82–50	27	780	11.7	4.3				66.0
(29) 82–62	27	910	10.3	2.2	4.6	+		96.0
(30) 82–56	27	1,020	16.5	2.1				30.0
(31) 82–106	27	1,100	2.7	<1.0				36.0
(32) 82–57	28	800	13.6	12.1			+	28.0
(33) 82–104	29	1,090	7.0	2.8		+		72.0
(34) 82–36	29	1,220	7.9	8.3				62.4
(35) 82–90	30	1,330	6.2	7.6	7.3	+	+	32.0
			10.4*	5.0†				

* Comparable (p = 0.16) to control-embryonic levels
† Comparable (p = 0.8) to control-embryonic levels
‡ Percentage volume of the spindle cell cytoplasm occupied by rough endoplasmic reticulum (RER)

TABLE 4–5 Treatment-Lag-Activation Infants Surviving From 4 to 20 Days

Infant	Gestational Age (wk)	Birth Weight (g)	Spindle Cell Volume of Nerve Fiber Layer (%)	Average Gap Junction Area (%)	RER (%)‡	Search for Endothelial Necrosis Performed	Life (days)
Treatment-lag Activation (N = 10)							
(36) 82–148	24	550	3.4	16.0	5.3		6.25
(37) 83–16	24	620	11.1	17.5			10.00
(38) 83–2	25	660	13.2	8.5			6.80
(39) 82–67	26	850	9.4	<1.0	8.9		10.25
(40) 83–8	26	770	10.4	4.8			15.60
(41) 82–52	27	910	9.9	<1.0			4.75
(42) 82–18	27	760	4.6	10.4	12.2	+	5.00
(43) 82–25	27	940	5.6	4.3			11.00
(44) 82–130	27	940	6.6	4.4			11.70
(45) 82–128	27	760	11.3	10.1	9.8	+	18.75
			8.6*	7.8†			

* Comparable (p = 0.2) to treatment-embryonic levels
† Comparable (p = 0.1) to treatment-embryonic levels
‡ Percentage volume of the spindle cell cytoplasm by rough endoplasmic reticulum (RER)

TABLE 4–6 Treatment-delayed Activation and Treatment-delayed Maturation Infants Surviving >15 Days

Infant	Gestational Age (wk)	Birth Weight (g)	Spindle Cell Volume of Nerve Fiber Layer (%)	Average Gap Junction Area (%)	RER (%)[#]	Search for Endothelial Necrosis Performed	Life (days)
Treatment-delayed Activation (N = 9)							
(46) 83–125¶	24	500	16.3	41.0	40.0	+	80.0
(47) 82–93	25	680	12.2	21.4	45.0		20.0
(48) 81–109	25	760	10.8	34.3			25.0
(49) 82–124	25	760	13.5	52.0	41.0	+	27.5
(50) 81–110	26	830	5.3	31.8			15.0
(51) 82–129	26	750	5.7	50.9	52.0		20.3
(52) 82–65	27	740	7.9	32.1		+	20.0
(53) 81–19	27	940	4.8	22.9			20.0
(54) 84–42	27	940	8.5	50.3	33.0	+	58.0
			9.0*	37.4†			
Treatment-delayed Maturation (N=1)							
(55) 84–55¶	26	790	46.8‡	6.3§	6.3	+	163.0

* Comparable to both treatment-embryonic (p = 0.4) and lag-activation (p = 0.8) levels
† Comparable (p = 0.8) to control-activation levels
‡ Comparable (p = 0.3) to control-maturation levels
§ Comparable (p = 0.6) to control-maturation levels
¶ ROP Stage 3
# Percentage volume of the spindle cell cytoplasm occupied by rough endoplasmic reticulum (RER)

TABLE 4–7 Treatment-suppressed Activation Infants Surviving >4 Days

Infant	Gestational Age (wk)	Birth Weight (g)	Spindle Cell Volume of Nerve Fiber Layer (%)	Average Gap Junction Area (%)	RER (%)‡	Search for Endothelial Necrosis Performed	Life (days)
Treatment-suppressed Activation (N = 18)							
(56) 83–43	27	850	4.3	<1.0	3.3		70.00
(57) 81–66	27	1,030	1.3	<1.0		+	133.00
(58) 82–51	28	980	8.1	<1.0			4.50
(59) 81–55	28	790	6.6	12.4			10.00
(60) 81–54	28	1,040	4.0	1.9		+	119.00
(61) 82–47	28	1,040	9.6	10.3			23.00
(62) 81–26	29	940	3.1	5.9			19.00
(63) 82–72	29	1,040	15.7	5.3	8.9		6.75
(64) 82–43	29	1,100	15.3	2.5			16.50
(65) 82–87	29	1,150	8.8	10.5			12.75
(66) 82–31	29	1,160	18.0	<1.0	8.2	+	56.00
(67) 83–33	29	1,180	5.6	<1.0			112.00
(68) 82–79	30	1,180	13.7	5.1	4.7		12.00
(69) 82–64	30	1,320	12.5	2.5	5.5	+	32.00
(70) 82–55	30	1,400	7.2	1.8			5.50
(71) 82–162	31	1,400	6.1	14.6	6.8	+	140.00
(72) 82–30	31	1,270	14.1	11.5		+	5.00
(73) 82–100	31	1,370	12.7	5.6			25.00
			9.3*	5.3†			

* Comparable (p = 0.5) to treatment-embryonic levels
† Comparable (p = 0.8) to treatment-embryonic levels
‡ Percentage volume of the spindle cell cytoplasm occupied by rough endoplasmic reticulum (RER)

+/− intramuscular supplementation (orally, 100 mg per kilogram per day of dl-alpha-tocopherol[10] or dl-alpha-tocopheryl acetate[11,12]; intramuscularly, 15, 10, 10, and 10 mg per kilogram of dl-alpha-tocopherol on days one, two, four, and six respectively.[12] These 73 pairs of whole-eye donations were analyzed for the percentage of the spindle cell plasma membrane that was differentiated into gap junctions and the percentage of the nerve fiber layer that was occupied by spindle cells. The percentage of the spindle cell, cytoplasmic volume that was occupied by rough endoplasmic reticulum was calculated in one eye each of 30 infants. In one eye each of 24 infants, the presence of endothelial necrosis was sought along continuous montages from the optic disc to the ora serrata. The dynamics of photoreceptor maturation, as related to ontogeny of the outer plexiform layer, the location of the peripheral edge of the spindle cell apron, and the location of inner retinal vessels and capillaries along the optic disc-ora serrata axis, was determined in one eye each of 11 infants who survived less than 4 days. Assays for angiogenic activity within hypotonic homogenates of the vanguard or rearguard retina, of one eye each from 12 infants, were determined by induced loop activation from the chorioallantoic membrane of the fertilized chicken egg, as per the technique of Glaser, et al.[13-16]

An additional 24 pairs of whole-eye donations were obtained from infants who survived less than 4 hours and were not enrolled in one of the three clinical trials. Immunocytochemical detection of interstitial retinol binding protein (IRBP) within the developing interphotoreceptor matrix was performed in one eye each of these 24 infants, as per the technique reported by Johnson, et al[17-18] (Table 4–8).

Clinically, most premature infants weighing 1,500 grams or less at birth, who survive, do not develop severe ROP. However, infants who are not likely to survive are also at greatest risk of developing ROP. Therefore, the data base is enriched with eyes from infants who, had they survived, most likely would have developed severe ROP.

EARLY RETINAL DEVELOPMENT

When the optic vesicle invaginates to form the optic cup, the central cavity is obliterated, and the cell layers of the developing retina and retinal pigment epithelium become apposed. As photoreceptors differentiate, a space separates the apical surfaces of the retinal pig-

ment epithelium, photoreceptors, and Müller cells. This subretinal space contains a mixture of glycoproteins and glycosaminoglycans,[19] which forms the interphotoreceptor matrix. The development of photoreceptors in the human retina is nearly complete at term, except in the macula.[20] Thus, to probe the ontogeny of the subretinal space in humans, it is necessary to study the retinas of preterm infants.

The retina begins its maturation centrally by repetitive mitosis, nuclear migrations, and sequential differentiation of ganglion, bipolar, and photoreceptor cells. Within the low in utero oxygen tension, oxygen freely diffuses across the primitive retina from the choroidal vessels. Since photoreceptors have not as yet developed, there is no barrier to halt the diffusion of oxygen from the choroid across the neuroblastic retina to the large cystoid spaces within the forming nerve fiber layer.

TABLE 4-8   Distribution of Interstitial Retinol Binding Protein

Gestational Age (wk)	Birth Weight (g)	Anti-IRBP Antibody Immunocytochemistry*
20	260	16
21	310	5
21	430	8
22	420	30
23	260	10
23	450	27
23	460	50
23	530	10
24	560	60
24	600	20
24	630	23
24	640	26
24	640	42
25	560	50
26	700	53
26	840	35
26	980	30
27	830	39
27	840	58
28	960	92
28	970	40
28	980	76
32	1,200	100
Term	2,400	100

* Data expressed as percentage distance from the optic disc to the ora serrata that has fluorescence within the subretinal space. This correlates precisely with the site where the transition from Stage II to Stage I photoreceptors occurs.

ONTOGENY OF THE INTERPHOTO-RECEPTOR MATRIX: RELATIONSHIP TO PHOTORECEPTOR DEVELOPMENT, RETINAL VITAMIN E LEVELS, AND OXYGEN DIFFUSION

Photoreceptors secrete IRBP, which spans the subretinal space.[21-24] Johnson, et al[17-18] have documented that the secretion of initial IRBP by photoreceptors is concomitant with the formation of nascent, random, tubular discs in the primitive outer segment. IRBP is a glycoprotein component of the interphotoreceptor matrix[25] that binds and shuttles vitamins A and E[26] between the retinal pigment epithelium and neural retina. Since vitamin E efficacy in suppressing the development of severe ROP is critically related to retinal uptake of the antioxidant[8-9;18], it is vital to understand the relationship between gestational age and the location of photoreceptors that have matured to the point of secreting IRBP.

Figures 4–1 to 4–5 demonstrate the ultrastructural spectrum of photoreceptors in the preterm retina, the comparable fluorescent micrographs of frozen sections that have been incubated with antiserum against purified bovine IRBP, and the parallel light microscopy morphology.

Figure 4–1 shows Stage I photoreceptor ultrastructure, in which no inner segments protrude beyond the outer limiting membrane. These immature photoreceptor precursors are not secreting IRBP, and immunocytochemically, there is no fluorescence of anti-IRBP antibody in the tiny, subretinal space. Figure 4–2 demonstrates Stage II photoreceptor ultrastructure, in which a nascent, balloon-shaped outer segment contains tubular discs (Fig. 4–3A). This is the earliest stage of photoreceptor maturation at which IRBP is secreted. There is a faint fluorescence to anti-IRBP antibody within the subretinal space. Figure 4–4 defines Stage III photoreceptor ultrastructure, in which the short, stubby outer segments contain stacks of discs oriented both parallel and at right axis to the outer limiting membrane (Fig. 4–3B). These photoreceptors are actively secreting IRBP. There is a wide and bright fluorescence of anti-IRBP antibody within the enlarging subretinal space. Figure 4–5 illustrates Stage IV photoreceptor ultrastructure, in which mature, long outer segments contain organized, stacked discs. The fluorescent image of anti-IRBP antibody in the subretinal space is bright, outlines the outer and inner segments, and spans the large

subretinal space between the retinal pigment epithelium and outer limiting membrane. Stage III and Stage IV photoreceptors have high oxygen-utilization requirements[27] and establish an oxygen sink that impedes the diffusion of oxygen from the choroid into the inner retina (Fig. 4–6). In the premature retina, Stage III and Stage IV photoreceptors, if they have developed centrally, are far removed from the demarcation line where neovascularization may occur. The demarcation line is always transretinal to Stage I and II photoreceptors, which create no barrier to the diffusion of oxygen from choroidal vessels to the nerve fiber layer. Thus, inner retinal hypoxia is not a parameter in the pathogenesis of ROP.

At 20-weeks gestational age, only the most central 10 percent of the retina around the optic disc has Stage II photoreceptors and IRBP within the subretinal space (Table 4–8). By 28-weeks gestational age, approximately 80 percent of the retinal distance from the optic disc to the ora serrata possesses IRBP (Table 4–8). Stage III photoreceptors have developed centrally, but Stage II photoreceptors have not yet reached the ora serrata. Between 28- and 32-weeks gestational age, Stage II photoreceptor development encroaches upon the ora serrata, and the maturing, far peripheral photoreceptors start to secrete IRBP (Table 4–8).

This relationship, Stage II photoreceptor development with secretion of IRBP, may explain vitamin E levels in the vanguard retina as a function of gestational age. Prior to 27-weeks gestational age, there are only trace levels of vitamin E (R. E. Anderson and J. Nielsen, personal communication) that correlate with the restricted domain of IRBP to the most central regions where Stage II photoreceptors have matured. After 28-weeks gestational age, there are significant levels of vitamin E (R. E. Anderson and J. Nielsen, personal communication). This correlates with the fact that Stage II photoreceptors have matured peripherally at loci closer to the ora serrata, Stage II and Stage III photoreceptors are secreting IRBP, and IRBP is shuttling vitamin E from the retinal pigment epithelium into peripheral, retinal membranes (Fig. 4–6).

The peripheral, preterm retina is structurally isolated from hydrophobic substances by the hydrophilic, subretinal space on one side and the paucity of inner retinal vessels on the other. The migrating apron of spindle cells is far in advance of the inner retinal capillaries, and only minimal amounts of vitamin E can reach the peripheral spindle cells from the physiologically vasoconstricted inner retinal vessels. In this situation, vitamin E carrier proteins in the hydrophilic subretinal space play a major role in the delivery of vitamin E to Müller cells, and ulti-

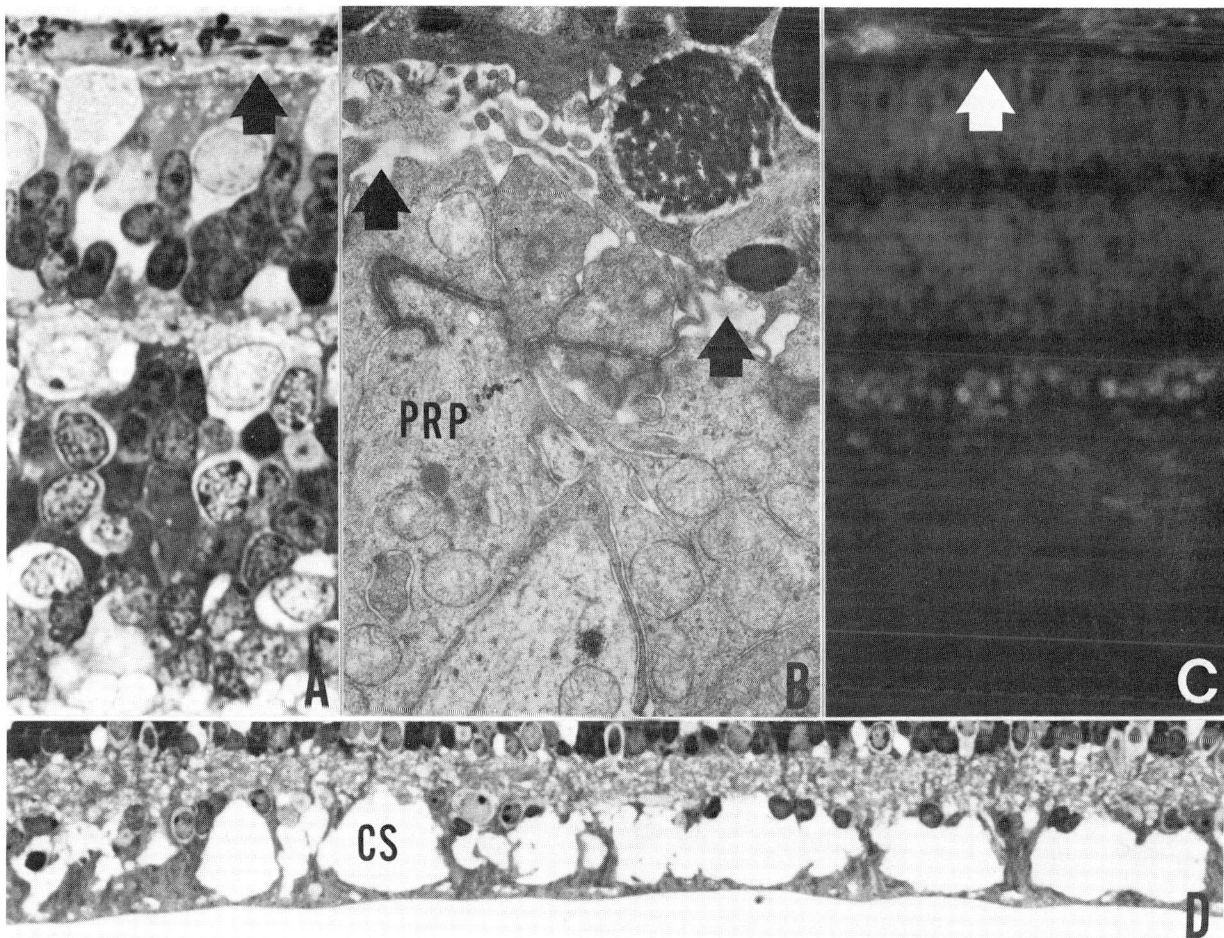

Figure 4–1   Stage I photoreceptors and subretinal space exemplified by light microscopy A (1,300×), transmission electron microscopy B (18,000×), and fluorescence microscopy of a frozen section incubated with rabbit antibovine IRBP antiserum C (310×). The tiny subretinal space (⬆) contains no IRBP, since the photoreceptor precursors (PRP) have no inner or outer segments and are not yet secreting IRBP into the subretinal space. Therefore, there is no potential to shuttle vitamin E from the retinal pigment epithelium to retinal membranes. Characteristically, the nerve fiber layer transretinal to Stage I photoreceptors D (470×) is composed of cystoid spaces (CS) that are devoid of spinal cells. However, in infants of 27-weeks gestational age or less, Stage I photoreceptors are transretinal to the majority of the spindle cell apron.

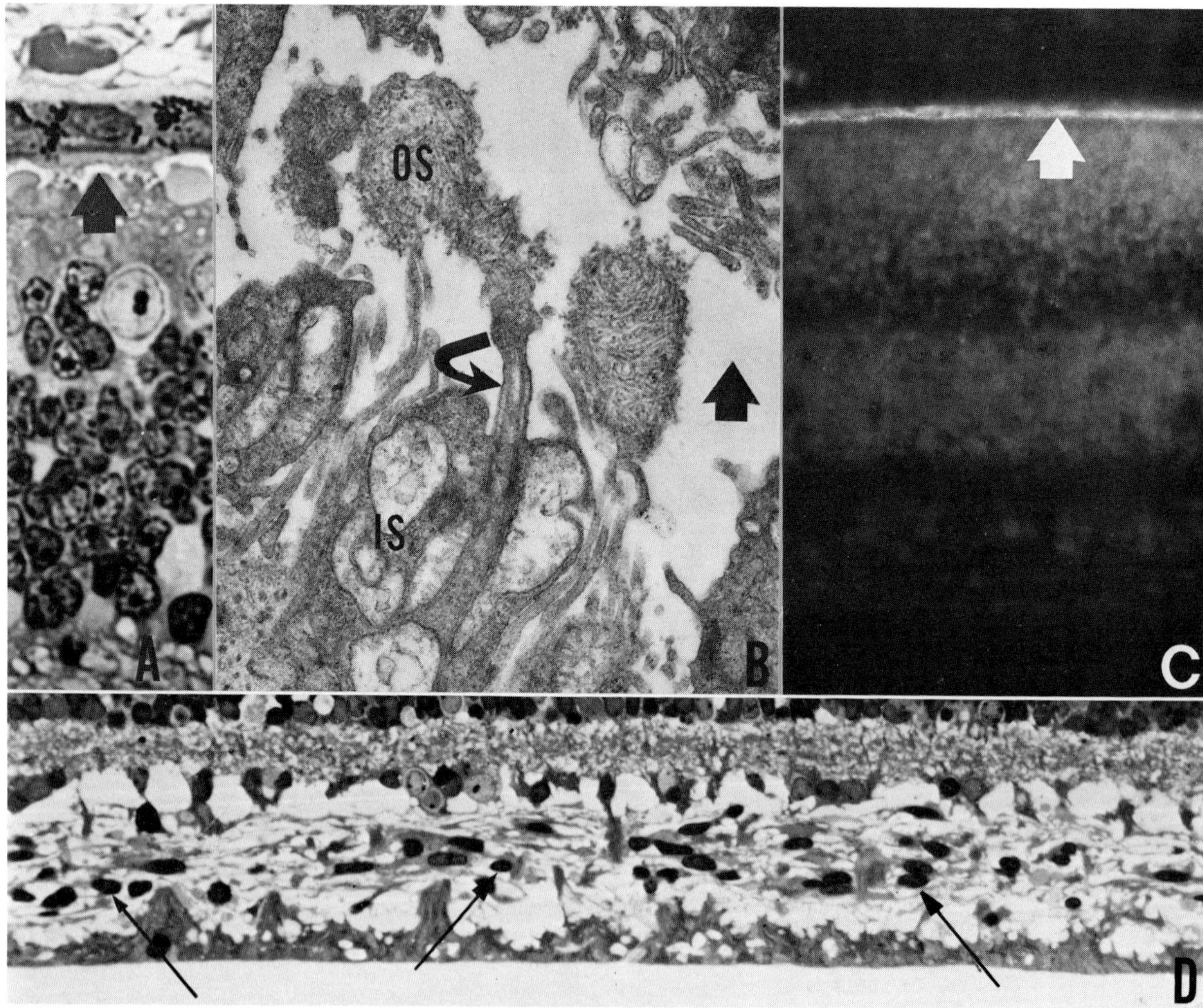

Figure 4–2 Stage II photoreceptors and subretinal space exemplified by light microscopy A (1,300×), transmission electron microscopy B (18,000×), and fluorescence microscopy of a frozen section incubated with rabbit antibovine IRBP antiserum C (310×). The enlarging subretinal space (⬆) contains a thin band of immunospecific fluorescence adjacent to the apical surface of the retinal pigment epithelium. Therefore, there is a potential to shuttle vitamin E from the retinal pigment epithelium to retinal membranes. Ultrastructurally, photoreceptor inner segments (IS) contain a few mitochondria. A connecting cilium (↰) links the inner segment to the balloon-shaped outer segment (OS) with random tubular membrane profiles. Characteristically, in infants of 28-weeks gestational age or more, the nerve fiber layer transretinal to Stage II photoreceptors D (470×) is composed of migrating spindle cells (⟵), such that the majority of the spindle-cell apron can be stabilized by a threshold antioxidant level. It is proposed that Müller cells are the connecting links between vitamin E in the subretinal space and vitamin E within the membranes of the nerve fiber layer.

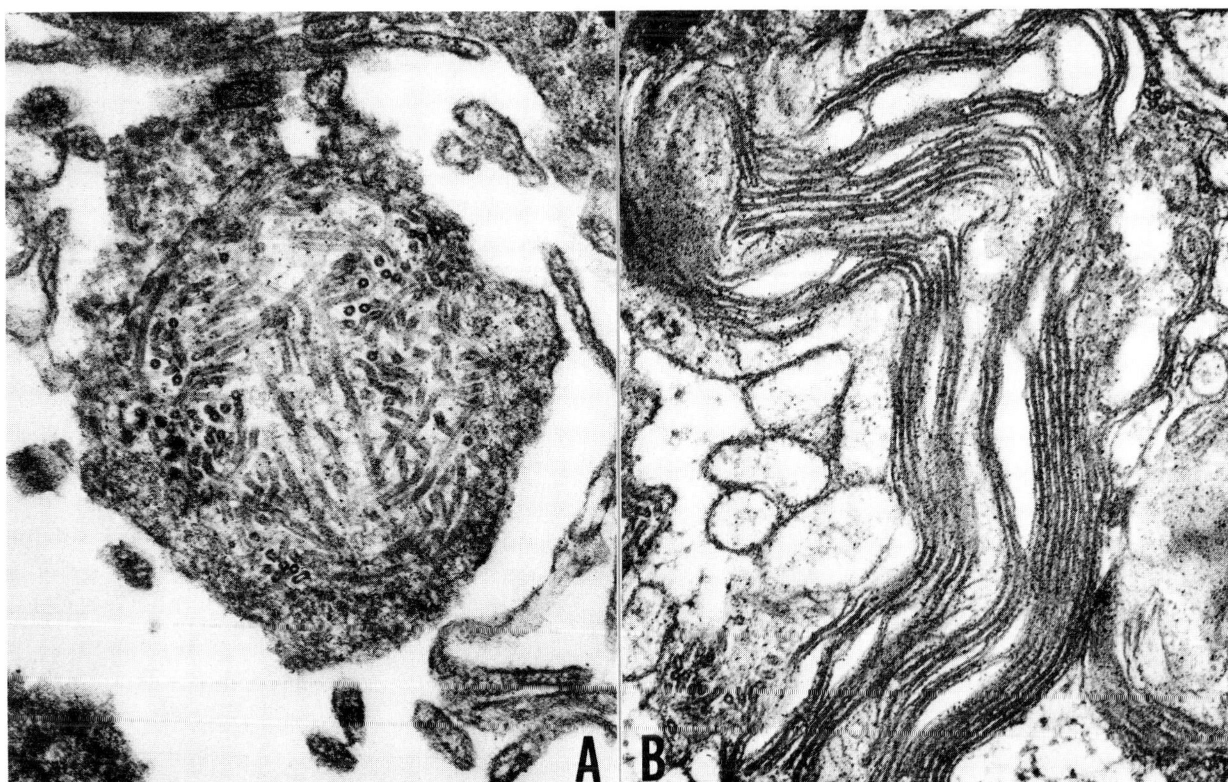

Figure 4–3 Transmission electron micrographs (49,500×) demonstrating the configuration of outer segment discs in Stage II photoreceptors A and Stage III photoreceptors B. Stage II photoreceptors have randomly oriented tubular membrane profiles with a diameter of 500A within the cytoplasm of the outer segment. Concomitant with this stage of morphological development, photoreceptors initiate secretion of IRBP. Stage III photoreceptors have stacked membrane discs oriented both parallel and at right angles to the outer limiting membrane within the cytoplasm of the outer segment.

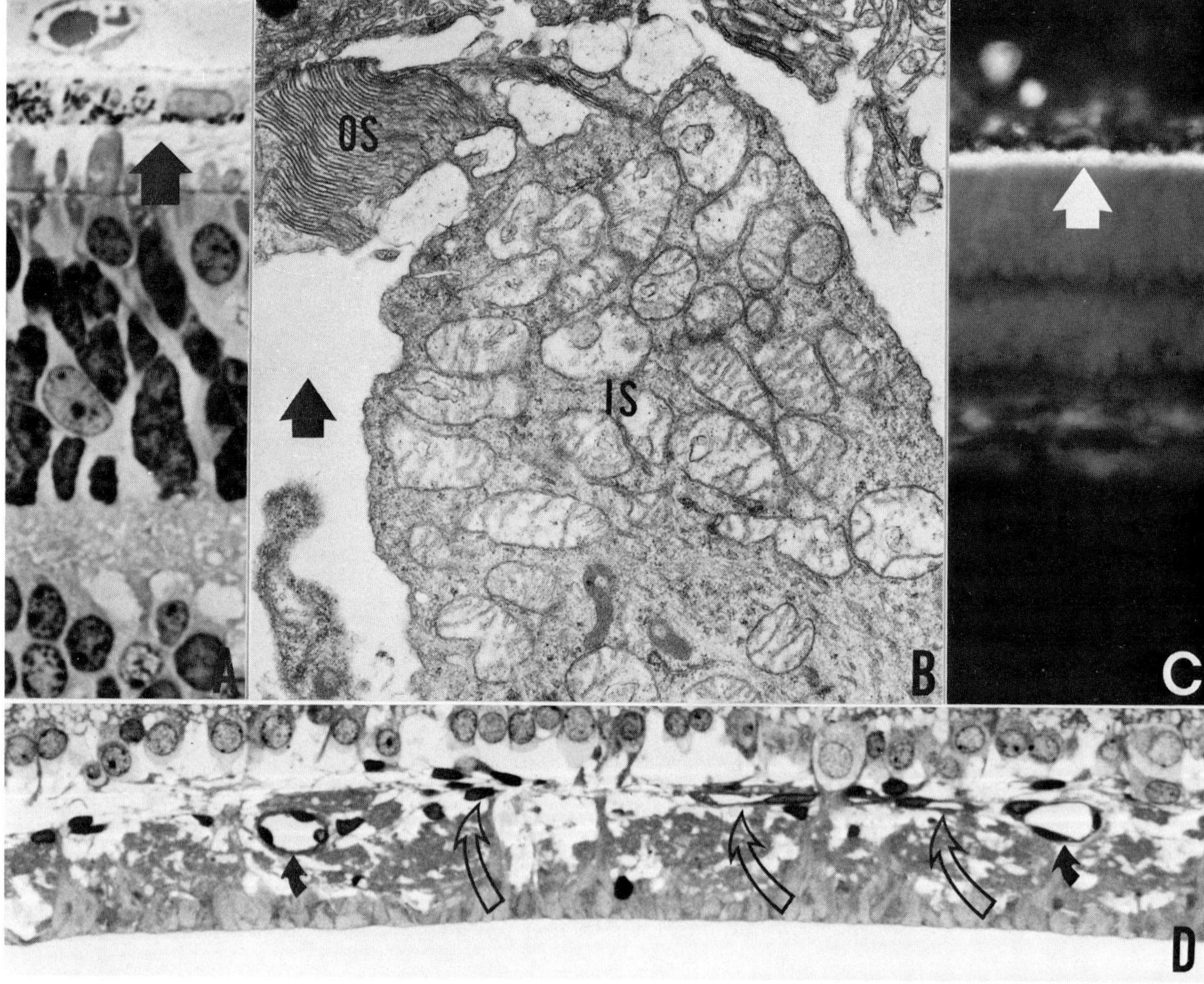

Figure 4–4   Stage III photoreceptors and subretinal space exemplified by light microscopy A (1,300×), transmission electron microscopy B (18,000×), and fluorescence microscopy of a frozen section incubated with rabbit antibovine IRBP antiserum C (310×). The large subretinal space (   ) contains a thick band of bright immunospecific fluorescence. Therefore, there is an operant shuttle system to transport vitamin E from the retinal pigment epithelium to the apical processes of Müller cells. Ultrastructurally, photoreceptors have inner segments (IS) with densely packed mitochondria. Morphologically, this suggests that Stage III photoreceptors have high metabolic rates that create a barrier to the diffusion of oxygen across the retina from the choroidal vessels. The outer segments (OS) contain stacked membrane profiles arranged randomly within the cytoplasm. The nerve fiber layer transretinal to Stage III photoreceptors D (470×) is composed of small capillaries (   ) and canalizing spindle cells (   ), creating a new vascular bed to counterbalance the oxygen deficit caused by maturing photoreceptors.

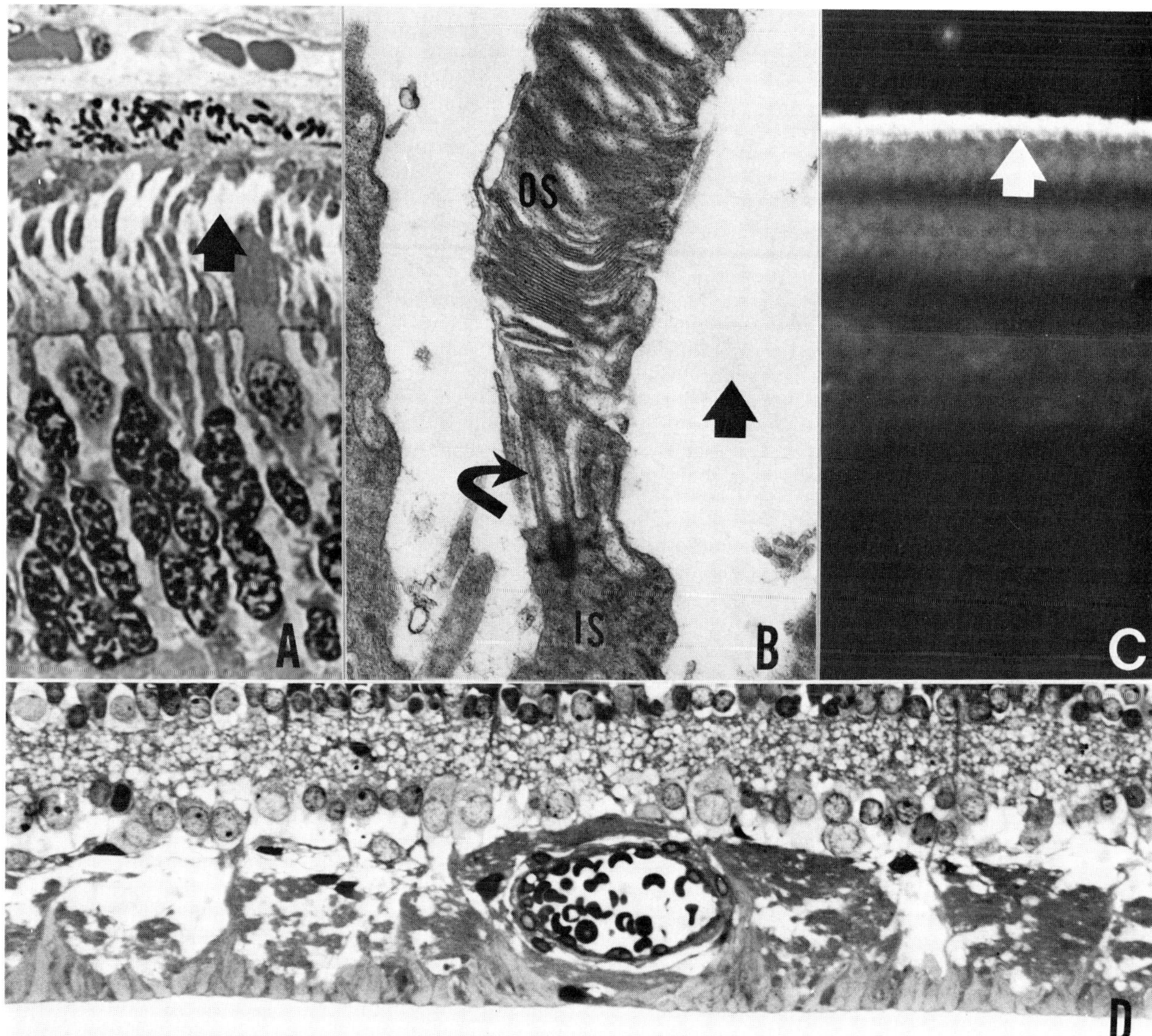

Figure 4–5 Stage IV photoreceptors and subretinal space exemplified by light microscopy A (1,300×), transmission electron microscopy B (18,000×), and fluorescence microscopy of a frozen section incubated with rabbit antibovine IRBP antiserum C (310×). The mature subretinal space ( ) contains a complex immunospecific fluorescence consisting of a bright line adjacent to the apical surface of the retinal pigment epithelium, a striated band in the region of the outer segments, and a faint band outlining the photoreceptor inner segments. Therefore, there is a operant shuttle system to transport vitamin E from the retinal pigment epithelium to the apical processes of Müller cells. Ultrastructurally, photoreceptor inner segments (IS) are longer and thinner than those of Stage III photoreceptors, possess an ellipsoid packing of mitochondria, and are connected by a cytoplasmic bridge containing a sensory cilium ( ) to the outer segment (OS) with uniformly stacked disc membranes. Mature photoreceptors have a high oxygen consumption that creates a formidable barrier to the diffusion of oxygen across the retina from the choroidal vessels. The nerve-fiber layer transretinal to Stage IV photoreceptors D (470×) is composed of large vessels that supply the metabolic needs of the inner retina.

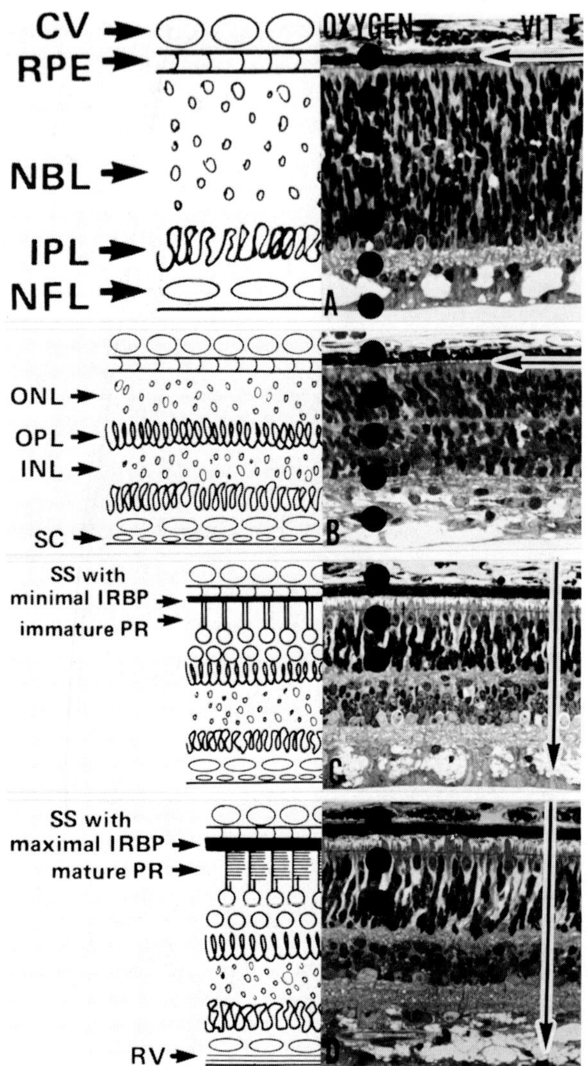

Figure 4–6   Oxygen flux (●●) and vitamin E (Vit E) transport (↓) across the developing, preterm retina as a function of the neuroblastic retina A, Stage I photoreceptors B, Stage III photoreceptors C, and Stage IV photoreceptors D. The line diagrams on the left show the choroidal vessels (CV), retinal pigment epithelium (RPE), neuroblastic layer (NBL), inner plexiform layer (IPL), nerve fiber layer (NFL), outer nuclear layer (ONL), inner nuclear layer (INL), spindle cells (SC), and retinal vessels (RV). These line drawings are aligned with light micrographs on the right (200×). There is an operant vitamin E transport system at Stage III photoreceptors with a subretinal space (SS) that contains interstitial retinal binding protein (IRBP). Stage III (immature) photoreceptors (PR) and Stage IV (mature) photoreceptors (PR) have inner segments packed with mitochondria. Their high metabolic rate creates an oxygen barrier to the diffusion of oxygen from the choroidal vessels. It is proposed that vitamin E is carried in the plasma by low-density lipoproteins, and then transferred sequentially to the retinal pigment epithelium, IRBP, apical surfaces of Müller cells, Müller cell cytoplasm, and inner retinal membranes.

Figure 4–7   Transmission electron micrograph demonstrating the intimate contact betwen Müller cell processes (M) and a spindle cell (SC) as it migrates through the cystoid spaces (CS) of the nerve fiber layer. The spindle cell plasma membrane is outlined with arrows as it is enshrouded by lateral processes of Müller cells. (11,520×)

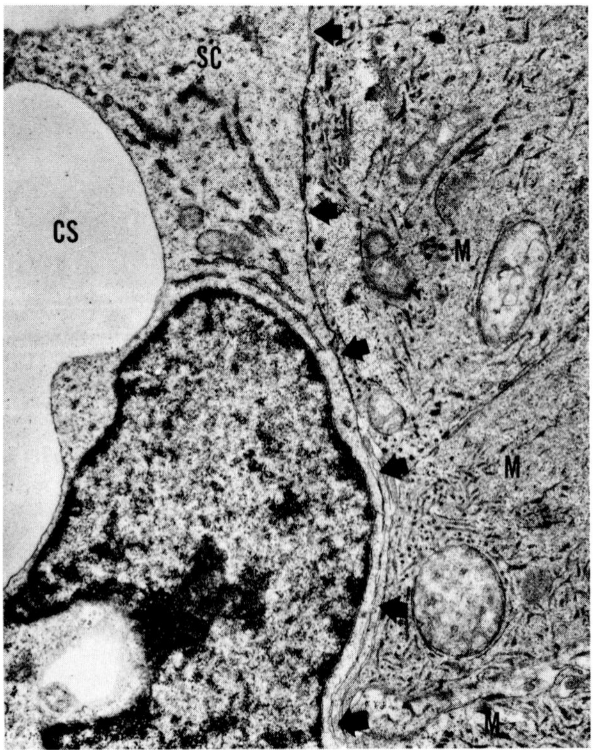

mately to the inner retina. The transretinal Müller cells, with their large surface area of apical processes within the subretinal space, and with their basal surfaces at the vitreous interface, are links between vitamin E carried across the subretinal space by IRBP and the spindle cells in the nerve fiber layer. Morphologically, there is a large contact area between Müller cells and spindle cells, supporting this concept (Fig. 4–7).

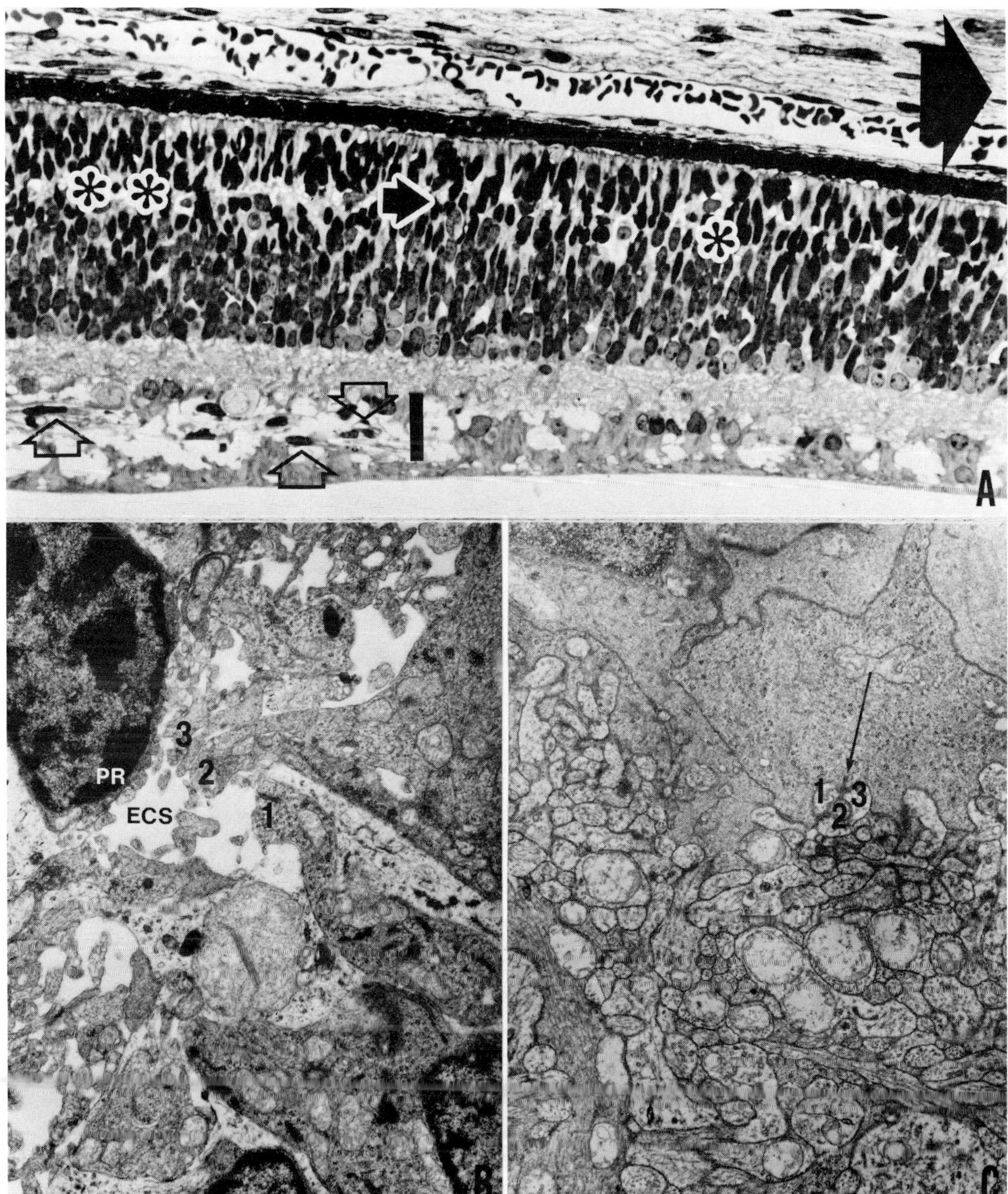

Figure 4–8 Micrographs demonstrating the migration of spindle cells into the nerve-fiber layer following a point of retinal development in which outer plexiform synapse formation first occurs (large arrow, direction of ora serrata). A, light micrograph (425×) showing the migration of spindle cells (⇦) to a peripheral point (▮) where the nascent outer plexiform layer disappears (➡). The choroid is patent, photoreceptors have not developed, and there is free diffusion of oxygen into the hyperoxic, vanguard inner retina. Two electron micrographs (B and C, 3,060×) demonstrate the critical point in outer plexiform synaptology that correlates with the peripheral migration of spindle cells. In B, the photoreceptor terminal (PR) is approached by three growth cones (1,2,3) that are separated by extracellular space (ECS). The ultrastructure in B correlates with area (✻) in A. In C, primitive synapse formation has occurred between three neuronal processes (1,2,3) and a photoreceptor terminal (PR) that contains a primitive synaptic ribbon (╱). The ultrastructure in C correlates with area (✻✻) in A.

SPINDLE CELL MIGRATION AND CANALIZATION: RELATIONSHIP TO OUTER PLEXIFORM DEVELOPMENT AND OXYGEN DIFFUSION

The inner retinal vasculature within the nerve fiber layer develops from spindle cell precursors that invade the nerve fiber layer, starting at the optic disc, and migrate peripherally along an advancing point of outer plexiform maturation (Fig. 4–8A). The critical stage of retinal development, which parallels the peripheral edge of the anastomosing apron of spindle cells, appears to occur when photoreceptor, bipolar, and horizontal processes first contact each other. There is subsequent obliteration of the extracellular spaces in the outer plexiform layer (Fig. 4–8B) and development of primitive synaptic ribbons (Fig. 4–8C).

Spindle cells migrate through the cystoid spaces of the forming nerve fiber layer (Fig. 4–9A). Posterior to this migrating apron, spindle cells form solid cords, with eventual lumen formation and metamorphosis of spindle cells into endothelial cells by a process of canalization (Fig. 4–9B). Spindle cells reach the ora serrata at about 29-weeks gestational age. In contrast, inner retinal vaso-

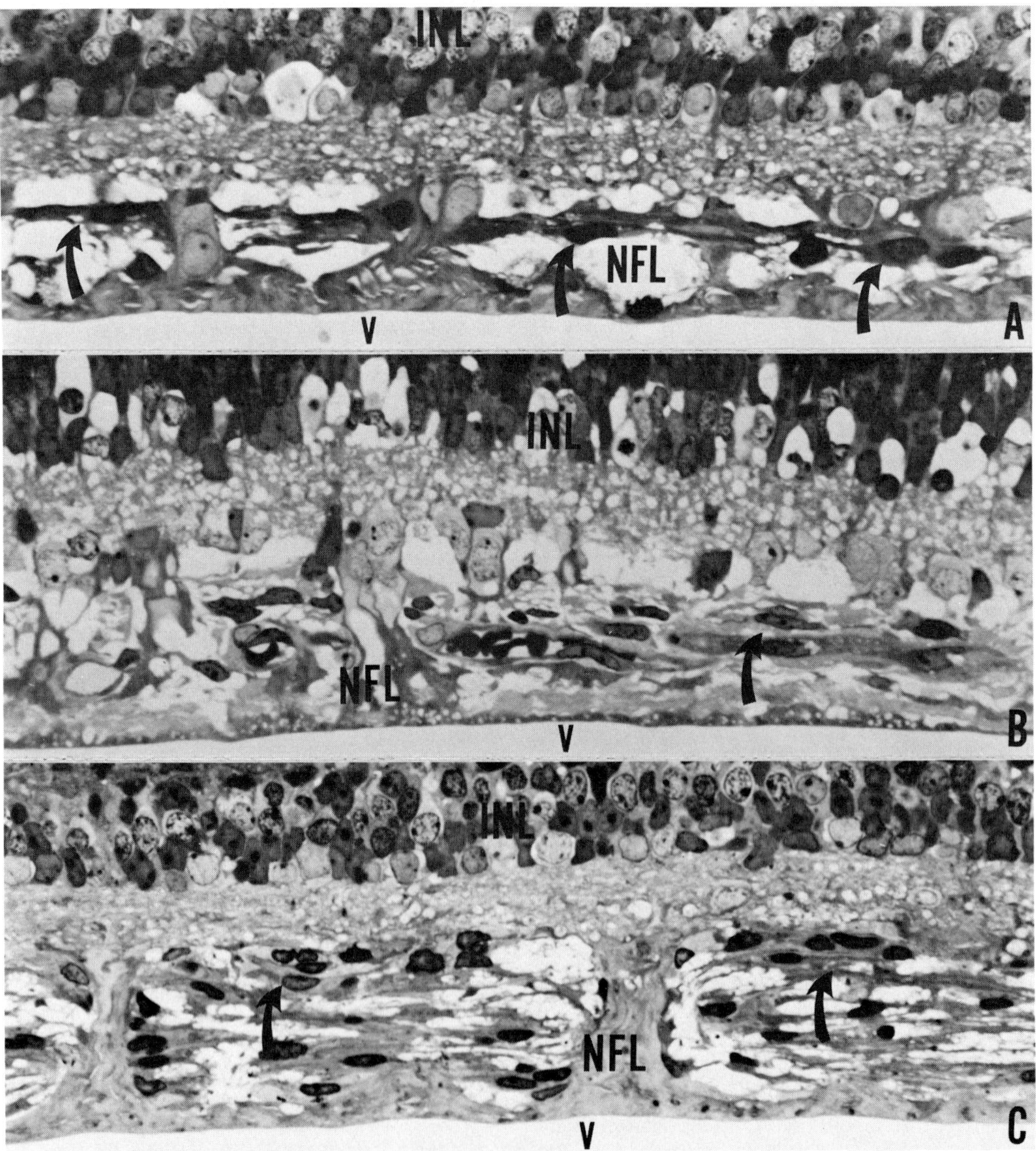

Figure 4–9 Light micrographs (680×) demonstrating the three configurations of spindle cells ( ) within the nerve fiber layer (NFL) of the preterm retina. A, migrating; B, canalizing; and C, stacked. (INL), inner nuclear layer; (V), vitreous.

formation lags far behind this advancing apron and reaches the temporal ora serrata only at term. Thus, the preterm infant is born with a 360-degree avascular, vanguard retina, which is larger in infants of lower gestational age.

The process of spindle cell migration and canalization occurs prior to the ontogeny of Stage III and Stage IV photoreceptors, and the human choroidal vasculature does not vasoconstrict with elevated oxygen tension. Thus, in the preterm human retina when the infant is given oxygen administration after birth (Fig. 4–6), the migrating and canalizing spindle cells and demarcation line are in hyperoxic environments.

In the developing human retina, there is a tight relationship between photoreceptor maturation and the composition of the nerve fiber layer. The high metabolic rate of Stage IV photoreceptors is counterbalanced by the transretinal development of large, inner retinal vessels (Fig. 4–5D). The lower metabolic rate of Stage III photoreceptors is associated with the ontogeny of small, inner retinal capillaries in the nerve-fiber layer (Fig. 4–4D). In contrast, the low metabolic rate of Stage II photoreceptors, as deduced by the scarce mitochondria within the developing inner segment, is transretinal to migrating spindle cells (Fig. 4–2D). The percentage of the total spindle cell apron that is transretinal to Stage II photoreceptors changes dramatically as a function of gestational age. Lastly, Stage I photoreceptors with few mitochondria within the precursor inner segment are transretinal to a nerve fiber layer with cystoid spaces devoid of spindle cells (Fig. 4–1D). In those infants of 27-weeks gestational age or less, a large percentage of the total spindle cell apron is transretinal to Stage I photoreceptors.

SPINDLE CELLS IN THE RETINAS OF CONTROL INFANTS

Control Embryonic

Based on the study of 14 control infants who survived less than 4 days (Table 4–2), spindle cells occupy a minimal volume of the nerve fiber layer, the adjacent plasma membranes have minimal gap junctions (Fig. 4–10A), and the cytoplasm contains scarce, rough endoplasmic reticulum (RER) (Fig. 4–11A). Morphologically, the scarce, rough endoplasmic reticulum reflects minimal protein synthesis and secretion. Homogenates of the vanguard retina do not stimulate neovascular loops from the chorioallantoic membrane (CAM) (Table 4–9, infant 2). Furthermore, spindle cells in the vanguard retina are transretinal to Stage I and II photoreceptors, the choroid is patent, and the vanguard, nerve fiber layer is, thus, hyperoxic. This morphological and physiological state of spindle cells is called *control embryonic*. Despite 2 hours (Table 4–2, infant 6) and 36 hours (Table 4–2, infant 13) of continuous oxygen administration, there is no ultrastructural evidence of endothelial cell necrosis, despite physiological vasoconstriction along the optic disc-ora serrata axis (Fig. 4–12A), and homogenates of the rearguard retina do not induce neovascular loops from the CAM (Table 4–9, infant 2). Therefore, physiologically vasoconstricted retinal vessels are not insulted by elevated oxygen tension and are not secreting angiogenic factors.

Control Activation

After the first 4 days of life (Table 4–3, infants 15 to 20), spindle cells are still an anastomosing apron, constituting a minimal volume within the nerve fiber layer that is comparable to control embryonic levels. There is a significant increase in gap junctions (Figs. 4–10B, C, and D) above the control embryonic levels. Gap junction increases occur as early as 4 days of life (Table 4–3, infants 15 and 18) and correlate with the cessation of migration and canalization and the increase in the cytoplasmic volume of rough endoplasmic reticulum. The latter morphologically equates with extensive protein synthesis and secretion (Fig. 4–11B). Homogenates from the vanguard retina induce prolific neovascular loops from the CAM (Table 4–9, infants 15 and 19). This morphological and physiological state of spindle cells is called *control activation*. These activated spindle cells in the vanguard retina are in a hyperoxic environment, since they are transretinal to low-oxygen-requiring Stage I and Stage II photoreceptors and a patent choroid. There is no ultrastructural evidence of endothelial cell necrosis after 5, 23, and 56 days of oxygen supplementation (Table 4–3, infants 16, 19, and 20; Fig. 4–12B), and homogenates of the rearguard retina do not promote neovascular loops from the CAM (Table 4–9, infants 15 and 19).

Thus, the inducers of the neovascularization associated with ROP are never the rearguard vessels, but rather gap-junction-linked spindle cells within the hyperoxic vanguard retina. The significant morphological increase in gap junctions reflects a transformation of spindle cells from endothelial cell precursors to sites of synthesis and secretion of angiogenic factors that induce

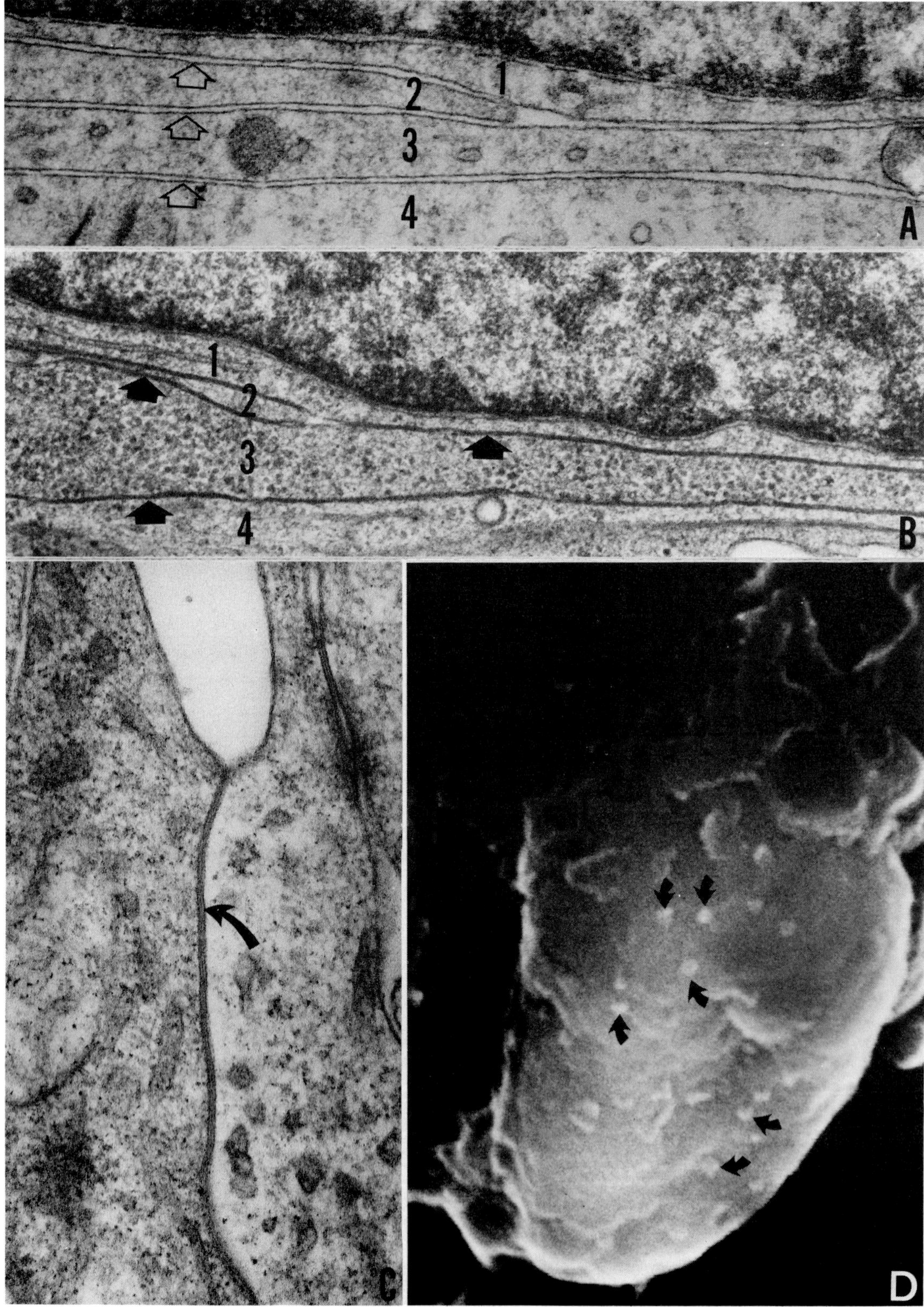

Figure 4–10   Electron micrographs demonstrating gap junctions between adjacent spindle cell, plasma membranes. The significant plasma membrane surface-area changes are demonstrated as the absence of close membrane appositions (⟁) in the four interdigitating processes (1,2,3,4) of control embryonic spindle cells A (40,800×), as contrasted with the extensive close membrane appositions (➡) of control activation spindle cells B (40,800×). The spindle cells in A continue to migrate and canalize and secrete no factors that activate the CAM angiogenic response. The spindle cells in B have ceased migration and canalization and secrete factors that activate the CAM angiogenic response. At higher magnification C (71,400×), the close membrane appositions are identified as gap junctions with substructure within the 20–30A gap (➤). With scanning electron microscopy, gap junctions appear as patches (✦) on the fractured plasma membrane surfaces of spindle cells D (24,650×).

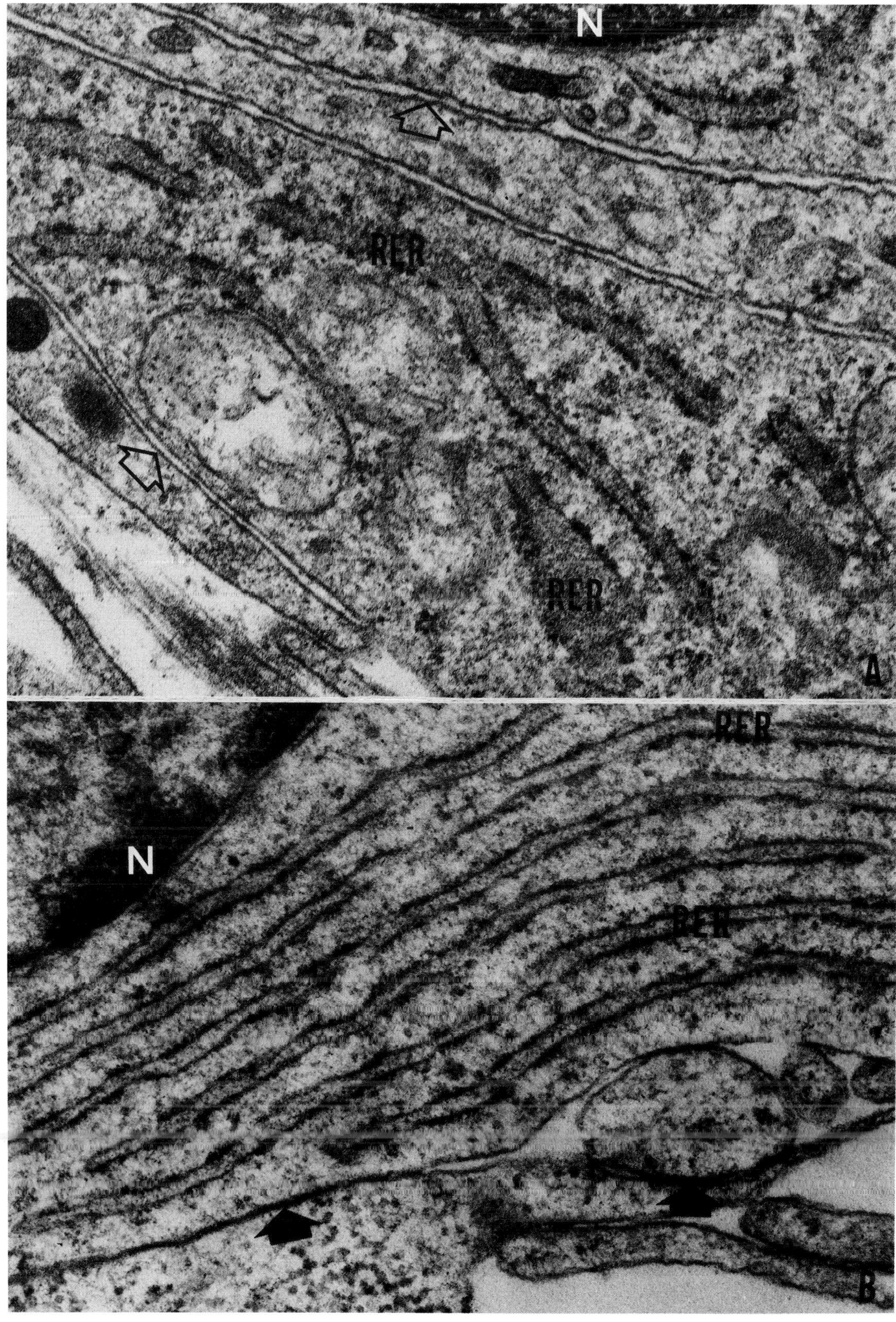

Figure 4–11   Electron micrographs (61,200×) demonstrating the proliferation of the rough endoplasmic reticulum (RER) after gap junction formation. A, control embryonic spindle cells with minimal gap junctions (⟩), scarce RER, and no activation of the CAM angiogenic response. B, control activation spindle cells with extensive gap junctions (►), abundant RER, and activation of the CAM angiogenic response. N, spindle cell nucleus.

TABLE 4–9 Assay for Angiogenic Factors in Homogenates of the Rearguard or Vanguard Retina by Induced Loop Formation from the Chorioallantoic Membrane

Infant	Gestational Age (wk)	Birth Weight (g)	Duration of Life	Stage of ROP	Number of Induced Loops*	
					Rearguard	Vanguard
Control Embryonic						
(2) 82–81	23	450	3 hours	---	0	2
Control Activation						
(15) 82–14	24	520	4.25 days	---	2	18
(19) 82–133	27	900	23 days	1	3	16
Control Maturation						
(22) 81–16	27	900	84 days	3	1	0
Treatment Embryonic						
(29) 82–62	27	910	96 hours	---	0	0
Treatment-lag Activation						
(42) 82–18	27	760	5 days	---	1	1
(45) 82–128	27	760	18.75 days	---	0	0
Treatment-delayed Activation						
(47) 82–93	25	680	20 days	---	1	17
(46) 83–125	24	500	80 days	3	1	18
Treatment-delayed Maturation						
(55) 84–55	26	790	163 days	3	0	1
Treatment-suppressed Activation						
(56) 83–43	27	850	70 days	1	0	1
(69) 82–64	30	1,320	32 days	1	0	3

* Saline pads induce 0–3 loops as insignificant background stimulation

neovascularization from the last-formed capillaries. These angiogenic factors have not been isolated, their molecular weights are unknown, and their activity can only be detected in homogenates of the vanguard retina that contain gap-junction-linked spindle cells. Spindle cells are the only retinal cell types that demonstrate such a cytoplasmic volume increase in rough endoplasmic reticulum.

Control Maturation

Two control infants (Table 4–3, infants 21 and 22) developed ROP Stage 3. At 70 and 84 days of life respectively, spindle cells have down-modulated gap junctions to control embryonic levels and contain scarce, rough endoplasmic reticulum, which morphologically indicates a cessation of extensive protein synthesis. The spindle cells occupy a large volume of the nerve fiber layer (Fig. 4–9C), which is statistically different from the average spindle cell volume of the entire control data base (Tables 4–2 and 4–3, infants 1 to 20). Homogenates of the vanguard retina with stacked spindle cells do not stimulate neovascular loops from the CAM (Table 4–9, infant 22). This morphological and physiological state of spin-

dle cells is called *control maturation*. At 70 and 84 days of life respectively, with continuous oxygen supplementation and the development of severe ROP, there is no ultrastructural evidence of endothelial cell necrosis (Fig. 4–12C). The proliferating vessels at the demarcation line are always transretinal to a patent choroid and immature, low-oxygen-consuming Stage I and Stage II photoreceptors. Thus, the neovascularization that develops in severe ROP occurs in hyperoxic retinal regions. Homogenates of the rearguard retina, with its tortuous and dilated vessels, do not stimulate loop formation from the CAM (Table 4–9, infant 22). The data presented here (Table 4–3) demonstrate that spindle cell stacking[28] is a late event that occurs only after the induction of neovascularization.

Myofibroblasts are oblong cells (Fig. 4–13A) that are distinct from spindle cells and Müller cells. Myofibroblasts contain dense cytoplasmic aggregations of 50A filaments throughout the cytoplasm[29] (Figs. 4–13B,C). These are distinct from the glial fibrillary acidic protein (GFAP) filaments (100A) that are diagnostic for Müller cells.[30,31] Myofibroblasts invade the vitreous through the dilated and tortuous neovascularization at the interface between the vascular and avascular retina. There are no myofibroblasts within the subretinal space, between reti-

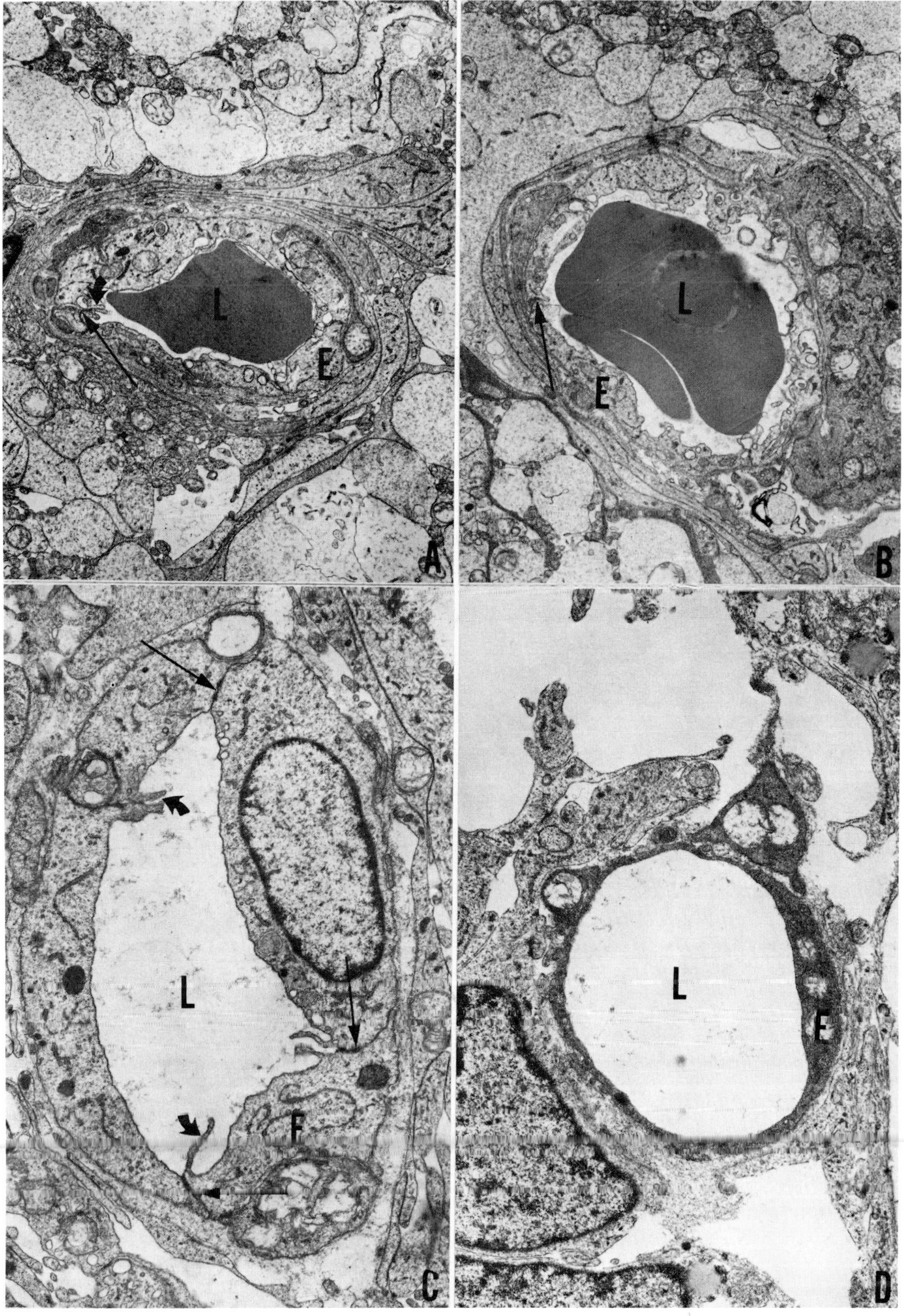

Figure 4-12 Electron micrographs demonstrating the absence of endothelial cell necrosis despite continuous oxygen administration for 36 hours (A, control embryonic, Table 4–2, infant 13, 6,800×); 5 days (B, control activation, Table 4–3, infant 20, 6,800×); 84 days (C, maturation, Table 4–3, infant 22, 10,200×); 80 days (D, delayed activation, Table 4–6, infant 46, 10,200×). E, endothelial cells; L, lumen; (▟), marginal flap; (◄———), tight junctions. At all time points, homogenates of the rearguard retina induce no activity within the CAM.

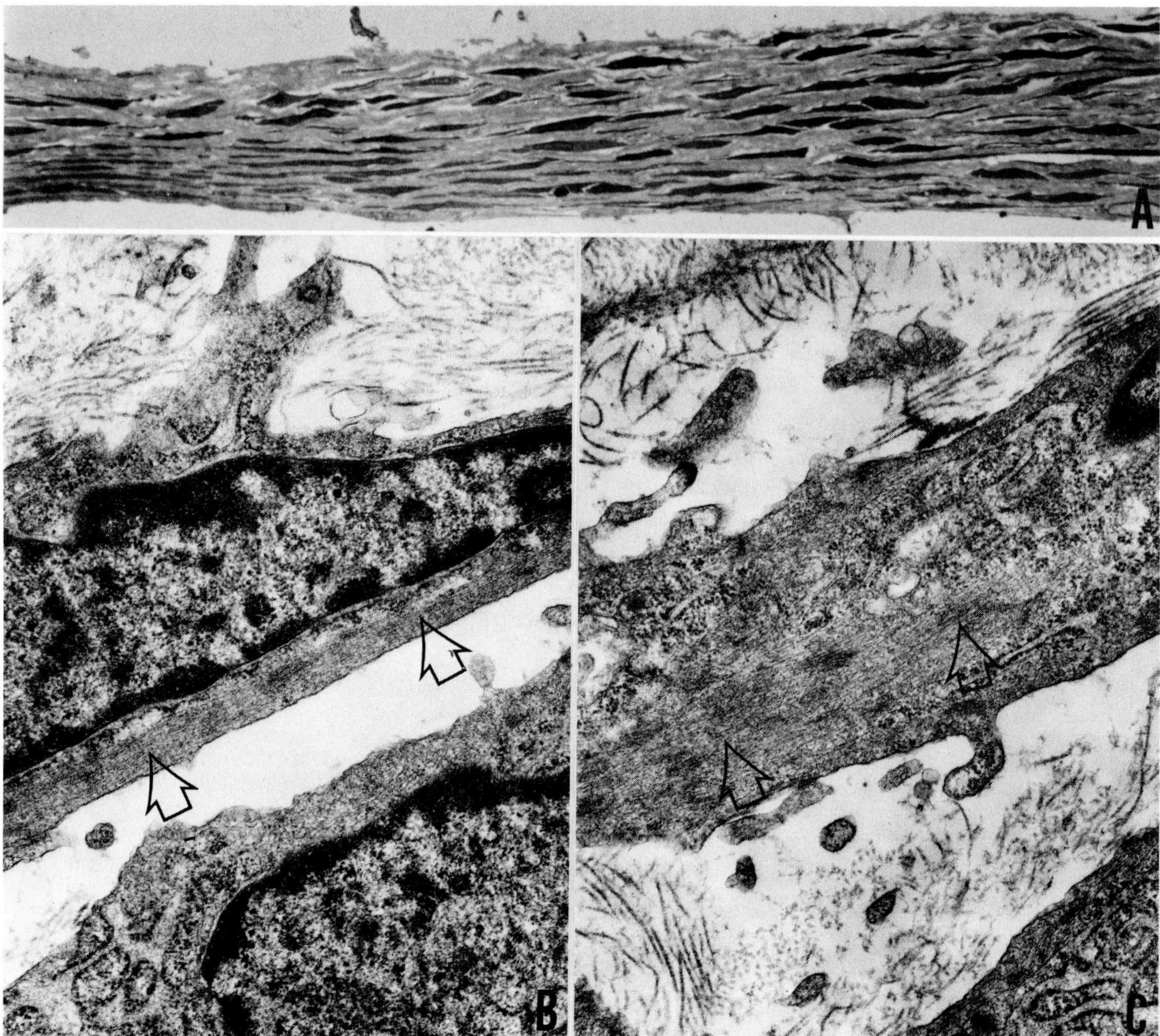

Figure 4–13   Light micrograph A (465×) and transmission electron micrographs B and C (25,110×) of myofibroblasts in the vitreous. Ultrastructurally, the myofibroblasts have a perinuclear ring of 50A filaments B ( ) that extend throughout the cytoplasm C of the fusiform cells.

nal neurons, or within the nerve fiber cystoid spaces. The myofibroblast invasion occurs simultaneously with the cessation of synthesis and secretion of angiogenic factors. The contractile filaments within the cytoplasm of the myofibroblasts provide a tractional force that results in retinal separation when myofibroblasts are present in sufficient numbers within the vitreous.

Summary of the Control Infant Population

The kinetics of gap junction formation in control infants is summarized in Figure 4–14A. The clinical implications deduced from this control population are fourfold:

Spontaneous Regression Does Occur. Unknown environment and physiologic parameters may at any time induce a down modulation of gap junctions. The synthesis and secretion of angiogenic factors then ceases, and spontaneous regression of ROP is observed clinically.[32]

Early Cryotherapy is Rationalized in Terms of Spindle Cell Activity. Ben-Sira, et al[33], Nissenkorn, et al[34], Hindle[35], and Hindle and Leyton[36], have demonstrated that early 360-degree cryoablation of the vanguard retina (± shunt) triggers regression of severe ROP. Late cryotherapy is not efficacious when it is applied solely to the vanguard retina[37] and is disastrous when the tortuous and dilated polar vessels are frozen.÷– The "cryotherapy debate" is resolved when spindle cells are identified as the inducer of ROP. For consistent efficacy, gap-junction-linked spindle cells, which are still secreting angiogenic factors, must be cryoablated prior to their maturation and before a significant invasion of myofibroblasts occurs. If early cryotherapy is directed at the proliferating vessels, severe hemorrhage occurs, and neovascularization continues [39], since the source of angiogenic stimulus is still operant in the vanguard retina. If peripheral cryotherapy is delayed[38], the procedure must include the shunt, since spindle cell maturation has occurred and extensive myofibroblasts have invaded the vitreous body. It must be remembered that ROP is not a disease of completed vascularization, such as occurs in diabetes mellitus and sickle cell disease, but an embryologic vasculopathy induced by activated spindle cells.

Case Reports of ROP in Term Infants Do Not Contradict the Spindle Cell Pathogenesis of ROP. Gap junction formation can also be triggered by hypoxia[40], low pH[41], or low temperature.[42] Thus, a multitude of early in utero catastrophies can trigger gap junction formation between adjacent spindle cells, as well as priming the development of severe ROP in the term infant.[43] Likewise, premature birth into ambient air with no oxygen supplementation can trigger gap junction formation, rough endoplasmic reticulum proliferation, and synthesis and secretion of angiogenic factors. Thus, there is nothing magically safe about 40 percent oxygen.

The Numerous Risk Factors of ROP are Unified by the Spindle Cell Pathogenesis. A. *Immaturity.* The most consistently identified risk factor is immaturity. This correlates with extensive retinal areas containing immature photoreceptors that are not secreting IRBP. Thus, retinal levels of vitamin E are low, and spindle cells are not completely protected against gap junction formation. Immaturity also correlates with a larger vanguard retina that contains more spindle cells to potentially synthesize and secrete large quantities of angiogenic factors. Historically, infants weighing more than 1,500 grams at birth have been at high risk of developing severe ROP. However, with current judicious curtailment of oxygen supplementation, the small spindle cell apron is not activated to secrete a threshold level of angiogenic factors, so that blinding ROP is not triggered in these large infants.

B. *Oxygen.* Another consistent risk factor is the cumulative amount of oxygen administered. The pathological response of spindle cells in the induction of ROP is triggered by oxygen tension greater than the hypoxic, intrauterine environment. Risk factors such as patent ductus arteriosus, bronchopulmonary dysplasia, hyaline membrane disease, pneumothorax, and apnea are associated with the therapeutic use of supplemental oxygen, which potentiates gap junction formation between adjacent spindle cells. The amount of oxygen administered is not the sole cause of ROP but is merely one unavoidable factor if the infant is to survive with an intact central nervous system. There is no safe, minimal level of oxygen that can be administered. All extrauterine levels are hyperoxic challenges to the immature, peripheral retina, because the choroidal vasculature does not vasoconstrict, and immature photoreceptors create no barrier to transretinal diffusion of oxygen (Fig. 4–6).

C. *Shift in Oxygen Dissociation Curve by Adult Hemoglobin.* Spindle cells are also activated by other risk factors that alter the amount of oxygen carried in the blood. Transfusion of packed, red blood cells from an adult shifts the oxygen dissociation curve, because adult hemoglobin releases more oxygen than fetal hemoglobin, and as a result, more oxygen is released to the retina. The very sick premature infant receives relatively large quantities of adult blood in replacement transfusions.

D. *Sepsis.* Sepsis is also identified repeatedly as a risk factor for ROP. Macrophages release a large quantity of oxygen radicals concomitantly with the ingestion of bacteria. This burst of oxygen presumably overloads the antioxidant systems of the preterm infant and potentiates gap junction formation between adjacent spindle cells.

E.*High Light Intensity.* Prolonged high light intensity increases the risk of ROP.[44] Light damages photoreceptors which results in decreased utilization of oxygen by even the most immature photoreceptor precursors. Thus, this minimal oxygen barrier becomes further reduced and permits a greater oxygen flux across the retina to potentially damage spindle cell plasma membranes.

F.*Hypoxia and Hypothermia.* Still other risk factors related to difficult stabilization of infants, such as asphyxia with a resultant low pH, or postnatal transport with a resultant low temperature, cause irreversible gap junction formation. Thus, the initial stabilization period of the infant may delineate the course of retinal pathology. In such cases, administration of antioxidants may have no effect. Severe ROP in an infant who has suffered extreme birth asphyxia or hypothermia almost always occurs 8 weeks following birth, despite vitamin E supplementation from the first hours of life.

SPINDLE CELLS IN THE RETINAS OF TREATMENT (VITAMIN E SUPPLEMENTED) INFANTS

Treatment Embryonic

For the first 4 days of life, with early and continuous vitamin E supplementation (Table 4–4, infants 23 through 35), spindle cells continue to migrate and canalize, occupy a minimal volume of the nerve fiber layer comparable to control embryonic levels, contain minimal gap junctions comparable to control embryonic levels, have scarce, rough endoplasmic reticulum, and secrete no angiogenic factors, as detected by the absence of neovascular loop formation from the CAM (Table 4–9, infant 29). Spindle cells are transretinal to Stage I and Stage II immature photoreceptors, the choroid is patent, and the vanguard nerve fiber layer is, thus, hyperoxic. Such spindle cells are called *treatment embryonic*. Despite 9 to 84 hours of continuous oxygen administration, there is no ultrastructural evidence of endothelial cell necrosis (Table 4–4, infants 24, 27, 32, and 35), and homogenates of the rearguard retina do not stimulate loop formation from the CAM (Table 4–9, infant 29). Thus, elevated oxygen tension after birth does not compromise or insult inner retinal vessels.

Treatment-Lag Activation

For the first 20 days of life, spindle cells in treatment infants of 27-weeks gestational age or less (Table 4–5, infants 36 through 45) continue to migrate and canalize, occupy a minimal volume of the nerve fiber layer comparable to treatment embryonic levels, have minimal gap junctions comparable to treatment embryonic levels and scarce, rough endoplasmic reticulum. Again, homogenates of the vanguard retina do not activate loop formation from the CAM (Table 4–9, infants 42 and 45). This phase of the spindle cell response to vitamin E and oxygen is called *treatment-lag activation*. There is no ultrastructural evidence of endothelial cell necrosis (Table 4–5 infants 42 and 45), and homogenates of the rearguard retina do not stimulate loop formation from the CAM (Table 4–9, infants 42 and 45).

Treatment-Delayed Activation

In the group of treatment infants of 27-weeks gestational age or less, who survived more than 15 days (Table 4–6, infants 46 through 54), spindle cells are a

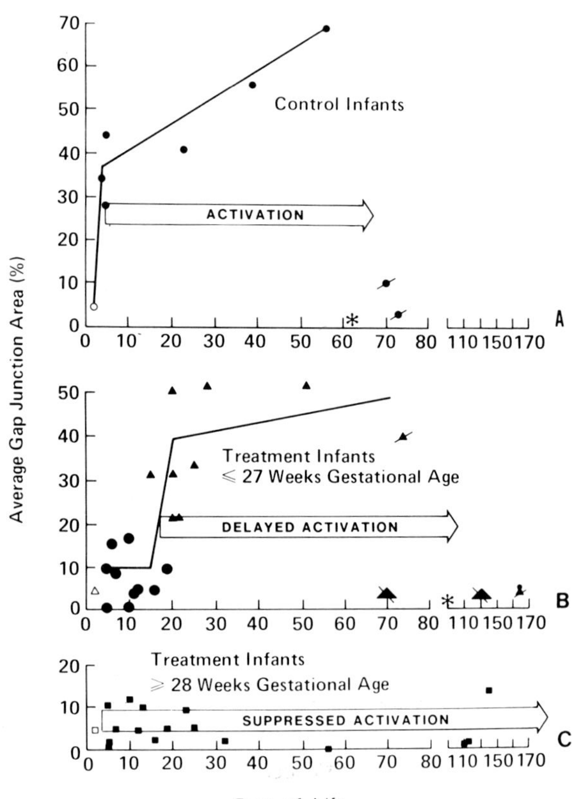

Figure 4–14 Average gap junction area (%) as a function of days of life. A, control infants, n=8 (●). B, treatment infants of 27-weeks gestational age or less, n=22 (● , lag activation; ▲ , delayed activation; ♟ , delayed maturation). C, treatment infants of 28-weeks gestational age or more, n=16 (■). For each group, the average gap junction area in equivalent infants who survived for less than 4 days is plotted (○ , n=14 infants; △ , n=9 infants; and □ , n=4 infants). Four infants with clinically documented severe ROP are represented by ✔ , ✔ , and ♟ . Two infants of 27-weeks gestational age or less with minimal ROP risk factors are represented by ▲ . The average time when severe ROP develops (∗) for each group is based on the results of clinical studies that enrolled 418 high-risk preterm infants.[10-12]

minimal component of the nerve fiber layer, comparable to both treatment embryonic and treatment-lag activation levels. However, spindle cells are now extensively gap junction linked to a level that equates to control activation and contain abundant, rough endoplasmic reticulum, which m orphologically indicates extensive protein synthesis and secretion. Homogenates of the vanguard retina induce extensive, neovascular loops from the CAM (Table 4–9, infants 46 and 47). This phase of the spindle cell response to vitamin E supplementation and oxygen is called *treatment-delayed activation*. Again, there is no ultrastructural evidence of endothelial cell necrosis, despite the fact that the infants were on continuous oxygen administration for 20 days (Table 4–6, infant 52), 27.5 days (Table 4–6, infant 49), 58 days (Table 4–6, infant 54), and

80 days (Table 4–6, infant 46; Fig. 4–12D) respectively. Homogenates of the rearguard retina do not activate loop formation from the CAM (Table 4–9, infants 46 and 47).

Treatment-Delayed Maturation

One treatment infant (Table 4–6, infant 55) developed ROP Stage 3 at 84 days of life but was too ill to undergo cryotherapy of the avascular vanguard retina. When the infant died at 163 days of life, spindle cells had down-modulated gap junctions to control maturation levels and contained scarce, rough endoplasmic reticulum, which m orphologically indicated a cessation of extensive protein synthesis. The spindle cells formed stacked profiles and occupied a large volume of the nerve fiber layer equivalent to control maturation levels. This phase of the spindle cell response to vitamin E and oxygen is called *treatment-delayed maturation*. There is no evidence of endothelial cell necrosis, despite 163 days of continuous oxygen administration. This infant can be equated to the two control maturation infants (Table 4–3, infants 21 and 22) except that the continuous vitamin E supplementation delayed the clinical onset of severe ROP and the theoretical time of down modulation of gap junctions, as exemplified by infant 46 (Table 4–6).

Treatment-Suppressed Activation

Two treatment infants (Table 4–7, infants 56 and 57) survived for 70 and 133 days respectively and developed only transient ROP Stage 1, despite their gestational age, 27 weeks each. These two infants had minimal ROP risk factors. Their spindle cells were less vulnerable to oxidative damage, few gap junctions formed, there was minimal proliferation of rough endoplasmic reticulum, a low level of angiogenic factors was secreted (Table 4–9, infant 56), and only transient intraretinal neovascularization developed clinically.

Sixteen treatment infants of 28-weeks gestational age or more (Table 4–7, infants 58 through 73) developed only ROP Stage 1. Spindle cells continued to migrate and canalize, occupied a minimal volume within the nerve fiber layer comparable to treatment embryonic levels, had minimal gap junctions comparable to treatment embryonic levels, and contained scarce, rough endoplasmic reticulum. Homogenates of the vanguard retina did n ot activate loop formation from the CAM (Table 4–9, infant 69). Ultrastructurally, these older, high-risk infants had retinas with developed interphotoreceptor matrices that approach the ora serratas. IRBP maximally shuttled vitamin E into retinal membranes, retinal vitamin E levels were above the critical threshold, and spindle cells were protected against oxidative induction of gap junction formation, despite severe ROP risk factors. This state of spindle cells is called *treatment-suppressed activation*. No endothelial cell necrosis is evident at 5 days (Table 4–7, infant 72), 32 days (Table 4–7, infant 69), 56 days (Table 4–7, infant 66), 119 days (Table 4–7, infant 60), 133 days (Table 4–7, infant 57), and 140 days (Table 4–7, infant 71) despite continuous oxygen administration and physiological vasoconstriction. At no time in the preterm retina does oxygen trigger endothelial cell necrosis, and homogenates of the rearguard retina do not activate loop formation from the CAM (Table 4–9, infant 69).

Summary of Treatment-Infant Population

The kinetics of gap junction formation in treatment infants is summarized in Figures 4–14B and 4–14C. The clinical implications deduced from this treatment population are sixfold:

Vitamin E Supplementation Must Begin Within the First Hours of Life. Oxidative insults impinge on spindle cells at birth and result in morphologically-detectable, gap junction increases as early as 4 days of life (Fig. 4–14A). These early, subclinical events prime the neovascularization that begins weeks later. Thus, antioxidant protection is needed immediately at birth. The clinical data of Finer, et al[45] regarding the efficacy of early supplementation versus late onset support the concept that antioxidant protection of spindle cells is required immediately after birth.

The Route of Vitamin E Administration Must Be Optimal for Immediate Retinal Uptake. The optimal vitamin E preparation for retinal uptake is an oral form[46] with an efficient vehicle for maximal absorption from the premature gut. The poorest retinal uptake follows rapid intravenous supplementation (delayed uptake to low levels).[47] This explains why the clinical trials of Phelps, et al[48] demonstrated vitamin E's nonefficacy in suppressing the development of severe ROP, because the initial rapid intravenous infusion on days 1 and 2 of life left spindle cells vulnerable to early oxidative damage.

Continuous Vitamin E Supplementation From the First Hours of Life Is Not A Panacea for Suppressing the Development of Severe ROP in Infants of 27-Weeks Gestational Age or Less.[7] In the 19 infants of 27-weeks gestational age or less (Tables 4–5 and 4–6), plasma vitamin E is elevated to the adult physiological range, but the restricted domain of IRBP (Table 4–8) is apparently not sufficient to shuttle a threshold level of the antioxidant into peripheral retinal membranes. Only trace levels of vitamin E are transported into the retina. There is minimal antioxidant protection afforded the spindle cells against the high oxygen tension, which diffuses transretinally into the vanguard inner retina. This explains why severe ROP may develop in infants of 27-weeks gestational age or less, despite continuous vitamin E supplementation from the first hours of life. This result also stresses the fact that vitamin E efficacy in suppressing the development of severe ROP must be determined by multivariate analysis, because clinical failures predictably develop in the smallest infants.

In infants of 27-weeks gestational age or less, vitamin E supplementation does delay both the clinical development of severe ROP (8 to 10 weeks for control-infants versus 10 to 12 weeks for treatments) and the down modulation of gap junctions (Fig. 4–14; compare control infants 21 and 22 in Tables 4–3 and 4–9 with treatment infant 46 in Tables 4–6 and 4–9). There is a 15 to 20 day lag in gap junction formation, but the ultimate magnitude of gap junction formation is comparable to control activation infants, if sufficient risk factors are operant. The subthreshold retinal levels of vitamin E delay the clinical development of severe ROP, allow more time in which to contemplate the option of cryotherapy in a larger eye with thicker sclera, and enhance the possibility of spontaneous regression, which may occur with improving health and maturity.

The changing relationship between the overlap of spindle cells within the nerve fiber layer and the trans-retinal appearance of IRBP in the subretinal space explains why vitamin E is maximally efficacious in infants of 28-weeks or more gestation. At around 28 weeks the overlap between IRBP in the subretinal space and spindle cells in the nerve fiber layer increases. Now only a small percentage of the vulnerable spindle cell apron is not transretinal to the expansion of the IRBP pool within the subretinal space, and most spindle cells are protected by sufficient antioxidant levels.

If secretion of IRBP into the subretinal space would occur prior to the peripheral migration of spindle cells toward the ora serrata, or if spindle cells were restricted to regions around the last-formed inner retinal blood regions around the last-formed inner retinal blood vessels, vitamin E would eliminate ROP in all viable infants not experiencing hypoxia or hypothermia. It would be possible to transport sufficient vitamin E from the plasma to retinal membranes and so protect spindle cells from gap junction formation in infants of all gestational ages. Unfortunately, vitamin E uptake into peripheral retinal membranes is dependent upon retinal maturation. Perhaps supplementation with selenium, a water-soluble antioxidant, can circumvent this maturation dependency and offer antioxidant protection to spindle cells in the smallest, viable, preterm infants.

Early Intramuscular Supplementation of Vitamin E Does Not Suppress the Development of Severe ROP More Efficaciously Than Early Oral Supplementation.[12] A rapid rise (intramuscular) versus a slower rise (oral) in plasma vitamin E is not a critical factor in suppressing the development of severe ROP and does not alter the kinetics of gap junction formation between adjacent spindle cells. The critical parameter is the development of a sufficient interphotoreceptor matrix to transport a threshold level of antioxidant into retinal membranes. It is the IRBP component of the interphotoreceptor matrix that most likely limits the efficacy of vitamin E in suppressing the development of severe ROP. The bottom line is that plasma vitamin E must impact on spindle cells and suppress gap junction formation.

There Is No Justification to Exceed a Mean Plasma Vitamin E Level of 3.5 mg per Deciliter. If the retina has a developed interphotoreceptor matrix with IRBP that overlaps the majority of the spindle cell apron (infants of 28-weeks gestational age or more) retinal vitamin E uptake will occur to threshold levels and protect spindle cells. If the interphotoreceptor matrix is restricted to central regions (27-weeks gestational age or less), retinal vitamin E uptake is minimal, spindle cells are poorly protected, and delayed activation can ensue. Under all circumstances, megadose therapy is futile and produces only toxicity (sepsis and necrotizing enterocolitis).[49]

Vitamin E Supplementation Must Continue Until the Inner Retinal Vessels Reach the Ora Serrata. As long as spindle cells are in the vanguard retina, ambient oxygen tension diffusing across the retina is sufficient to trigger gap junction formation. Spindle cells are absent from the nerve fiber layer only when the inner retinal vessels reach the ora serrata in both the nasal and temporal hemispheres. Thus, vitamin E supplementation must not be interrupted or halted prematurely.[7]

FOUR BASIC CONCEPTS

The spindle cell pathogenesis of ROP embraces four basic concepts, derived from 97 pairs of whole-eye donations that have been processed for morphological analyses, immunocytochemical localization of IRBP within the developing subretinal space, and detection of angiogenic factors in homogenates of the rearguard or vanguard retina.

1. Hyperoxia, hypoxia, pH decrease, or temperature depression impinge on spindle cells in the avascular vanguard retina and trigger gap junction formation (Table 4–1). These events remove spindle cells from the normal, vasoformative process and transform them into sites for synthesis and secretion of angiogenic factors. These spindle cells are the peripheral inducers of the central neovascularization that may develop at the demarcation line.

2. With judicious oxygen administration, no endothelial cell necrosis occurs, despite physiological vasoconstriction.

3. In the preterm infant, the demarcation line and vanguard retina are hyperoxic when neovascularization is developing.

4. The levels of retinal vitamin E, which provide antioxidant protection to spindle cells, are related to the development of the interphotoreceptor matrix with its IRBP.

This research has been supported by grants and contributions from the Retina Research Foundation, Research to Prevent Blindness, Farish Foundation, Roy H. Cullen, and Hoffmann-La Roche. The three clinical trials were possible only through the support of Arnold J. Rudolph and the neonatal staff, pediatric house staff, and nurses in the neonatal units of Texas Children's and Jefferson Davis Hospitals. The Lion's Eyes of Texas Eye Bank (Robert Fort and E. J. Farge) and the house staff at Texas Children's and Jefferson Davis Hospitals sensitively encouraged whole-eye donations. The ultrastructural analyses included data generated by Rekha Mehta, A. Tim Johnson, David Hunter, Evelyn Brown, Pat Glazebrook, Chaula Rana, and Donna Goad.

A. Tim Johnson and David Hunter were M.D./Ph.D students on stipends supported by the NIGMS Medical Scientist Training Program and McGlothlin-Andress Physician Scientist Fund respectively, and by the National Retinitis Pigmentosa Foundation Fighting Blindness. Chaula Rana and Donna Goad were medical students at Baylor College of Medicine who opted for research rotations. The immunocytochemical studies were performed in collaboration with C. D. B. Bridges and D. M. K. Lam, with rabbit antibovine IRBP antibody kindly provided by Shao-Ling Fong and Gregory Liou. We acknowledge the photographic expertise of Alexander Kogan and Gilma Miranda, the editorial talents of Dorothy Carr, and the manuscript critique of Michael Osato. F. K. dedicates this chapter to his beloved parents, who instilled within him an eagerness to probe the elegant structure function relationships of life's mysteries.

REFERENCES

1. Patz A. Current therapy of retrolental fibroplasia. Ophthalmology 1983; 90:425–427.
2. Patz A. Current concepts of the effects of oxygen on the developing retina. Curr Eye Res 1984; 3:159–163.
3. Patz A. Retinal neovascularization: early contributions of Professor Michaelson and recent observations. Br J Ophthalmol 1984; 68:42–46.
4. Kretzer FL, Hittner HM, Johnson AT, Mehta RS, Godio LB. Vitamin E and retrolental fibroplasia: ultrastructural support of clinical efficacy. Ann NY Acad Sci 1982; 393:145–166.
5. Kretzer FL, Hunter DG, Mehta RS, Brown ES, Blifeld C, Johnson AT, Hittner HM. Spindle cells as vasoformative elements in the developing human retina: vitamin E modulation. In: Coates PW, Markwald RR, Kenny AD, eds. Developing and regenerating vertebrate nervous systems. New York: Alan R Liss, 1983; 199–210.
6. Kretzer FL, Mehta RS, Johnson AT, Hunter DG, Brown ES, Hittner HM. Vitamin E protects against retinopathy of prematurity through action on spindle cells. Nature 1984; 309:793–795.
7. Hittner HM, Rudolph AJ, Kretzer FL. Suppression of severe retinopathy of prematurity with vitamin E supplementation: ultrastructural mechanism of clinical efficacy. Ophthalmology 1984; 91:1512–1523.
8. Hittner HM, Kretzer FL. Retinopathy of prematurity: pathogenesis, prevention, and treatment. In: Chiswick ML, ed. Recent advances in perinatal medicine. London: Churchill Livingston, 1985; (2):145–163.
9. Kretzer FL, Hittner HM. Initiating events in the development of retinopathy of prematurity. In: Silverman WA, Flynn JT, eds. Retinopathy of prematurity. Boston, Massachusetts: Blackwell Scientific Publications, 1985; 121–152.
10. Hittner HM, Godio LB, Rudolph AJ, Adams JM, Garcia-Prats JA, Friedman Z, Kautz JA, Monaco WA. Retrolental fibroplasia: efficacy of vitamin E in a double-blind clinical study of preterm infants. N Engl J Med 1981; 305:1365–1371.
11. Hittner HM, Godio LB, Speer ME, Rudolph AJ, Taylor MM, Blifeld C, Kretzer FL. Retrolental fibroplasia: further clinical evidence and ultrastructural support for efficacy of vitamin E in the preterm infant. Pediatrics 1983; 71:423–432.
12. Hittner HM, Speer ME, Rudolph AJ, Blifeld C, Chadda P, Holbein MEB, Godio LB, Kretzer FL. Retrolental fibroplasia and vitamin E in the preterm infant: comparison of oral versus intramuscular: oral administration. Pediatrics 1984; 73:238–249.
13. Glaser BM, D'Amore PA, Seppa H, Seppa S, Schiffmann E. Adult tissues contain chemoattractants for vascular endothelial cells. Nature 1980; 288:483–484.
14. Glaser BM, D'Amore PA, Michels RG, Patz A, Fenselau A. Demonstration of vasoproliferative activity from mammalian retina. J Cell Biol 1980; 84:298–304.
15. Glaser BM, D'Amore PA, Lutty GA, Fenselau AH, Michels RG, Patz A. Chemical mediators of intraocular neovascularization. Trans Ophthalmol Soc UK 1980; 100:369–373.
16. Glaser BM, D'Amore PA, Michels RG, Brunson SK, Fenselau AH, Rice T, Patz A. The demonstration of angiogenic activity from ocular tissues. Ophthalmology 1980; 87:440–446.
17. Johnson AT, Kretzer FL, Hittner HM, Glazebrook PA, Bridges CDB, Lam DMK. Development of the subretinal space in the preterm human eye: ultrastructural and immunocytochemical studies. J Comp Neurol 1985; 233:497–505.
18. Johnson AT, Kretzer FL. Interstitial retinol binding protein in the developing human retina: a proposed explanation for vitamin E suppression of retinopathy of prematurity. In: Bridges CDB, Alder AJ, eds. The interphotoreceptor matrix in health and disease. New York: Alan R. Liss, 1985; 251–277.
19. Berman ER, Bach G. Acid mucopolysaccharides of cattle retina. Biochem J 1968, 100:75–80.
20. Abramov I, Gordon J, Hendrickson A, Hainline L, Dobson V, LaBossiere E. The retina of the newborn human infant. Science 1982; 217:265–267.
21. Gonzalez-Fernandez F, Landers RA, Glazebrook PA, Fong SL, Liou GI, Lam DMK, Bridges CDB. An extracellular retinol-binding glycoprotein in the eyes of mutant rats with retinal dystrophy—development, localization, and biosynthesis. J Cell Biol 1984; 99:2092–2098.
22. Hollyfield JB, Fliesler SJ, Rayborn ME, Fong SL, Landers RA, Bridges CDB. Synthesis and secretion of interstitial retinol-binding protein by the human retina. Invest Ophthalmol Vis Sci 1985; 26:58–67.
23. Nir I, Cohen D, Papermaster DS. Immunocytochemical localization of opsin in the cell membrane of developing rat retinal photoreceptors. J Cell Biol 1984; 98:1788–1795.

24. Carter-Dawson L, Alvarez RA, Sperling HG, Bridges CDB. Rhodopsin, interstitial retinol binding protein and retinyl ester isomers in developing mouse retinas. Invest Ophthalmol Vis Sci 1984; 25 (Suppl):275.

25. Fong SL, Liou GI, Landers RA, Alvarez RA, Gonzalez-Fernandez F, Glazebrook PA, Lam DMK, Bridges CDB. Characterization, localization, and biosynthesis of an interstitial retinol-binding glycoprotein in the human eye. J Neurochem 1984; 42:1667–1676.

26. Liou GI, Bridges CDB, Alvarez RA, Fong SL. Binding specificity of interstitial retinol-binding protein—possible physiological consequences of competition between vitamins A and E. Invest Ophthalmol Vis Sci 1983; (Suppl) 24:42.

27. Weiter JJ, Zuckerman R, Schepens CL. A model for the pathogenesis of retrolental fibroplasia based on the metabolic control of blood vessel development. Ophthalmol Surg 1982; 13:1013–1017.

28. Foos RY. Acute retrolental fibroplasia. Graefes Arch Clin Exp Ophthalmol 1975; 195:87–100.

29. Soong HK, Eller AW, Hirose T, Hanninen L, Kenyon KR. In situ actin distribution in excised retrolental membranes in retinopathy of prematurity. Arch Ophthalmol 1985; 103:1553–1556.

30. Hiscott PS, Grierson I, Trombetta CJ, Rahi AHS, Marshall J, McLeod D. Retinal and epiretinal glia—an immunohistochemical study. Br J Ophthalmol 1984; 68:698–707

31. Eisenfeld AJ, Bunt-Milam AH, Sarthy PV. Müller cell expression of glial fibrillary acidic acid protein after genetic and experimental photoreceptor degeneration in the rat retina. Invest Ophthalmol Vis Sci 1984; 25:1321–1328.

32. Koerner FH. Retinopathy of prematurity: natural course and management. Metab Ophthalmol 1978; 2:325–329.

33. Ben-Sira I, Nissenkorn I, Grunwald E, Yassur Y. Treatment of acute retrolental fibroplasia by cryopexy. Br J Ophthalmol 1980; 64:758–762.

34. Nissenkorn I, Kremer I, Ben-Sira I, Cohen S, Garner A. Br J Ophthalmol 1984; 68:36–41.

35. Hindle NW. Cryotherapy for retinopathy of prematurity to prevent retrolental fibroplasia. Can J Ophthalmol 1982; 17:207–211.

36. Hindle NW, Leyton J. Prevention of cicatricial retrolental fibroplasia by cryotherapy. Can J Ophthalmol 1978; 13:277–282.

37. Mousel DK, Hoyt CS. Cryotherapy for retinopathy of prematurity. Ophthalmology 1980; 87:1121–1127.

38. Kingham JD. Acute retrolental fibroplasia. II. Treatment by cryosurgery. Arch Ophthalmol 1978; 96:2049–2053.

39. Payne JW, Patz A. Treatment of acute proliferative retrolental fibroplasia. Trans Acad Ophthalmol Otolaryngol 1972; 76:1234–1246.

40. Yee AG, Revel JP. Loss and reappearance of gap junctions in regenerating liver. J Cell Biol 1978; 78:554–564.

41. Turin L, Warner AE. Intracellular pH in early Xenopus embryos: its effect on current flow between blastomeres. J Physiol (Lond) 1980; 300:489–504.

42. Picard-Schneider G, Cartentier JL, Girardier L. Quantitative evaluation of gap junctions in rat brown adipose tissue after cold acclimation. J Membr Biol 1984; 78:85–89.

43. Hittner HM. Retinal and central nervous system abnormalities: syndromes which resemble retrolental fibroplasia. Metab Pediatr Syst Ophthalmol 1985; 8:5–10.

44. Glass P, Avery GB, Subramanian KNS, Keys MP, Sostek AM, Friendly DS. Effect of bright light in the hospital on retinopathy of prematurity. N Engl J Med 1985; 313:401–404.

45. Finer NN, Schindler RF, Peters KL, Grant GD. Vitamin E and retrolental fibroplasia: improved visual outcome with early vitamin E. Ophthalmology 1983; 90:428–435.

46. Pantoja A, Ukrainski C, Belenky D, Grinberg A, Hulac P, Mathis J. Vitamin E (VE) kinetics in infants <1,500 grams: intramuscular (IM) vs oral administration. Pediatr Res 1984; 18:157A.

47. Bhat R, Braum RJ. Retinal and tissue vitamin E kinetics in the newborn kitten following vitamin E administration. Pediatr Res 1984; 18:149A.

48. Phelps DL. Symposium on Ephynal. Washington, D.C.: January 19, 1984.

49. Johnson L, Bowen FW, Abbasi S, et al. Relationship of prolonged pharmacologic serum levels of vitamin E to incidence of sepsis and necrotizing enterocolitis in infants with birth weight 1,500 grams or less. Pediatrics 1985; 75:619–638.

Differential Diagnosis of Retinopathy of Prematurity   5

Helen M. Hittner, M.D.
Frank L. Kretzer, Ph.D.

With the recent understanding of normal inner retinal vasoformation and the spindle cell pathogenesis of retinopathy of prematurity (ROP),[1-5] the differential diagnosis of ROP is no longer a baffling assortment of bilateral neovascularization with or without leukocoria. Multiple genetic and environmental factors can affect the process of inner-retinal vasoformation prior to the time when the vessels reach the ora serrata.

NORMAL INNER RETINAL VASOFORMATION RELATED TO THE DIFFERENTIAL DIAGNOSIS OF ROP

The process of inner retinal vasoformation occurs as an orderly sequence of migration, canalization, and differentiation of spindle cells into endothelial cells at a predictable time (Fig. 5–1).[1,5] Müller's cells (glial elements) are present very early in ocular development. Differentiation of the retina occurs from the inner to the outer layers, ganglion cells to bipolar cells to photoreceptors, and from the central to the peripheral retina, optic disc to ora serrata. Differentiated ganglion cells encroach on the ora serrata by the sixteenth-week gestational age (Fig. 5–1A). From the neuroblastic layer bipolar cell and photoreceptor nuclei are separated by the outer plexiform layer. This process begins at the optic disc at the sixteenth-week gestational age and reaches the ora serrata by the twenty-ninth-week gestational age. The peripheral migration of spindle cells parallels the formation of the outer plexiform layer from the optic disc to the ora serrata (Chapter 4, Fig. 8).[2] Thus these precursors of inner retinal vessels migrate in the nerve fiber layer from the sixteenth- to the twenty-ninth-week gestational age (Fig. 5–1B). Maturation of photoreceptor outer segments occurs from the eighteenth- to the fortieth-week gestational age as a changing relationship of Stage 1 to 4 photoreceptors (Chapter 4, Figs. 1 to 5).[4-5] As photoreceptors differentiate and mature, their energy and oxygen requirements create a metabolic sink that utilizes more and more oxygen from choroidal vessels. The formation of inner retinal capillaries and vessels parallels the maturation of Stage 3 and 4 photoreceptor outer segments respectively. This late-developing vascular system supplies the inner retina with oxygen that can no longer diffuse from choroidal vessels. Stage 4 photoreceptors and inner retinal vessels reach the temporal ora serrata at 40-weeks gestational age (Fig. 5–1C).[4-5]

SPINDLE CELL PATHOGENESIS RELATED TO THE DIFFERENTIAL DIAGNOSIS OF ROP

ROP develops when premature birth presents the immature retina with environmental challenges (Fig. 5–2). The environmental challenges cluster into two major groups. Hyperoxia is created by oxygen administration; transfusion of adult hemoglobin, which delivers more oxygen to the retina; release of oxygen by macrophages during sepsis; or high light intensity, which increases oxygen flux by damaging photoreceptors. Hypoxia and/or hypothermia can occur when stabilization of a premature infant is difficult. When any of these environmental challenges develop, migration of spindle cells ceases, gap junctions form between adjacent spindle cells, the cytoplasmic volume of the rough endoplasmic reticulum increases, spindle cells synthesize and secrete angiogenic factors, and neovascularization is induced at the interface between the central vascularized

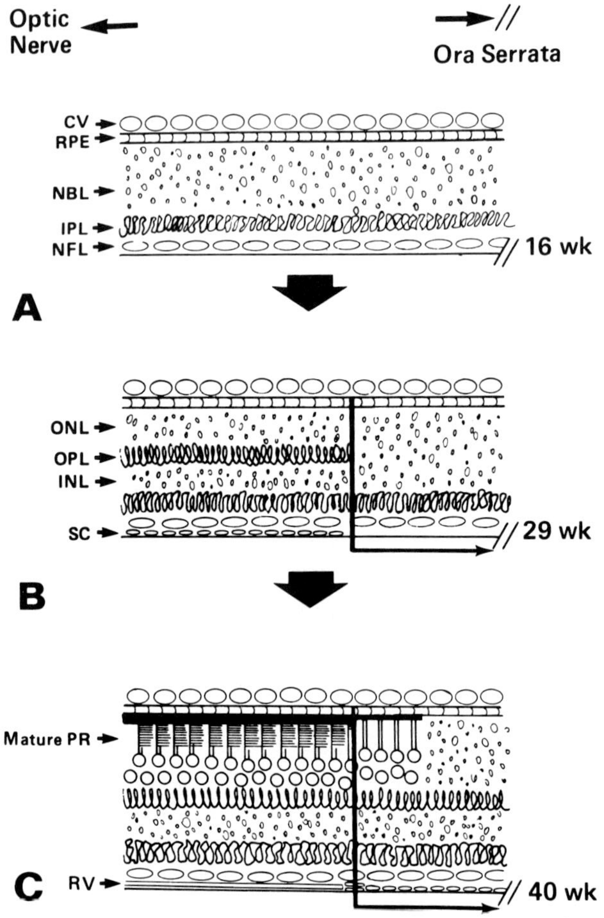

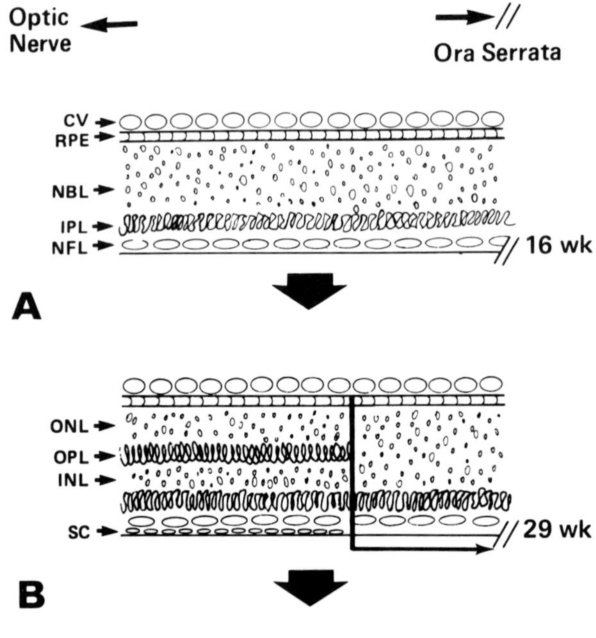

Figure 5–1   Normal inner retinal vasoformation: A, Retinal development demonstrating formation of choroidal vessels (CV), retinal pigment epithelium (RPE), neuroblastic layer (NBL), inner plexiform layer (IPL), and nerve fiber layer (NFL) with ganglion cells to the ora serrata by the sixteenth-week gestational age. B, Spindle cell (SC) migration in the nerve fiber layer parallels division of the neuroblastic layer into an outer nuclear layer (ONL) and an inner nuclear layer (INL) by the formation of the outer plexiform layer (OPL) to the ora serrata by the twenty-ninth-week gestational age. C, Retinal-vessel (RV) formation in the nerve fiber layer parallels maturation of Stage 3 and 4 photoreceptors (mature PR) with formation of outer segments with organized stacked discs to the ora serrata by the fortieth-week gestational age. These data are extrapolated from the 97 pairs of whole-eye donations studied by Kretzer, et al (Chapter 4).

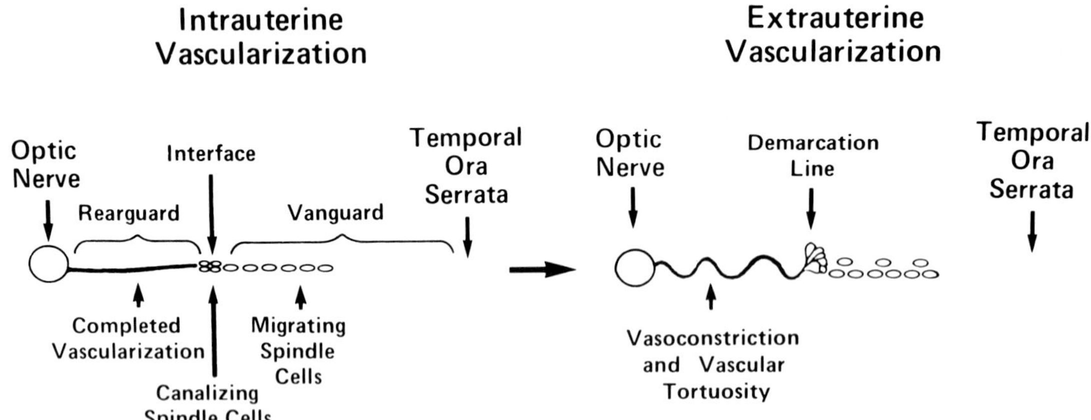

Figure 5–2   Spindle cell pathogenesis of ROP: Comparison of intrauterine normal inner retinal vasoformation (left) and extrauterine development of severe ROP in an immature infant with maximal risk factors operant (right). Left: Intrauterine vascularization with migrating (in vanguard retina) and canalizing (at interface) spindle cells that are minimally gap junction-linked and contain a small, cytoplasmic volume of rough, endoplasmic reticulum. Differentiation of spindle cells into endothelial cells is complete in rearguard retina. Right: Extrauterine vascularization with cessation of normal retinal vasoformation. This results from spindle cells that are gap junction-linked, contain a large cytoplasmic volume of rough endoplasmic reticulum (in vanguard retina), and are synthesizing and secreting angiogenic factors that induce neovascularization at the demarcation line. This triggers vascular tortuosity of the physiologically vasoconstricted inner retinal vessels in the rearguard retina. These data are extrapolated from the 97 pairs of whole-eye donations studied by Kretzer, et al (Chapter 4).

(rearguard) and peripheral nonvascularized (vanguard) retina.[1-3]

RELATIONSHIP BETWEEN CENTRAL NERVOUS SYSTEM AND OCULAR DEVELOPMENT AND PATHOLOGY

Central nervous system and ocular development have parallel processes of neuroectodermal histiogenesis, cell migration, and cell differentiation. This sequence occurs prior to the invasion of vascular elements in both the brain and the eye.[6-7] This sequence is detailed in relation to multiple embryonic parameters in Figure 5–3.

Central nervous system neuroectodermal histiogenesis starts prior to the seventh week of gestation. Cell migration occurs between the seventh and thirteenth weeks, and cell differentiation continues between

the tenth week and the post-term period. Vascular formation occurs after early neuronal differentiation. Gyri of the brain become well defined between the twelfth and twenty-sixth weeks. Cortical layers appear in the following sequence: I at 10 to 11 weeks, VI at 11 to 13 weeks, V at 20 weeks, IV at 28 weeks, III at 29 weeks, II at 30 weeks. The mesenchymal precursors of the central nervous system vasculature migrate between the eighth and the fourteenth weeks and differentiate between the ninth week and the post-term period.[6]

By comparison, retinal, neuroectodermal histiogenesis starts prior to the seventh week of gestation. Cell migration occurs between the seventh and ninth weeks, and cell differentiation begins at the optic disc at 9 weeks and reaches the temporal ora serrata just prior to term.[7] Retinal vascularization develops from the migration of mesenchymal spindle cells within the nerve fiber layer. Spindle cell migration starts at the optic disc at 16 weeks and reaches the temporal ora serrata at

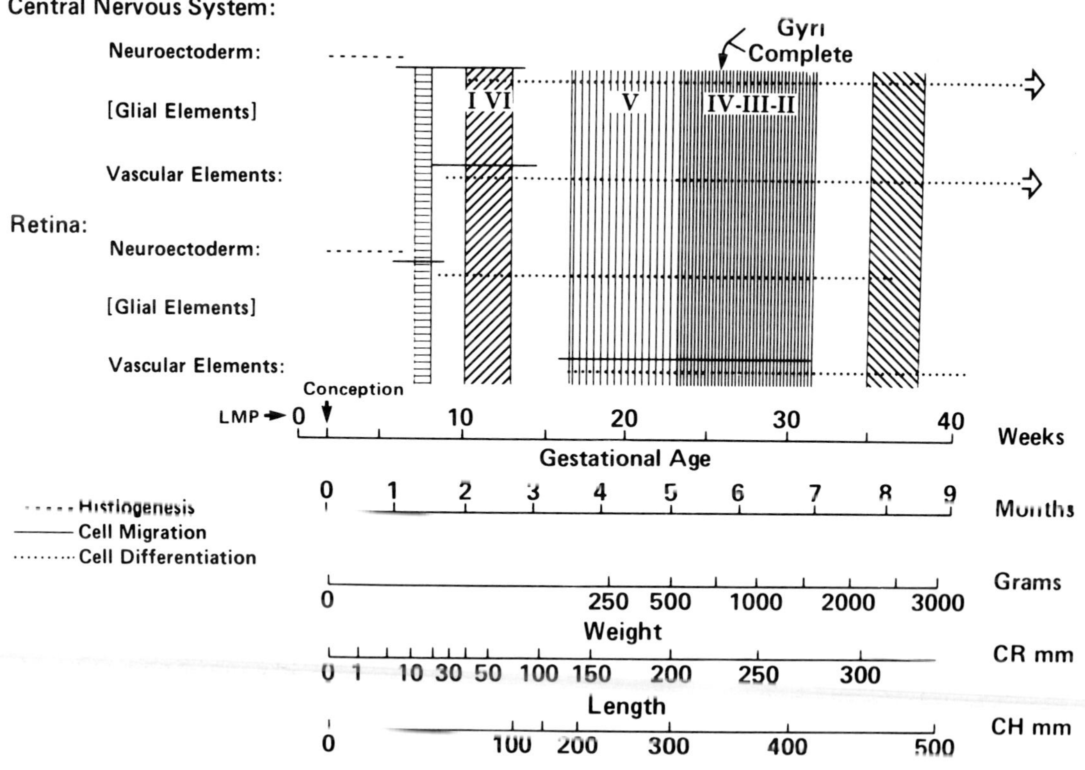

Figure 5–3 Diagrammatic representation of neuroectodermal histiogenesis (- - - - -), cell migration (———), and cell differentiation (· · · · · ·) concomitantly in the central nervous system[6] and retina.[7] Horizontal axes represent gestational age in weeks from the last menstrual period (LMP), lunar months from conception, birth weight in grams, crown to rump (CR) length in millimeters, and crown to heel (CH) length in millimeters.
≡ =Norrie's syndrome (Group A); //// =Walker-Warburg syndrome (Group B);
||||||| =clinical occurrence of ROP in preterm survivors (between 23- and 31-weeks gestational age, from 501 to 1,500 grams birth weight) (Group C);
|| || | =additional period of vulnerability of migrating spindle cells between 16- and 23-weeks gestational age, from 100 to 500 grams birth weight, i.e., nonviable fetuses) (Group C);
\\\\\ =Familial exudative vitreoretinopathy and incontinentia pigmenti (Group D).
I–VI=cortical layers.

29 weeks. The differentiation of spindle cells into endothelial cells begins at the optic disc at 17 weeks and terminates at the temporal ora serrata at 40 weeks.

GROUPS OF DISORDERS CLINICALLY RESEMBLING ROP

Recognizing the time at which the processes of spindle cell migration, canalization, and inner retinal vasoformation occur allows a rational understanding of the clinical association between central nervous system and ocular anomalies (Fig. 5–3). Thus severe central nervous system abnormalities usually accompany altered formation of the inner and outer retina, with interruption of spindle cell migration. In contrast, the central nervous system can be normal, if only the final stages of inner retinal vasoformation are altered.

This concept is exemplified by four distinct groups of disorders that illustrate the interplay between genetic and environmental factors, producing constellations resembling ROP clinically. They can all be explained by understanding the spindle cell pathogenesis of ROP (Fig. 5–2) and the time course of normal inner retinal vasoformation (Fig. 5–3). The four groups, A to D, cluster as follows:

Group A. Defective formation of the inner retina, the ganglion cells. This results in a lack of cystoid spaces in the nerve fiber layer, through which spindle cells usually migrate toward the ora serrata (Fig. 5–4).

Group B. Abnormal differentiation of the outer retina, the bipolar cells and photoreceptors. This causes an absence of metabolically active photoreceptors, which usually stimulate spindle cell migration toward the ora serrata (Fig. 5–5).

Group C. Initiation of gap junction formation between adjacent spindle cells by intrauterine hypoxia or hyperoxia. Therefore, spindle cell migration toward the ora serrata ceases (Figs. 5–6 and 5–7).

Group D. Abnormal retinal antioxidant systems. As a result, gap junctions form between adjacent spindle cells in the peripheral retina, with cessation of the final phases of normal inner retinal vasoformation (Figs. 5–8 and 5–9).

THEORETICAL EXPLANATION OF THE GROUPS OF DISORDERS CLINICALLY RESEMBLING ROP

Groups A and B. Syndromes with abnormal central nervous system and ocular neuroectodermal migration and/or differentiation may be caused by abnormal glycoprotein complexes,[8] and these syndromes may be marked by abnormal layering in the central nervous system (lissencephaly) and in the retina (retinal dysplasia). Theoretically, such abnormal complexes are genetically derived in a recessive manner from a single gene.

Group C. Later, in embryogenesis, vascular precursors in the central nervous system and retina can be damaged. Patients with abnormal central nervous system vascularization or vascular accidents include those with hydranencephaly, porencephalic cysts, and pseudoporencephalic cysts. Patients with ocular damage related to abnormal retinal vessels include those with retinal neovascularization that is pathologically indistinguishable from ROP. Oculocerebral vascular abnormalities can result from intrauterine hypoxia or environmental factors related to genetic factors in a multifactorial, hereditary manner.

Group D. In the final stages of embryogenesis, syndromes that have abnormal, retinal antioxidant systems can allow the highly vulnerable process of inner retinal vasoformation to be damaged in its final stages in the far peripheral retina, with or without causing similar central nervous system devastation. Familial exudative vitreoretinopathy is an example of a syndrome with a deficient, endogenous antioxidant system.[9] Incontinentia pigmenti is an example of a syndrome with an altered potential of melanin to sequester oxygen radicals.[10] Both syndromes occur in the final stages of embryogenesis. In such syndromes, the central nervous system can be normal, as in familial exudative vitreoretinopathy, or abnormal, as in incontinentia pigmenti. Theoretically, such syndromes are related to abnormal structural proteins that are genetically transmitted in a dominant manner— autosomal dominant, in the case of familial exudative vitreoretinopathy; X-linked dominant, in the case of incontinentia pigmenti.

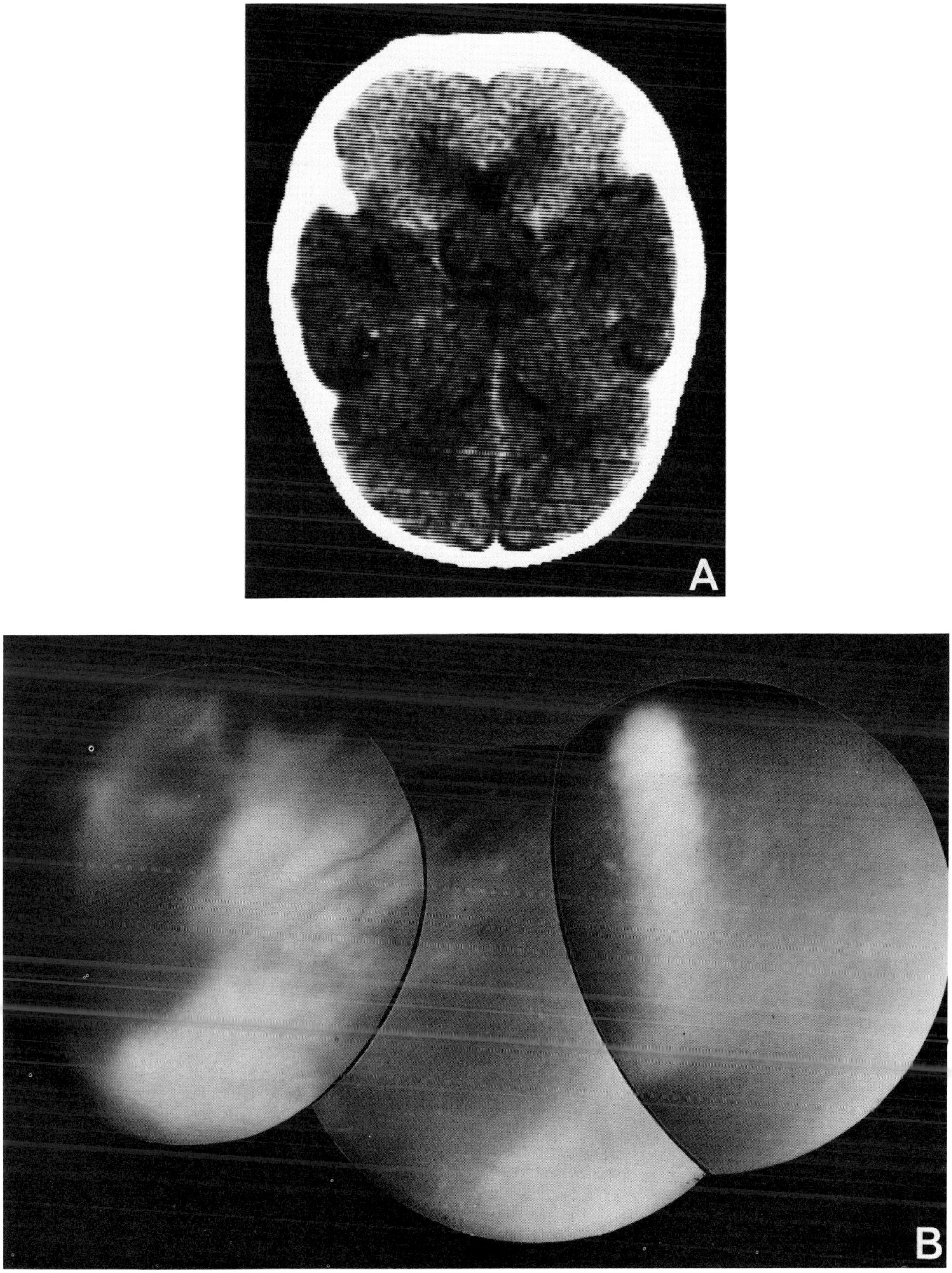

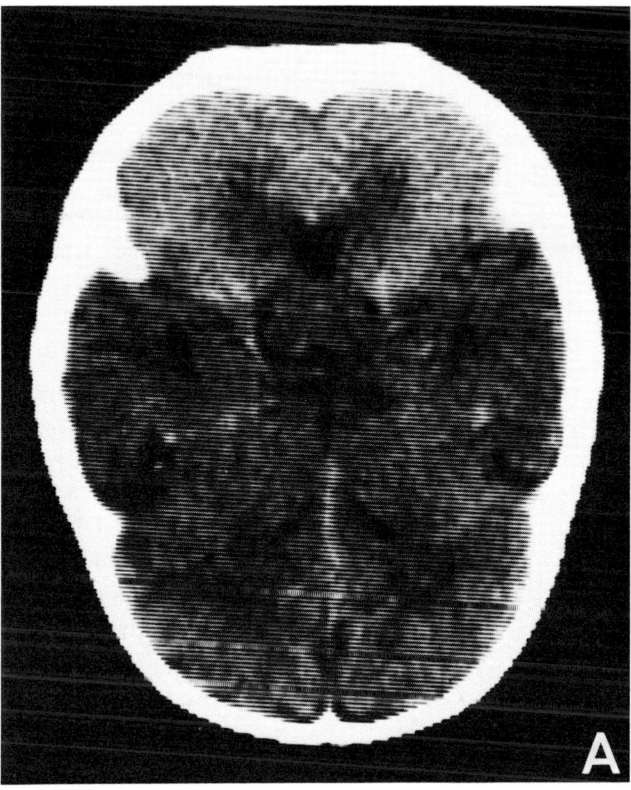

Figure 5–4   Example of Group A disorder, Norrie's syndrome: defective formation of the inner retina. A, CT scan of brain that demonstrates minimal, incomplete lamination often seen in Norrie's syndrome. B, Retinal montage of the left eye at age 9 weeks. The preretinal membranes associated with hemorrhage are demonstrated.

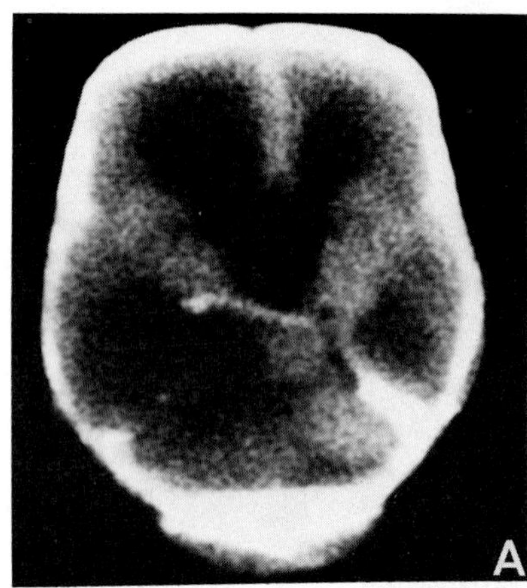

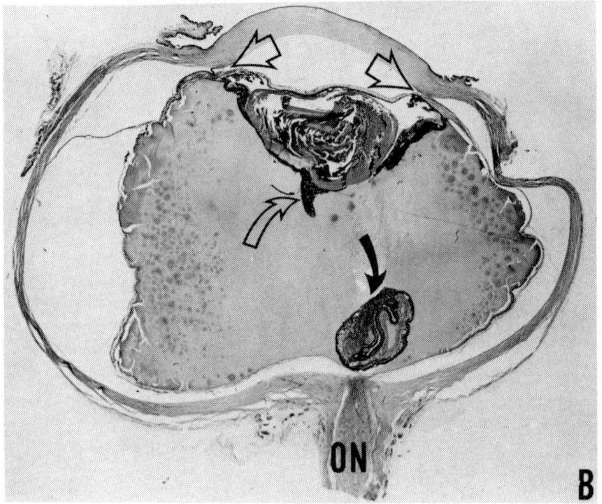

Figure 5–5 Example of Group B disorder, Walker-Warburg syndrome: abnormal outer retinal differentiation. A, CT scan of brain with lissencephaly of cortical areas of scan. B, Light micrograph of the pathological appearance of the left eye at age 2 weeks. The dysplastic retinal elements are reduced to a small mass behind the lens ( ) and at the optic nerve ( ). There is also incomplete cleavage of the anterior chamber angle ( ) and an atrophic optic nerve (ON). Light micrograph is courtesy of Dr. Ramon Font.

DEFECTIVE FORMATION OF THE INNER RETINA (GROUP A)

Norrie's Syndrome

Norrie's syndrome, which is sex-linked recessive, is an example of defective formation of the inner retina, with resultant lack of cystoid spaces through which spindle cells migrate toward the ora serrata (Fig. 5–4).[11,12] The abnormal gene must be manifest very early in embryogenesis, probably at about the seventh-week gestational age. Usually, the lamination of the central nervous system is only minimally affected (Fig. 5–4A). The retinal defect is the absence of ganglion

cells,[13] which results in a malformation of all retinal layers, since retinal development occurs sequentially from ganglion cells to bipolar cells to photoreceptors. Furthermore, with the absence of ganglion cells, there is no differentiation of a nerve fiber layer with cystoid spaces through which spindle cells arising in the adventitia of the hyaloid artery can migrate toward the ora serrata. Spindle cells surge into the vitreous, producing the characteristic neovascularization that superficially resembles ROP clinically (Fig. 5–4B). This congenital neovascularization is coupled with an atrophic optic nerve and optic radiations to the lateral geniculate body and correlates with the absence of third-order neurons. Furthermore, the dysplastic retina triggers proliferation of the retinal pigment epithelium.

The differential diagnosis is made because the pathology is present at birth in term infants; there is a typical genetic pattern of affected males and carrier females; there is incomplete lamination of the cerebral cortex, often demonstrable by CT scan; and there is an absent electroretinogram at birth because of the absence of retinal differentiation and retinal detachment.

Norrie's syndrome, reported as nonoxygen-induced retinopathy in full-term infants, can be found, in hindsight, in the literature. For example, case five of Stefani and Ehalt probably represents a case of Norrie's syndrome.[14]

ABNORMAL DIFFERENTIATION OF THE OUTER RETINA (GROUP B)

Walker-Warburg Syndrome

The Walker-Warburg syndrome, or lissencephaly, is an example of a genetic syndrome with abnormal differentiation of the outer retina (autosomal recessive, Fig. 5–5).[15,16] This syndrome occurs at about the tenth-week gestational age, when the central nervous system gyri are beginning to form. Thus abnormal layering of the cortex is a prominent feature of this syndrome (Fig. 5–5A). Abnormal differentiation of the outer retina is accompanied by a metabolic block of spindle cell migration toward the ora serrata, since the formation of a normal outer retina provides the stimulus for spindle cell migration. In lissencephaly, the ganglion cells, bipolar cells, and photoreceptors are present. However, there is an absence of inner retinal vessels or their precursors, the mesenchymal spindle cells, because the photoreceptors never mature and create an oxygen

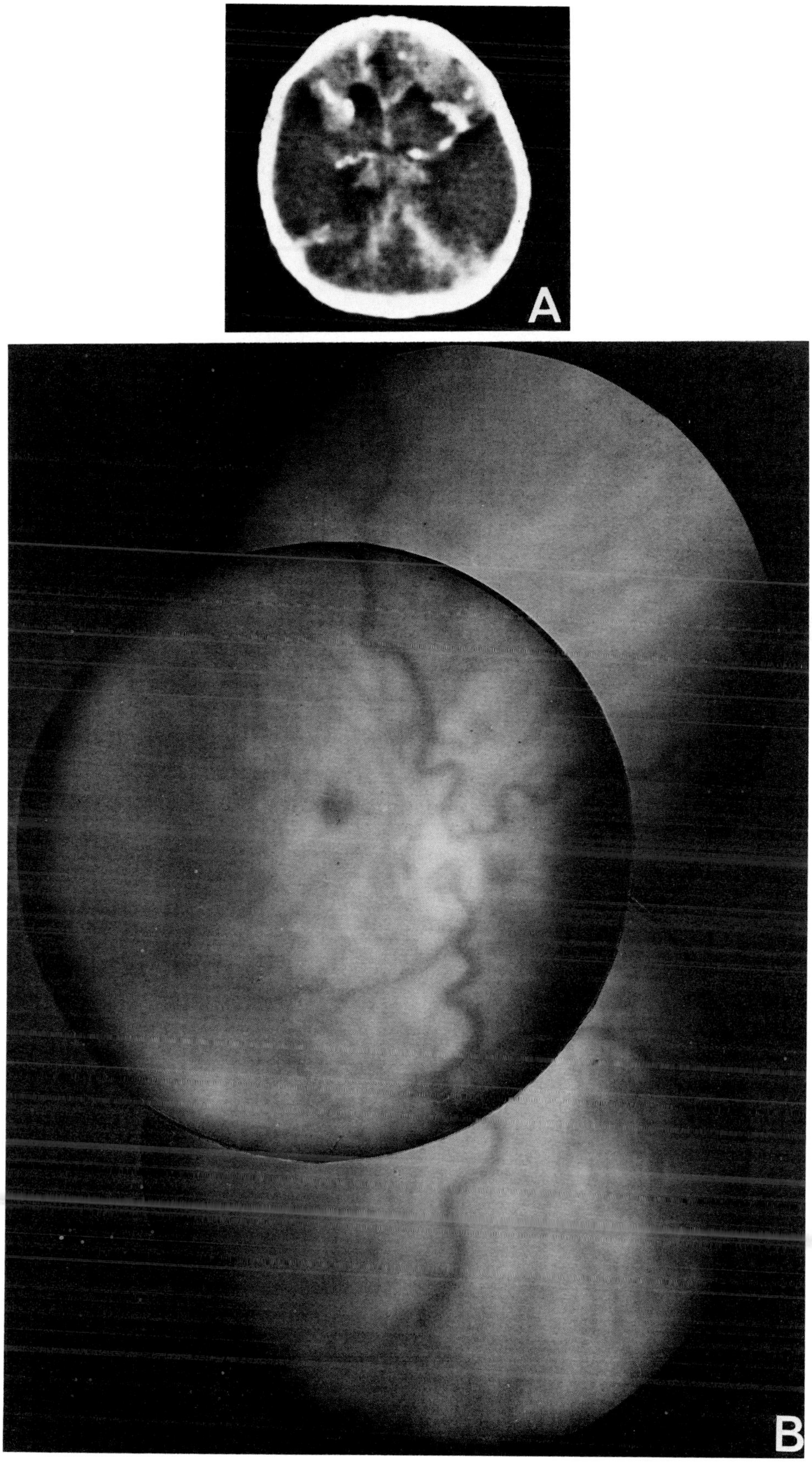

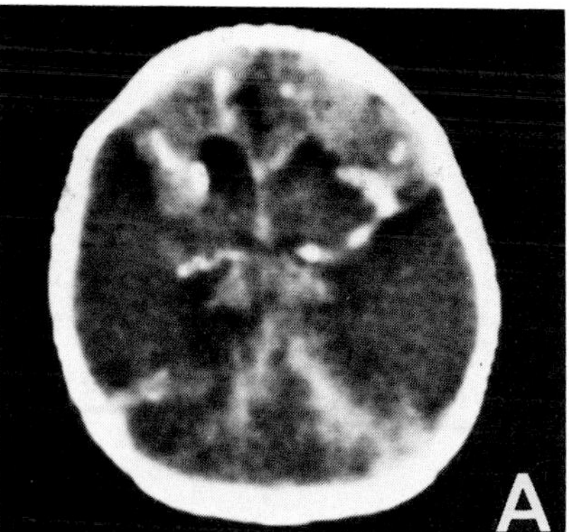

Figure 5–6 Example of Group C disorder, spontaneous infarction of both middle cerebral arteries: intrauterine initiation of gap junction formation between adjacent, retinal spindle cells. A, CT scan of brain with absence of cerebral mantle. B, Retinal photograph of the right eye at age 8 weeks. The optic nerve reflects the central nervous system atrophy, the retinal vessels are tortuous, and the peripheral retina is detached.

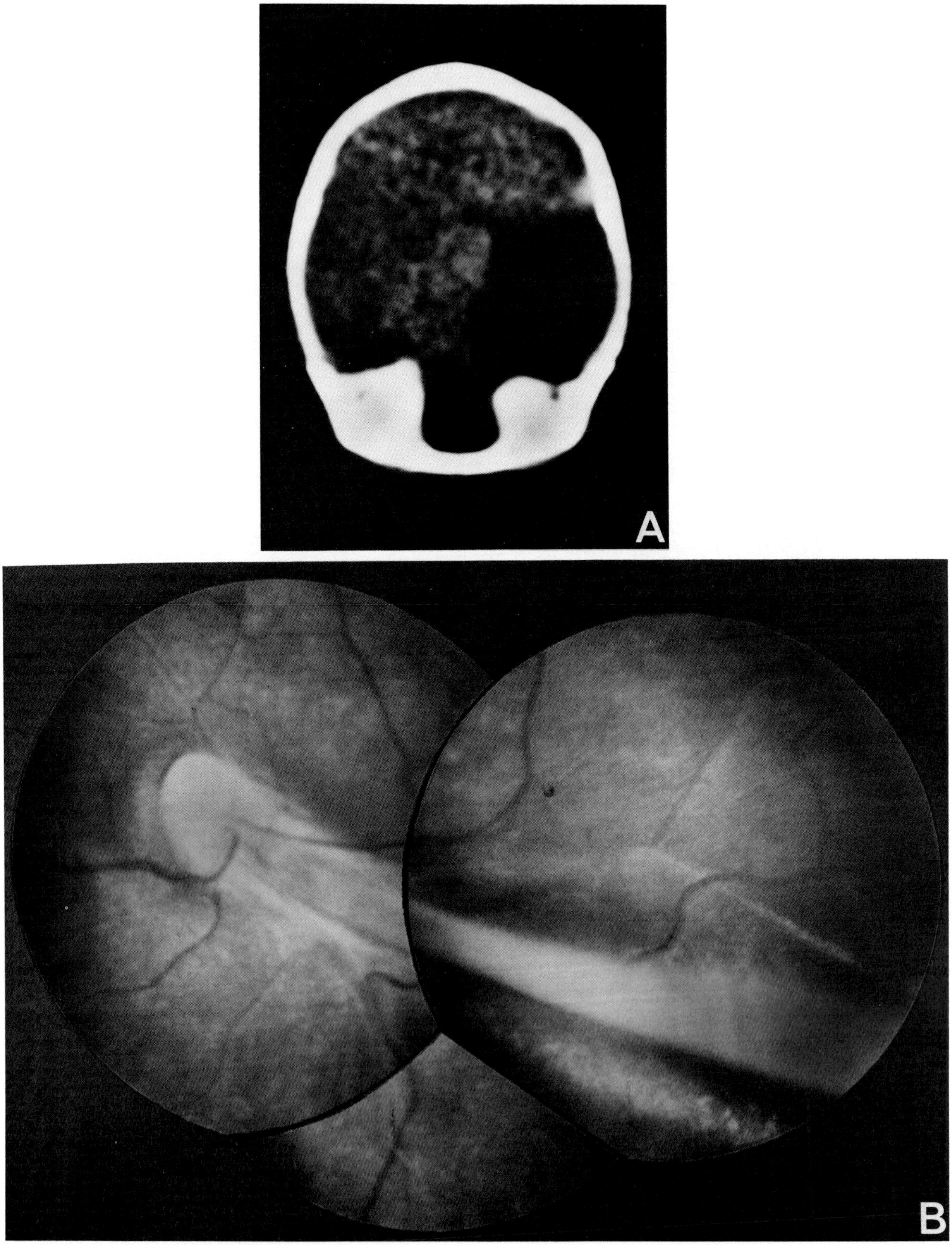

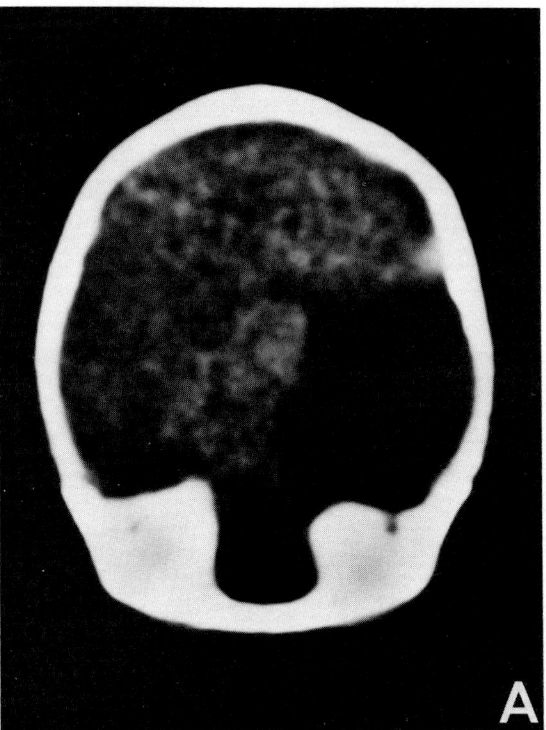

Figure 5–7 ˙ Example of Group C disorder, sincipital Vietnamese syndrome; intrauterine initiation of gap junction formation between adjacent, retinal spindle cells. A, CT scan of brain with porencephalic cyst. B, Retinal montage of the left eye at age four weeks. The retinal vessels are typical of cicatricial Grade III RLF.

sink. There is also incomplete cleavage of the anterior chamber angle, persistence of the anterior tunica vasculosa lentis, and ganglion cell dropout in the optic nerve (Fig. 5–5B).[17-19] Ultrastructurally, there is bloated, rough, endoplasmic reticulum, with dense lumen content in corneal endothelium and photoreceptor inner segments. This bloated, rough endoplasmic reticulum may indicate that the secretion of abnormal glycoprotein complexes prevents normal neuroectodermal (neuroblastic) differentiation.[19]

Differential diagnosis is made because of the following: retinal detachment is present at birth in term infants; there may be a history of consanguinity; the CT scan will reveal lissencephaly with agyria; and there will be an abnormal electroretinogram at birth owing to the blockage of photoreceptor differentiation and retinal detachment. There is generalized cessation of cellular migration, resulting in incomplete stratification of the cerebral cortex,[16] absence of spindle-cell migration in the nerve fiber layer, as deduced from Figure 5–5 in the publication of Yanoff, et al,[17] and incomplete cleavage of the anterior chamber angle owing to a suppression of the first axial migration of neural crest derivatives.[20]

Multiple cases of nonhyperoxic term births with ROP in the literature may be examples of lissencephaly. Lissencephaly is reported occasionally as hydrocephaly or hydranencephaly. Halsey, et al[21] reported retinopathy that resembled ROP in term infants with hydranencephaly and agyria, cases five and six.

INITIATION OF GAP JUNCTION FORMATION BETWEEN ADJACENT SPINDLE CELLS (GROUP C)

Syndromes that occur as a result of the intrauterine initiation of gap-junction formation between adjacent spindle cells are pathologically indistinguishable from ROP. They occur between the sixteenth- and thirty-second-week gestational age and constitute the majority of ROP syndromes observed in term infants. Environmental stress or multifactorial genetic syndromes trigger gap-junction formation in spindle cells that are migrating through a normally differentiating retina. Intrauterine catastrophies occurring after spindle cells have invaded the nerve-fiber layer, i.e., in the second trimester, or affecting infants with genetic predisposition to anterior encephalocoeles constitute the vast majority of nonhyperoxic term infants who have a retinal appearance resembling ROP clinically. These cases are generally congenital, because they develop approximately 8 weeks following the intrauterine episode of hypoxia or hyperoxia. This is the exact timing of the occurrence of ROP in preterm infants not receiving vitamin E supplementation.[22] The pathogenetic sequence is identical to ROP, and spontaneous regression or retinal separation can ensue.[1] Misdiagnosis is common if an inadequate history of the pregnancy is taken or if there are no external central-nervous-system abnormalities that would prompt an early, postpartum ocular examination.

Intrauterine Catastrophies

Often intrauterine central nervous system vascular accidents in the second trimester result in infants with hydranencephaly, hydrocephaly, anencephaly, or porencephaly (Fig. 5–6A). Many episodes of second trimester bleeding with acute fetal hypoxia, severe maternal anemia with chronic fetal hypoxia, maternal-fetal intrauterine transfusions, and amnionitis can produce conditions with the retinal appearance of ROP (Fig. 5–6B).[23-25]

Differential diagnosis is made only by examination of a term infant at birth, when a history of intrauterine catastrophe is obtained. The time at which the catastrophe occurs can be deduced, as a function of gestational age, by the extent of the central retinal vascularization present. The CT scan is usually abnormal. The electroretinogram at birth is recordable if retinal detachment has not developed.

Examples of nonhyperoxic term infants who have ROP that is associated with porencephaly, hydranencephaly, hydrocephaly, anencephaly, and encephalocoeles can be found repeatedly in the literature.[26-31]

Anterior Encephalocoeles in Asians

Familial syndromes, such as anterior encephalocoeles in Asians, occur at this time in gestation.[32-34] The genetics are that of a multifactorial syndrome, since the sincipital region of the skull is particularly susceptible to internal pressure secondary to environmental stress (Fig. 5–7A).[35] The resultant fetal hypoxia produces a retinal appearance of ROP (Fig. 5–7B).

Differential diagnosis is made only by examination of an Asiatic infant when an anterior encephalocoele is noted. The CT scan is abnormal. The electroretinogram at birth is recordable if retinal detachment has not developed.

An example of this disorder has been described by Hittner.[33]

ABNORMAL RETINAL ANTIOXIDANT SYSTEMS (GROUP D)

Some syndromes express themselves near the end of fetal life, usually after the thirty-fourth-week gestational age. These patients have abnormal retinal vasculature in the far peripheral retina (Figs. 5–8 and 5–9).[36-38] This correlates with spindle cells that are vulnerable to complete normal vasoformation to the ora serrata. This condition is owing to late-onset, oxidative stress, for which there is inadequate retinal antioxidant protection, concomitant with increasing metabolic demands by the differentiating central retina. Often there are no retinal vessels beyond a certain demarcation line, indicating that the oxidative stress is not a transient postnatal event. Such a development is distinct from cases of ROP that have undergone spontaneous regression, in which retinal vessels grow anterior to the demarcation line. This reflects the transient, postnatal, oxidative stress related to prematurity.

Autosomal-Dominant, Familial Exudative Vitreoretinopathy

Recent data suggest that there is a deficient, endogenous, antioxidant system in autosomal-dominant, familial exudative vitreoretinopathy. There is apparently a basic defect in platelet aggregation, deduced by altered arachidonic acid metabolism in the prostaglandin cascade.[9] Pathological examination of an eye from such a patient reveals incomplete vascularization of the peripheral retina.[36] This defect is similar to the canine vasculature's vulnerability to complete peripheral differentiation, rendered vulnerable by a process of endothelial budding in the presence of aspirin, which interferes with the prostaglandin cascade.[39]

Differential diagnosis is made because retinal pathology is present at birth, there is a family history consistent with dominant inheritance and complete penetrance, there is normal central nervous system development, and there is recordable electroretinogram if retinal detachment has not occurred.

Spontaneous mutation or inadequate family history may lead to an incorrect diagnosis of ROP, since diagnosis is usually made on the basis of a family history. In cases of nonhyperoxic term infants with ROP, studies of endogenous, antioxidant systems are warranted to establish this diagnosis.

Incontinentia Pigmenti

The primary etiology of incontinentia pigmenti is dysplasia and proliferation of the retinal pigment epithelium,[40-42] concomitant with abnormal melanin[38] and an altered potential to sequester oxygen radicals.[10] Many cases have been reported with reference to an avascular peripheral retina.[38]

Differential diagnosis is made by evaluating the following: the characteristic skin appearance that is present early in life; a family history consistent with an X-linked dominant trait, lethal in males; central nervous system manifestations, especially motor abnormalities in approximately 30 percent of cases;[45] and a recordable electroretinogram if retinal detachment has not occurred.

Cases have been reported as ROP especially if a family history of abnormalities of the skin, teeth, eye, and central nervous system is absent or not elicited, and if the retina is examined later in life when most of the characteristic skin lesions have faded.[42]

IMPORTANCE OF ESTABLISHING THE CORRECT DIAGNOSIS

Because of litigation involving infants with ROP, approximately 200 case reports are emphasized in the literature. These reports stress ROP in term infants, ROP not associated with oxygen administration, and congenital ROP. The incidence of such "atypical" ROP cases is extremely low. Their occurrence should not obscure the fact that ROP is generally a disease of very-low-birth-weight infants—those of 1,500 grams or less at birth and 31 weeks or less gestational age—who require oxygen administration, have other neonatal complications, and develop the disease at a predictable postnatal age.[22]

The four groups of disorders studied in this chapter are far from complete; however, each case of bilateral neovascularization, with or without leukocoria, can be placed along the gradient of neuroectodermal histiogenesis, cell migration, and cell differentiation (Fig. 5–3). The four groups emphasize the need for early retinal examinations when severe complications of pregnancy or severe central nervous system anomalies occur, as well as when there is a family history of bilateral neovascularizations with or without leukocoria. Only early retinal examinations can distinguish some cases of nonhyperoxic ROP in term infants from classic ROP, since such cases can have identical pathology in the final cicatricial stages. Similarly, only early ophthalmic evalua-

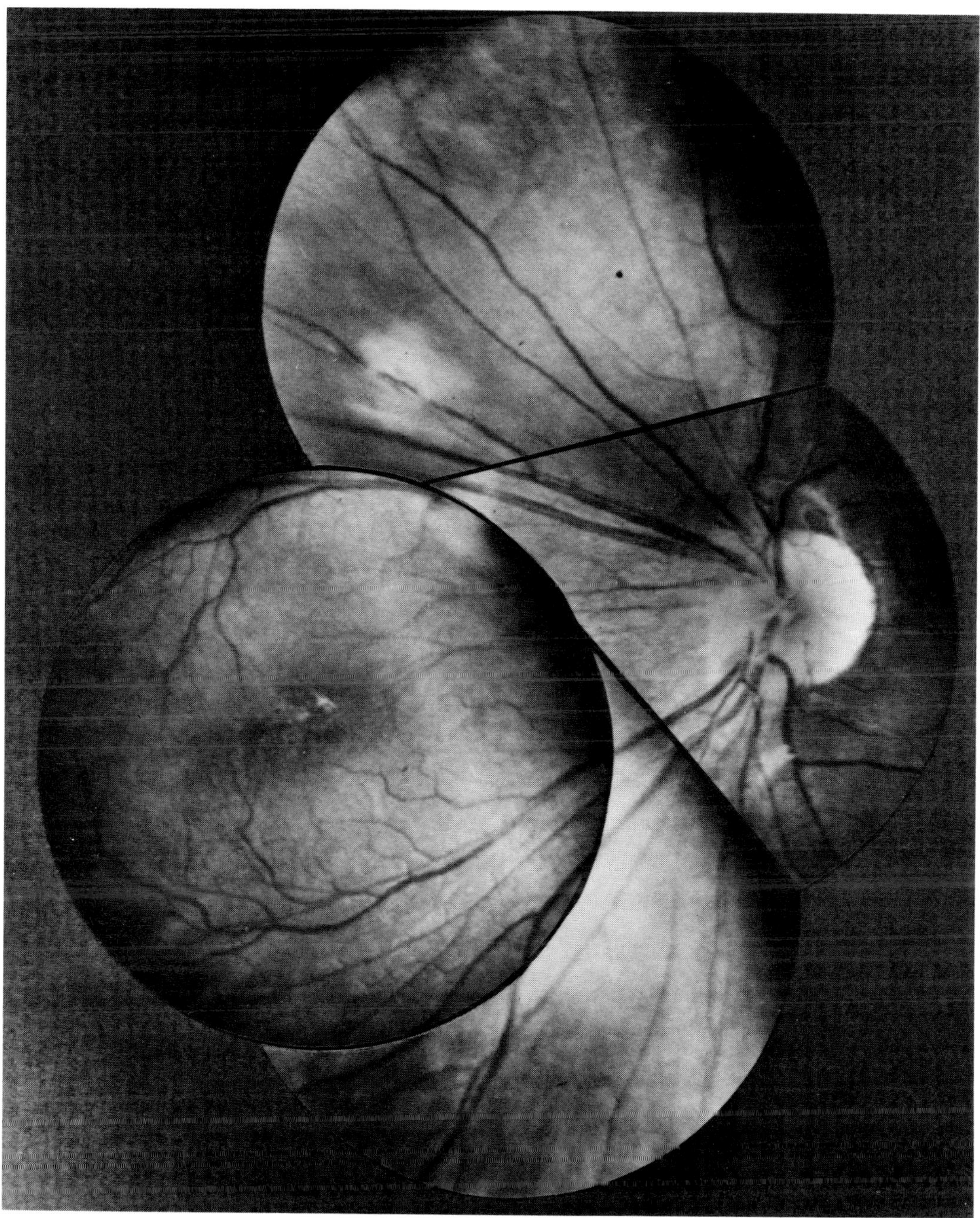

Figure 5–8 Example of Group D disorder, familial exudative vitreoretinopathy: deficient, endogenous, retinal antioxidant systems. Retinal montage of the right eye at age 13 years. The retinal vessels are typical of cicatricial Grade II RLF. Other family members have similar retinal abnormalities.

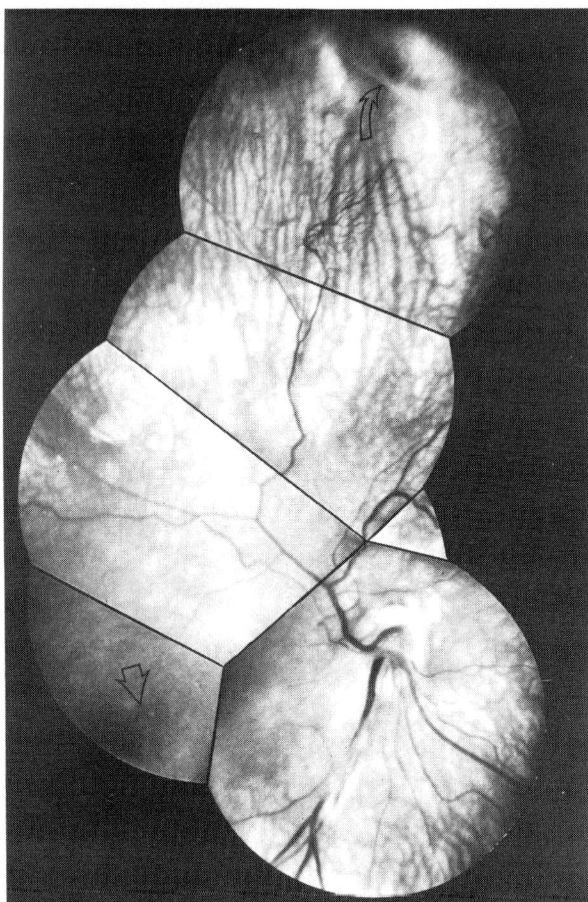

Figure 5–9 Example of Group D disorder, incontinentia pigmenti: altered potential via abnormal melanin to sequester oxygen radicals. Retinal montage of the right eye at age 3 years. White preretinal tissue (⇧) separates the peripheral, avascular retina from irregular, kinked vessels. The macula appears intact (⇩) with dragging of the retinal vessels inferiorly.

tions can identify those cases that occur late enough in gestation to be amenable to medical, i.e., glasses and patching, and surgical, i.e., cryotherapy, therapy. Eliminating unwarranted litigation, instituting adequate ophthalmic therapy, and providing appropriate genetic counseling in these congenital cases that resemble ROP can only be accomplished through a high index of suspicion.

Alexander Kogan and Lisa Emmit-Khan provided photographic assistance and assembled the retinal montages. Dr. Ramon Font kindly provided the light micrograph of the eye from the infant with Walker-Warburg syndrome. The Lion's Eyes of Texas Eye Bank (Robert Fort and E.J. Farge) sensitively encouraged whole-eye donations.

REFERENCES

1. Kretzer·FL, Mehta RS, Johnson AT, Hunter DG, Brown ES, Hittner HM. Vitamin E protects against retinopathy of prematurity through action on spindle cells. Nature 1984; 309:793–795.

2. Kretzer FL, Hunter DG, Mehta RS, Brown ES, Blifeld C, Johnson AT, Hittner HM. Spindle cells as vasoformative elements in the developing human retina: vitamin E modulation. In: Coats PW, Markwald RR, Kenny AD, eds. Developing and regenerating vertebrate nervous systems. New York: Alan R. Liss, 1983; 199–210.

3. Kretzer FL, Hittner HM, Johnson AT, Mehta RS, Godio LB. Vitamin E and retrolental fibroplasia: ultrastructural support of clinical efficacy. Ann NY Acad Sci 1982; 393:145–166.

4. Johnson AT, Kretzer FL, Hittner HM, Glazebrook PA, Bridges CDB, Lam DMK. Development of the subretinal space in the preterm human eye: ultrastructural and immunocytochemical studies. J Comp Neurol 1984; 233:497–505.

5. Johnson AT, Kretzer FL. Interstitial retinol binding protein in the developing human retina: a proposed explanation for vitamin E suppression of retinopathy of prematurity. In: Bridges CDB, Adler AJ, eds. The interphotoreceptor matrix in health and disease. New York: Alan R. Liss, 1985; 251–277.

6. Warkany J, Lemire RJ, Cohen MM. Hydranencephaly; Encephalocoeles; Porencephaly; Lissencephaly; agyria and pachygyria. In: Warkam J, Lemire RJ, Cohen MM, eds. Mental retardation and congenital malformations of the central nervous system. Chicago: Year Book Medical Publishers, 1981; 83–100; 158–175; 191–199; 200–210.

7. Ozanics V, Jakobiec FA. Prenatal development of the eye and its adnexa. In: Jakobiec FA, ed. Ocular anatomy, embryology, and teratology. Philadelphia: Harper & Row Publishers, 1982; 11–96.

8. Liu HM. Axon-sheath cell interaction mediated by a neurotropic substance. Exp Neurol 1979; 66:123–134.

9. Chaudhuri PR, Rosenthal AR, Goulstein DB, Rowlands D, Mitchell VE. Familial exudative vitreoretinopathy associated with familial thrombocytopathy. Br J Ophthalmol 1983; 67:755–758.

10. Pietronigro DD, McGinness JE, Koren MJ, Crippa R, Seligman ML, Demopoulos HB. Spontaneous generation of adriamycin semiquinone radicals at physiologic pH. Physiol Chem Phys 1979; 11:405–414.

11. Norrie G. Causes of blindness in children: twenty-five years' experience of Danish institutes for the blind. Acta Ophthalmol (Kbh) 1927; 5:357–386.

12. Warburg M. Norrie's disease: a new hereditary bilateral pseudotumor of the retina. Acta Ophthalmol 1961; 39:757–772.

13. Apple DJ, Fishman GA, Goldberg MF. Ocular histopathology of Norrie's disease. Am J Ophthalmol 1974; 78:196–302.

14. Stefani FH, Ehalt H. Non-oxygen induced retinitis proliferans and retinal detachment in full-term infants. Br J Ophthalmol 1974; 58:490–513.

15. Walker AE. Lissencephaly. Arch Neurol 1942; 48:13–29.

16. Warburg M. The heterogeneity of microphthalmia in the mentally retarded. Birth Defects 1971; 7:136–154.

17. Yanoff M, Rorke LB, Allman MI. Bilateral optic system aplasia with relatively normal eyes. Arch Ophthalmol 1978; 96:97–101.

18. Bordarier C, Aicardi J, Goutieres F. Congenital hydrocephalus and eye abnormalities with severe developmental brain defects: Warburg's syndrome. Ann Neurol 1984; 16:60–65.

19. Dobyns WB, Kirkpatrick JB, Hittner HM, Roberts RM, Kretzer FL. Syndromes with lissencephaly. II. Walker-Warburg and cerebro-ocular-muscular syndromes and a new syndrome with type II lissencephaly. Am J Med Genet 1985; 22:157–196.

20. Hittner HM, Kretzer FL, Antoszyk JH, Ferrell RE, Mehta RS. Variable expressivity of autosomal dominant anterior segment mesenchymal dysgenesis in six generations. Am J Ophthalmol 1982; 93:57–70.

21. Halsey JH, Allen N, Chamberlin HR. The morphogenesis of hydranencephaly. J Neurol Sci 1971; 12:187–217.

22. Hittner HM, Rudolph AJ, Kretzer FL. Suppression of severe retinopathy of prematurity with vitamin E supplementation: ultrastructural mechanism of clinical efficacy. Ophthalmology 1984; 91:1512–1523.

23. Bruckner HL. Retrolental fibroplasia: associated with intrauterine anoxia? Arch Ophthalmol 1968; 80:504–505.

24. Johnson L, Schaffer D, Boggs TR. The premature infant, vitamin E deficiency and retrolental fibroplasia. Am J Clin Nutr 1974; 27:1158–1173.

25. Johnson L, Schaffer DB, Blesa MI, Boggs TR. Factors predisposing to RLF: complications of pregnancy. Pediatr Res 1978; 12:527.
26. Reese AB, Blodi FC, Locke JC. The pathology of early retrolental fibroplasia: with an analysis of the histologic findings in the eyes of newborn and stillborn infants. Am J Ophthalmol 1952; 35:1407–1454.
27. Hill K, Cogan DG, Dodge PR. Ocular signs associated with hydranencephaly. Am J Ophthalmol 1961; 51:267–275.
28. Andersen SR, Bro-Rasmussen F, Tygstrup I. Anencephaly related to ocular development and malformation. Am J Ophthalmol 1967; 64:559–566.
29. Manschot WA. Eye findings in hydranencephaly. Ophthalmologica 1971; 162:151–159.
30. Addison DJ, Font RL, Manschot W. Proliferative retinopathy in anencephalic babies. Am J Ophthalmol 1972; 74:967–976.
31. Ehrenkranz RA, Puklin JE. Letters to the editor: RLF and vitamin E. Ophthalmology 1982; 89:988–989.
32. Flatz G, Sukthomya C. Fronto-ethmoidal encephalomeningocoeles in the population of Northern Thailand. Hum Genet 1970; 11:1–8.
33. Hittner HM. Retinal and central nervous system abnormalities: syndromes which resemble retrolental fibroplasia. Metab Pediatr Syst Ophthalmol 1985; 8:5–10.
34. Suwanwela C. Geographical distribution of fronto-ethmoidal encephalomeningocoele. Br J Prev Soc Med 1972; 26:193–198.
35. Suwanwela C, Suwanwela N. A morphological classification of sincipital encephalomeningocoeles. J Neurosurg 1973; 36:201–211.
36. Criswick VG, Schepens CL. Familial exudative vitreoretinopathy. Am J Ophthalmol 1969; 68:578–594.
37. Brockhurst RJ, Albert DM, Zakov ZN. Pathologic findings in familial exudative vitreoretinopathy. Arch Ophthalmol 1981; 99:2143–2146.
38. Watzke RC, Stevens TS, Carney RG. Retinal vascular changes of incontinentia pigmenti. Arch Ophthalmol 1976; 94:743–746.
39. Flower RS, Blake DA, Wajer SD, Egner PG, McLeod DS, Pitts SM. Retrolental fibroplasia: evidence for a role of the prostaglandin cascade in the pathogenesis of oxygen induced retinopathy in the newborn beagle. Pediatr Res 1981; 15:1293–1302.
40. Berbich A, Dhermy P, Majbar M. Ocular findings in a case of incontinentia pigmenti (Bloch-Sulzberger syndrome). Ophthalmologica 1981; 182:119–129.
41. Rosenfeld SI, Smith ME. Ocular findings in incontinentia pigmenti. Ophthalmology 1985; 92:543–546.
42. Carney RG. Incontinentia pigmenti: a world statistical analysis. Arch Dermatol 1976; 112:535–542.

Medicolegal Aspects of Retinopathy of Prematurity

Jerome W. Bettman, M.D.

In the fall of 1942, I had my first experience as associate examiner on the American Board of Ophthalmology. While waiting for the first candidate, the board member in charge of the pathology section showed me a slide of a condition that I had never seen before; that board member was Dr. Terry, who originally described retrolental fibroplasia (RLF).[1] The number of cases of RLF increased at an alarming rate until this condition had become the largest cause of blindness in pre-school children. There were no medicolegal claims based upon RLF for a number of years succeeding Terry's publication, because the etiology was unknown.

The suspicion that oxygen was the etiology first arose with Kate Campbell's publication in 1951.[2] The significance of oxygen in a premature infant was the subject of a large number of articles, but medicolegal claims were not filed, because there was no indication of the unacceptable amount of oxygen.

PERMISSIBLE OXYGEN LIMIT

The alarming incidence of RLF stimulated authorities to attempt to define a permissible limit to the amount of oxygen that should be used. July 1, 1955, the California Department of Public Health issued a directive that the supplemental oxygen in the incubator's ambient air should not exceed 40 percent, attorneys now had a definite figure on which to base claims. A relatively large number of medicolegal claims arose, based upon premature infants being in an atmosphere greater than 40 percent oxygen and developing what was then called RLF. If a premature infant was born after July 1 and received more than 40 percent oxygen in the ambient air, a suit might be filed, because the amount exceeded that in the directive.

After the presumption that oxygen was the impor-tant factor in the RLF etiology, the oxygen use was drastically diminished in an attempt at prevention. The incidence of cerebral palsy, respiratory distress syndrome, and death increased; the incidence of medicolegal claims diminished. The dictum then changed—the premature infant was to be given the amount of oxygen that was necessary, but no more. This created problems related to the risk/benefit ratio, but these claims could be defended, since the amount of oxygen needed was a matter of judgment, except for a few cases in which there was little attempt to curtail the oxygen given to a healthy infant.

OTHER INFANTS IMPLICATED

The number of claims based upon what is now called the retinopathy of prematurity (ROP) has increased in recent years, to approach the incidence of claims that followed the directive of July 1, 1955. There are several reasons for this increase, some medical and some socio-economic. More premature infants in the high-risk group weighing less than one kilogram are being saved, and therefore, there is a larger group that stands at risk. The survival rate of infants less than one kilogram at birth rose from 8 percent in 1950 to 35 percent in 1980.[3,4] In some centers (personal communication from Philip Sunshine, M.D., Stanford Medical Center) the survival rate of the 750- to 1,000-gram birth-weight group is approaching 80 percent.[5] As Arnall Patz pointed out, ROP is now occurring despite meticulous monitoring of oxygen therapy.[3] It is possible that prematurity per se may be responsible for many of the current cases, in contrast to the overuse of oxygen, which was the major cause years ago.

So many very premature infants are being saved, and so many of these develop ROP despite excellent care and full realization of the risk of ROP that the estimated number of new ROP-blind, 546, is close to that of the "epidemic" of 1943 to 1955.[4] It has been estimated that 40,000 premature infants survive each year in this country, and approximately 4,000 of these have ROP (personal communication from Philip Sunshine, M.D.).

PHYSICIAN LIABILITY DIFFICULT TO DEFINE

The problem of medicolegal culpability is complicated by problems in diagnosis. It is probable that some cases were incorrectly diagnosed as ROP; not all patients with the familiar morphological picture of ROP have that disorder. Familial exudative vitreoretinopathy (autosomal-dominant exudative vitreoretinopathy) can appear to be identical in every morphological feature to ROP. The patient may have a dragged disc, a demarcated peripheral avascular zone and arteriovenous anastomoses, and other features that can occur in ROP.[5] The only differences are an absence of a familial history, absence of prematurity, and the absence of the administration of oxygen.[6] The absence of familial history might not be a reliable guide, because the gene can exhibit different expressibility.[7] The two conditions cannot be distinguished by the funduscopic appearance. Conditions such as persistence and hyperplasia of the primary vitreous (PHVP), Coat's disease, and occasional others may be misdiagnosed as ROP.

A number of claims involve the group of very premature infants. The claims are unjustified, as will be discussed below. Some have been based upon misdiagnosis. In retrospect, one must seriously question the validity of those claims in instances of infants who are nearly mature or have received little or no oxygen.

Some of the claims are unjustified. In these claims, oxygen administration was required, the oxygen level was properly monitored, and the oxygen was not used longer or in higher concentration than necessary. The ROP developed despite expert medical care and without evidence of substandard care. It is a risk that must be accepted.

Occasionally oxygen is given when it is not required, and continued longer than can be justified. A few such cases of substandard care are still seen.

In rare instances, older patients who have impaired vision from ROP file a claim. They maintain that they only recently became aware of the diagnosis and the role of oxygen, and therefore, the statute of limitations had not lapsed.

LEGAL ACTION BASED ON ROP

The number of medicolegal claims based upon ROP is significant. I analyzed 500 from all classifications in ophthalmology, and 29 (5.8 %) were based upon ROP.

Suits are filed for more reasons than the medical. The role of oxygen and the degree of prematurity are only part of the problem. Several socioeconomic facts also contribute to making ROP a target for claims, one of which is poor communication. After a successful struggle to keep a tiny premature infant alive, the parents are permitted to take home a live and apparently healthy child. They might be unaware of the risk of blindness, the need for supplemental oxygen, or do not fully understand this. The unpleasant surprise of possible blindness results in anger that, in turn, brings the thought of suit to their minds.

The timing of communication is important. If the risk of blindness is mentioned soon after birth, the parents can have a feeling of rejection. They might say, "I would rather have the baby dead than blind." Instead of stating the risk then, the physician should stress that the eyes will have to be carefully examined. The parents *must* be told of the threat of blindness, but this can be done two or three weeks after birth, at which time they will want the infant.

A plaintiff's attorney always considers the impact his client has upon the jury. The sight of a blind child who has enophthalmos can influence a jury to award large sums—even though they have been presented with little or no evidence of substandard care. The premature infant is often the only surviving child of a mother who has habitually aborted; this increases the jury's sympathy.

There has been a history of large awards in ROP cases. The plaintiff's attorney can claim the need for lifetime care, with many related embellishments that can move a jury to be very generous. This, plus the sympathy factor, has encouraged some attorneys to file claims and to persevere, even though there has been no evidence of substandard practice. These claims are occasionally successful. The court's rulings are not always based upon what might be substandard practice. Consider the following quotation from an associate justice of the Washington State Supreme Court: there is "a strong and growing tendency, where there is blame on neither side, to ask, in view of the exigencies of social justice, who can best bear the loss and hence to shift the loss by creating liability where there has been no fault."[8]

The medicolegal problems of ROP have become

more difficult as our knowledge of the subject increases. In the 1950s, a suit might have been successful if the premature infant had received more than 40 percent oxygen in the ambient air; in the ensuing years, the suit might have been successful if a newborn at whatever stage of maturity, including full-term birth, had been given oxygen in amounts greater—or duration longer—than might have been essential for survival. We know now the problem is not that simple.

CONTRIBUTORY CAUSES OF ROP

The etiology of ROP is multifactorial. We know of some contributory causes, but there are unknown or poorly understood causes. As examples: the brain of the tiny premature, approximately 800 grams, is essentially unmyelinated and is easily damaged by short periods of apnea, but an 1,800-gram infant's brain is partially myelinated and not as easily damaged (C. Hoyt, M.D., personal communication).

The small infant with apnea is at great risk. The oxygen level diminishes when the infant stops breathing, then suddenly increases when breathing is resumed. The CO_2 level varies in a similar manner; however, its role is not well understood.

The role of vitamin E is only beginning to be understood.

The oxygen concentration in the retinal tissue is determined by many factors that control the blood supply to the eye. These include the type and amount of hemoglobin present, as well as the effect that CO_2 and pH have upon the oxygen-dissociation curve. Other factors such as prostaglandin synthetase inhibitors can dilate the retinal vasculature.[9] The degree of influence of these is unknown.

In light of the above, it is not surprising that we have no way to establish, with any degree of precision, the duration or concentration of oxygen required so that this might be considered the principal cause of ROP. In some instances, we cannot be certain that oxygen was an important contributory factor. We cannot accurately define the degree of prematurity that makes ROP likely.

Some medicolegal questions remain unanswered. In the past, full-term infants and infants who received no oxygen have been reported to have ROP; in retrospect, these were probably instances of misdiagnosis. How long does oxygen have to be administered for it to be considered the important etiological factor in the development of ROP? What degree of prematurity is needed for us to diagnose ROP, rather than an ophthalmologically identical condition such as familial exudative vitreoretinopathy?

ATTEMPT TO ESTABLISH PROBABLE CAUSE

There is no way to establish the exact duration or concentration of oxygen as causative of ROP, nor can we establish with any certainty the degree of prematurity that makes this disorder likely. In the case of a 1,200- to 1,500-gram infant given oxygen for a few hours or a day or two, I do not know how to determine whether oxygen is the cause or a significant factor in the development of ROP.

Because we do not have definite answers, we must be guided by what is probable—in medicolegal terminology,"probable" is more than 50 percent. It is medically probable that infants who are not definitely premature do not have ROP, but rather a condition that can be ophthalmoscopically identical. It is also probable that oxygen would have to be administered for a significant length of time to be considered the etiology. A medicolegal claim in the name of one who has apparent ROP should only be pursued if there is a history of oxygen having been used, in a significantly premature infant, for periods or in amounts not required.

It is not within the legal definition of "probable" that an infant of 2,000 grams or more would have ROP, nor is it probable that a very short administration of oxygen at birth could be the cause. A 750-gram infant having the fundus picture associated with ROP probably does have ROP. Oxygen administered for several days to an infant of low birth weight is probably important as the cause of the ROP, but the marked prematurity itself might be the principal cause.

GUIDELINES FOR PHYSICIANS

If a premature infant is in the weight group that is more likely to develop ROP, and he was given oxygen, the decision regarding medicolegal culpability rests upon an evaluation of the risk/benefit ratio. We have learned that some require oxygen if an unacceptable risk of respiratory distress syndrome, cerebral palsy, and death is to be avoided. This is in the realm of the neonatologist and pediatrician.

I found no claims in my series based upon failure to perform surgery in an attempt to prevent or to correct retinal detachment, nor upon failure of such therapy when performed. The prognosis for this type of treatment is very guarded; therefore, failure can hardly be a legitimate reason for suit.

The incidence of medicolegal claims can be reduced by the following:

1. Render good pediatric care with careful evaluation of oxygen need and proper monitoring of oxygen, pH, and CO_2.
2. Give full disclosure to the family with an open discussion of risks and alternatives.
3. Complete documentation of the above. Documentation in cases in which there is a high risk of medicolegal claim is best accomplished by the following methods: *a* fully explain the risks, reasons for the risks, and the alternatives; *b* ask for feedback to be certain that this is understood; *c* hand the patient's chart to the parents and have them write on the chart what they do understand; *d* correct any misunderstandings. This is documentation that cannot be denied.

4. Refer the high-risk pregnant mother to a tertiary care center before delivery, or the neonate to such a center if the circumstances permit.

REFERENCES

1. Terry RL. Extreme prematurity and fibroplastic overgrowth of persistent vascular sheath behind each crystalline lens. Am J Ophthalmol 1942; 25:203-204.
2. Campbell K. Intensive oxygen therapy as a possible cause of retrolental fibroplasia. A clinical approach. Med J Aust 1951; 2:48-50.
3. Patz A. Current therapy of retrolental fibroplasia. Ophthalmology 1983; 90:425-427.
4. Phelps DL. Vision loss due to retinopathy of prematurity. Lancet 1981; 1:606.
5. Hittner HM, Rudolph AJ, Kretzer FL. Suppression of severe retinopathy of prematurity with vitamin E supplementation: Ultrastructural mechanism of clinical efficacy. Opthalmology 1984; 91:1512–1523.
6. Criswick VG, Schepens CL. Familial exudative vitreoretinopathy. Am J Ophthalmol 1969; 68:564–578.
7. Ober RR, Bird AC, Hamilton AM, Sehmi K. Autosomal dominant exudative vitreoretinopathy. Br J Ophthalmol 1980; 64:112-120.
8. Helling V. Carey, 83 Wash 2nd 514, 519 P 2nd 981, 1974.
9. Bigland AW, Brown DR, Reynolds JD, Milley JR. Risk factors associated with retrolental fibroplasia. Ophthalmology 1984; 91:1504–1511.

Medicolegal Issues Presented through Retinopathy of Prematurity: The Standard of Care Issue

Jim M. Perdue, J.D.

Significant medicolegal issues are presented through instances of retinopathy of prematurity. The devastating, lifelong effects of this condition often result in serious questions and challenges to the care of the infant, who is enduring a devastating existence of darkness, impairment, and dependence upon others. As has been indicated by other chapters in the work, this condition may be avoided, in some instances, by various regimens of treatment, including prophylaxis (vitamin E) and therapy (cryotherapy). The medical risk versus benefit debate that arises in these cases may ultimately lead to legal claims on behalf of specific patients, which must be resolved by the courts.

Unfortunately, experience has demonstrated that the lack of communication between the legal and medical professions has brought about confusion and misunderstanding between these honored disciplines. Admittedly, these medicolegal issues must be resolved with the benefit of the most recent, objective and accurate medical information available. Likewise, the medical profession has the inherent right to understand by what standard medical decisions will be judged. It may be gainsaid that medical knowledge and scientific information are now advancing at a rate that would have been inconceivable a generation ago; yet the recent advances in the understanding and prevention of retinopathy of prematurity are a classic example that proves this premise.

As the body of scientific knowledge expands exponentially, the medical clinician's crucial decision-making process may become more difficult. Likewise, the resolution of the legal rights of infants who are injured or impaired as a result of these medical decisions becomes more complex. The most common medicolegal questions raised by the medical clinician are:

At what point does a regimen of prophylaxis or therapy become accepted or "standard," such that the physician may be held legally liable, in the form of damages, for the failure to make such standard treatment available to the infant?

To what extent is the physician held responsible for making available to the patient the benefits of new, albeit not established in the traditional sense, medical procedures?

This chapter attempts to address these and the corollary questions that are presented by the recent advances in the treatment and prevention of retinopathy of prematurity. It should be recognized that the law supports no special rules for any given disease entity. To attempt to do so would be to impose an intolerable burden on the courts and juries. Thus, the resolution of the medicolegal issues presented through cases of retinopathy of prematurity must be decided by legal principles and rules that would apply to and govern, with equal effect and vigor, other similar areas of medical practice.

THE STANDARD OF CARE

Expert testimony on the ultimate issue, negligence of the physician, is essential to the successful prosecution of the medical negligence case.[1] Unfortunately, the rules surrounding expert medical testimony are, to a degree, confusing. A physician is held to a standard of good medical practice or to that degree of skill that a reasonable and prudent physician would use. A major consideration in establishing the standard of care to which a physician is held is the degree to which customary practice supercedes good medical practice.

A physician in Texas must use the degree of care and skill that a reasonable and prudent physician would use.[2] Courts, however, have required the reasonable and prudent physician to use only the care and skill practiced within the physician's locality. Texas arguably still follows the "same or similar community" rule.[3]

Whether the locality rule is followed or not, the question of custom is critical. If the standard of care is judged exclusively by usual and standard practice, the custom of the profession either locally, regionally, or nationally becomes conclusive. In effect, the issue of a physician's negligence turns on custom. This result is contrary to well-established principles of tort law, which state that custom is not conclusive on the negligence issue.[4] A standard of care based on customary medical practice is subject to criticism, because customary medical practice is not necessarily synonymous with good medical practice.[5]

Standard Medical Practice

While custom should not be conclusive in determining care, neither should it be essential to a finding of negligence. It merely aids the jury in evaluating the defendant's conduct. As stated by the supreme court: "Evidence as to such customs is not controlling and must not be taken as the legal standard of care and negligence, but is merely evidence to be considered along with other circumstances in determining what the ordinary reasonable man would do under the circumstances."[8] The ultimate inquiry for the jury is whether the defendant failed to act as a reasonably prudent person would.

The rules concerning custom apply beyond individual tortfeasors to cases involving the negligence of businesses and industries.[9] An industry or profession may not establish its own standards of conduct and escape liability by merely showing that it adhered to those standards.[10] If the standard does not meet the ordinary care requirement, the conduct will be found negligent.

Negligence and Custom in Medical Negligence Cases

Custom occupies a much more prestigious position in medical negligence cases than in other tort cases. Traditionally, testimony showing that the defendant deviated from the usual and customary practices of the medical profession establishes negligence in those cases.[11] Although the law establishes the standard of care in all negligence cases, only in medical negligence cases does a particular group's professional standards greatly influence the legal standard.[12]

The law generally holds the physician to the standard of care of a reasonable and prudent physician exercising ordinary care.[13] This standard is consistent with traditional tort principles, which require a person of exceptional skill or knowledge to act as a reasonable and prudent person, possessing the same or similar skill or knowledge, would.[14] Texas has judicially qualified the standard of care applicable in medical cases. The most notable qualification is the so-called locality rule.[15] In *Hood v. Phillips*,[16] however, the Texas Supreme Court recently reaffirmed the reasonable and prudent physician standard and made no mention of the locality rule.[17] It is unclear whether the court inadvertently omitted discussing the locality rule, or whether the court has implicitly abandoned it. Given the wide dissemination of medical information and the fact that there is no assurance that local, customary practice comports with good medical practice,[18] the locality rule should have little, if any, vitality as a rule of law.[19]

THE ADVENT OF "GOOD MEDICAL PRACTICE" AS THE STANDARD OF CARE

Even with the demise of the locality rule in Texas, the continued use of customary practice to show the standard of care tends to inhibit further modernization of the standard, because reliance upon custom may cause courts to ignore suggested, improved medical practice standards. The appropriate standard of care conforms to good medical practice.[20]

Helling v. Carey[21] held that custom was only one factor in determining good, prudent medical care. In 1959, the defendant ophthalmologist prescribed contact lenses for the plaintiff. Complaining of eye irritation, she consulted the ophthalmologist in September, 1963. Throughout the next five years, the ophthalmologist treated her as though her continuing problems related soley to the contact lenses. Finally, in October, 1968, he tested her eye pressure and field of vision for the first time and discovered that she had glaucoma.[22] By that time, the thirty-two-year-old patient had lost all peripheral vision and her central vision was severely reduced.

Ms. Helling instituted a malpractice action against the ophthalmologist, alleging that he was negligent in failing to diagnose and treat the glaucoma before it had seriously impaired her vision. Medical experts for both sides testified at the trial that it was not the customary practice of ophthalmologists to administer pressure tests for glaucoma to patients under forty years of age, because the disease rarely afflicted persons in that age group. Following a jury verdict in his favor, the trial court entered a judgment for the ophthalmologist which the court of appeals affirmed. The Washington Supreme Court reversed, holding that a physician's compliance with the customary practice of his profession does not necessarily insulate him from liability for professional negligence.[23]

Predictably, the medical community and some members of the legal community viewed the *Helling* decision with outrage and indignation.[24] It was declared, apocryphally so, that the decision represented a revolutionary break with precedent. In truth, the courts of this country had begun many years earlier to mitigate or abolish this anachronism of tort law.[25]

Commentators have indicated that good medical practice is nothing more or less than what is customary or usual in the profession.[26] Some have suggested that reliance on medical custom gives the medical profession, and arguably other health care providers, the privilege, usually emphatically denied to others, of setting their own standards through the practices they adopt.[27] While this appears to be the majority rule,[28] courts have been willing to seriously limit the rule[29] or abolish it altogether.[30]

At one time, courts held that if *any* testifying doctor approved the defendant's care, there could be no malpractice.[31] Now it is argued that the profession must be permitted to set its own standards,[32] lest the standards of medical practice be established by unknowledgeable juries and courts.[33] Some assert, however, that courts and juries are indeed capable of reviewing complex medical facts and determining whether the defendant followed good practice.[34] More significantly, some courts express concern at the inequities that would result if doctors could set their own standards of practice with impunity.[35] And allowing custom as *inconclusive* evidence of the standard of care provides obvious advantages: (1) it is consistent with general tort law; (2) it prevents any group, by way of the same school or locality rules, from establishing substandard practices as the norm; and (3) it simplifies analyzing the form of expert testimony.

In recent years, the Texas Supreme Court has been cautious in describing a physician's standard of care. For example, in 1965, Justice Smith dissented in *Hart v. Van Zandt*,[36] stating: "Evidence of what is usually or customarily done is not expert evidence of what should have been done by the Defendant."[37] In the 1969 opinion of *Snow v. Bond*,[38] the court, while speaking of the "reasonable and prudent" physician and the "standards of practice," rejected testimony of what a hypothetical physician "similarly situated" might do.[39] In 1980, the supreme court held that expert testimony that established that particular medical conduct would be "bad" was sufficient to establish the requisite standard of medical care by which conduct could be judged.[40] Custom was not discussed.

A 1977 Texas Supreme Court case seems to foreclose the use of custom to control medical practice standards. *Hood v Phillips*[41] involved the standard of care applied in a negligence case. After discussing the various standards of care, the supreme court, relying upon *Snow v. Bond*,[42] stated the Texas rule as follows: "A physician who undertakes a mode or form of treatment which a reasonable or prudent member of the medical profession would undertake under the same or similar circumstances shall not be subject to liability for harm caused thereby to the patients."[43]

While the reasonable-and-prudent-physician rule was nothing new to Texas, the decision is intriguing because of the negligence standards it rejected. First, the court rejected the "respectable minority" standard that had been adopted by the Court of Civil Appeals.[44] Such a standard holds that a physician will not be held liable if the method of treatment employed is supported by a "reasonable minority" or a "considerable number" of the physician's professional peers.[45] The supreme court rejected that standard, because it "could convey to a jury the incorrect notion that the standard for malpractice is to be determined by a poll of the medical profession."[46] Second, the court also rejected the "any variance" standard, which renders a physician liable if the physician deviates from the particular mode of treatment upheld by a consensus of medical professionals.[47] The major problem with this standard is that it precludes a physician from exercising professional judgment or from conducting experiments that could benefit mankind.[48]

The vice common to each of these unacceptable standards is that each centers around what a given number of physicians advocate as proper care. The rejected standards focus on what is "a respectable minority," "a consensus of opinion," and "a considerable number" of physicians, rather than on what is good medical practice. Indeed, the *Hood* court expressly endeavored to prevent the standard of care from being determined by a poll of the medical community. Thus, the defendant cannot escape liability by merely following the standard of practice advocated by a given number of physicians. The court expressly favored a standard based on reasonable and prudent conduct or good medical practice over a standard based on practice customary to a certain number of physicians within a certain locality.[49]

The relevant issue, then, is what the reasonable and prudent physician would do, in keeping with standards of good medical practice. If the ultimate issue is indeed what is customary or standard medical practice, then a witness, to be qualified, must be knowledgeable and conversant with what is ordinarily done in the community[50] or the profession generally.[51] The witness's testimony, likewise, must address what constitutes "standard" or "customary" practice. If, on the other hand, the standard by which medical conduct is to be measured is that of "good," "prudent," "acceptable," or "safe" medical practice, then the witness is qualified to express an opinion when, by virtue of training, education, and experience, the witness is shown to be conversant with those principles.[52] Hence, the standard of care would be established by showing: 1) that the witness is familiar with good and accepted medical practices; and, 2) that after review of the medical records, good medical practice under those circumstances would require specific actions by the physician.

Having identified the ultimate issue and the direction of the witness's testimony, the court and jury are better equipped to perform their functions. Specifically, the trial court can better analyze those matters that may be used to buttress or attack an expert witness's opinions. When the witness is said to be testifying as to what constitutes "good" rather than "customary" practice, the following would be appropriate areas for direct or cross examination: 1) what medical texts say;[53] 2) what medical schools teach;[54] 3) what other physicians do in their practices;[55] 4) what various medical organizations or boards recommend; 5) what the witness recommends;[56] and 6) what the witness does in the witness's own practice.[57]

CONCLUSION

It is to be hoped that the foregoing analysis would lead the medical practitioner to conclude that the courts are struggling with the compromising of competing interests. These competing interests should be familiar to the clinician. On the one hand, the law does not want to impose legal liability on the physician for medical actions in circumstances whereby it would have been unreasonable to exact a specified medical performance. On the other hand, the formulation of a medical standard of care requires that physicians be given latitude, such that scientific advancement is not discouraged or penalized. Hence, the question of "good" medical practice becomes a jury determination that must be made with the assistance of the most qualified expert guidance. The traditional medical concept of risk versus benefits becomes the cornerstone of legal analysis.

In determining the issue of whether the defendant-physician violated the standards of good medical practice in his care of an infant, the jury would have to weigh the risks presented by the treatment involved with the relative benefits that might be gained. Such an analysis would apply whether the issue was one of omission, failure to provide specified treatment, or commission, providing allegedly improper care. The determination or weighing of a procedure's risks would involve the consideration of such matters as whether the hazards were known, predictable, or had been established statistically by empirical or heuristic evidence. Likewise, the relative benefit that may be inherent or presented by any procedure must be weighed and considered. To the same effect, the gravity of the risk or hazard must be weighed against the significance of the benefit that may be achieved. This is the essential lesson of *Helling v. Carey*.[58]Such considerations would determine the issue of good medical practice in the prevention of retinopathy of prematurity. The legal liability of physicians, hospitals, and the manufacturers of drugs and appliances involved in the treatment of infants would, for the most part, be determined through these principles.[59]

The implications of such a rule for dealing with legal cases involving retinopathy of prematurity should be pellucid. If qualified medical experts are willing to present the necessary scientific knowledge, a medical standard may be established to the law's satisfaction. In the area of retinopathy of prematurity, this could involve claims for damages arising from improper oxygen therapy;[60] withholding vitamin E prophylaxis; for death or hepatic failure as a result of using vitamin E not FDA approved; for late retinal screening, such that cryotherapy could not be properly applied; and for withholding cryotherapy. Whether liability should be imposed under the specific circumstances in any given case remains a question that only the chosen jury will resolve. Certainly it is the hope and desire of physicians and lawyers alike that these decisions will be as well-informed as possible and made on adequate and complete scientific information.

REFERENCES

For those unfamiliar with legal citation, the following footnote authorities are cited in the standard form. *Brown v. Jones* (this is known as the "style" of the case. The first name "Brown" is the last name of the appealing party. "v." is an abbreviation for versus or against. "Jones" is the last name of the appellee or party against whom the appeal was taken.) 517 S.W.2d 132 (this is what is called the "citation". The first number represents the volume of the legal reporter. The middle initials represent the particular legal reporter - for example S.W.2d would be the second edition of the Southwestern Reporter. The third number represents the page of that reporter on which the opinion begins. References to additional pages may direct the reader to a specific portion of the opinion.) "Tex. 1983" (this indicates the court which authored the opinion and the date of the opinion. For example, in the citation given, the opinion cited was written by the Supreme Court of Texas in 1983.)"

1. Bowles v. Bourdon, 148 Tex. 1, 5, 219 S.W.2d 779, 782 (1949). See generally 70 C.J.S. Physicians & surgeons §62(2), at 1006 (1951).
2. King v. Flamm, 442 S.W.2d 679, 681 (Tex. 1969); Snow v. Bond, 438 S.W.2d 549, 550-51 (Tex. 1969). See also Hood v. Phillips, 554 S.W.2d 160, 165 (Tex. 1977).
3. Wilson v. Scott, 412 S.W.2d 299, 302 (Tex. 1967). See generally Annot., 99 A.L.R.3rd 1133, 1176-77 (1980). Recent decisions, however, have spoken in terms of the locality rule being "discretionary" with the trial court. See Webb v. Jorns, 488 S.W.2d 407, 411 (Tex. 1972) (limited in application to certain kinds of cases); Johnson v. Hermann Hospital, 659 S.W.2d 124, 126 (Tex. App.-Houston [14th Dist.] 1983, writ ref'd n.r.e.); Dupree v. Palmarozzi, 596 S.W.2d 544, 547 (Tex. Civ. App.-Beaumont 1980, no writ).
4. See Williams, Abandoning medical malpractice, 5 J. Legal Med. 549, 570 (1985), in which the author argues that resort to custom tends to set professional standards too low.
5. See Keeton, Medical negligence—the standard of care, 10 TEX. TECH. L. REV. 351, 353 (1979).
6. 61 Tex. 3, 6 (1884).
7. See, e.g., Leadon v. Kimbrough Bros. Lumber Co., 484 S.W.2d 567, 569 (Tex. 1972); Stanley v. Southern Pac. Co., 466 S.W.2d 548, 551 (Tex. 1971); Brown v. Lundell, 162 Tex. 84, 88-89, 344 S.W.2d 863, 867-68 (1961); Horrea v. Coca Cola Bottling Co., 143 Tex. 272, 278, 183 S.W.2d 968, 971 (1944). The source of the rule in most jurisdictions is the legendary case, the T.J. Hooper, 60 F.2d 737, 740 (2nd Cir.), *cert. denied*, 287 U.S. 662 (1932).
8. Stanley v. Southern Pac. Co., 466 S.W.2d 548, 551 (Tex. 1971).
9. See Texaco, Inc. v. Joffrion, 363 S.W.2d 827, 831-32 (Tex. Civ App.-Texarkana 1962, writ ref'd n.r.e.); Kuemmel v. Vradenberg, 239 S.W.2d 869, 872 (Tex. Civ. App.-San Antonio 1951, writ ref'd n.r.e.).
10. These principles are best exemplified in the classic case of The T.J. Hooper, 60 F.2d 737 (2nd Cir.), *cert. denied*, 287 U.S. 662 (1932). In T.J. *Hooper*, the industry's practice of not having radios on its tugboats was held insufficient to preclude a finding of negligence. *Id.* at 740. See also South Austin Drive-In Theatre v. Thomison, 421 S.W.2d 933, 951 (Tex. Civ. App.-Austin 1967, writ ref'd n.r.e.), for the Texas version. See generally, W. Prosser & W. Keeton, Prosser and Keeton on the law of torts §33 at 194 (5th ed. 1984).
11. See, e.g., Simpson v. Gleen, 537 S.W.2d 114, 117 (Tex. Civ. App.-Amarillo 1976, writ ref'd n.r.e.); Christian v. Jeter, 445 S.W.2d 51, 54 (Tex. Civ. App.-Waco 1969, writ ref'd n.r.e.). See generally, W. Prosser & W. Keeton, *supra* note 163, §32 at 188-89; T. Regan, Doctor and patient and the law, at 30 (3rd. ed. 1956).
12. Such a result has been the subject of criticism. See James & Sigerson, Particularizing standards of conduct in negligence trials, 5 VAN. L. REV. 697, 710 (1952); Morris, Custom and negligence, 42 COLUM. L. REV. 1147, 1163 (1942).
13. King v. Flamm, 442 S.W.2d 679, 681 (Tex. 1969); Snow v. Bond, 438 S.W.2d 549, 550-51 (Tex. 1969). See also Speer v. United States, 512 F. Supp. 670, 675 (N.D. Tex. 1981); Hood v. Phillips, 554 S.W.2d 160, 165 (Tex. 1977).
14. W. Prosser & W. Keeton, *supra* note 10, §32 at 185.
15. See, Wilson v. Scott, 412 S.W.2d 299, 301 (Tex. 1967); Smith v. Guthrie, 557 S.W.2d 163, 167 (Tex. Civ. App.-Fort Worth 1977, writ ref'd n.r.e.); Burks v. Meredith, 546 S.W.2d 366, 370 (Tex. Civ. App. - Waco 1976, writ ref'd n.r.e.). The locality rule seems to have had its genesis in the century-old Kansas case, Tefft v. Wilcox, 6 Kan. 33, 42-43 (1870), which set forth the proposition that a physician could be held only to that degree of care ordinarily possessed by other physicians in the community, locality, or neighborhood. The rationale behind the rule reflected the obvious differences at that time between physicians practicing in more remote areas and those practicing in large metropolitan areas. This requirement necessarily led to two harsh results. First, the plaintiff was often unable to find such a witness, or one willing to testify, due to the "conspiracy of silence" among local practitioners. See Note, *Michigan abandons "locality rule" with regard to specialists*, 40 FORDHAM L. REV. 435, 438 (1971). The second potential result was the possibility that a small group of local doctors would establish an unsatisfactory local standard of care. See Comment, *Standard of care for medical practitioners—abandonment of the locality rule*, 60 KY. L.J. 209, 210 (1971). Thus, the "same locality" rule was superseded by the "similar locality" rule, which although it eliminated some of the practical difficulties inherent in the former rule, inevitably led to the problem of determining what constituted "similarity." *Id.* at 212. The locality rule became further liberalized as its original rationale ceased to exist. In recognition of changes in population distribution, improved medical technology, better transportation and communication, and increased standardization of medical practice through specialization, many courts gradually abandoned this rule, instead adopting locality as only one factor to be considered in determining the standard of care. See, e.g., Hodgson v. Bigelow, 335 Pa. 497, 7 A.2d 338 (1939); Viita v. Dolan, 132 Minn. 128, 155 N.S. 1077 (1916). See generally Note, *supra* at 439; Note, *Willingness to abrogate the locality rule in medical malpractice suits indicated*, 43 MISS. L.J. 587, 589 (1972). Accordingly, the Washington Supreme Court rejected the "same or similar locality" rule in Pederson v. Dumouchel, 72 Wash. 2d 73, 431 P.2d 973 (1967), noting that the "locality rule" has no present-day value, except as one element to be considered in determining the requisite degree of care and skills. See Note, *Expanded standards of care for Washington physicians, dentists and hospitals—Pederson v. Dumouchel*, 44 WASH. L. REV. 505 (1969). In particular, a number of courts have specifically rejected the locality standard for specialists. Thus, the Washington Supreme Court adhered to the *Pederson* standard in Douglas v. Bussabarger, 73 Wash.2d 476, 438 P.2d 829 (1968) (en banc), recognizing the uniformity of practice that exists throughout the nation today for specialists. For a case demonstrating the harshness of the locality rule see Henderson v. Heyer-Schulte Corp., 600 S.W.2d 844, 848 (Tex. Civ. App. - Houston [1st Dist.] 1980, no writ), where an expert described by the court as "highly qualified" was held not qualified to testify and his testimony insufficient on the issue of standard of care, since he could not state that the technique employed by the defendant-plastic surgeon was "nonstandard" for Houston at the time in question. This was the result, even though the witness taught his students not to employ the technique and knew of no surgeons in his area who did. For a discussion of the locality rule, see generally 61 Am. Jr. 2d Physicians, surgeons and other healers §218 (1981); Annot., 99 A.L.R.3d 1133, 1176–77 (1980).
16. 554 S.W.2d 160 (Tex. 1977).
17. *Id.* at 165.
18. See Jeffcoat v. Phillips, 534 S.W.2d 168, 174 (Tex. Civ. App. - Houston [14th Dist.] 1976, writ ref'd n.r.e.) (error to refuse to admit out-of-town physician's testimony as to standard of care.

19. See Christian v. Jeter, 445 S.W.2d 51, 54 (Tex. Civ. App. - Waco 1969, writ ref'd n.r.e.). But see Henderson v. Heyer-Schulte Corp., 600 S.W.2d 844, 847 (Tex. Civ. App. - Houston [1st Dist.] 1980, writ ref'd n.r.e.).

20. The Texas Supreme Court has rejected a standard of care based on a "poll" of what a certain number of physicians do. Hood v. Phillips, 554 S.W.2d 160, 165 (Tex. 1977).

21. 83 Wash.2d 514, 519 P.2d 981 (1974).

22. The defendant-ophthalmologist testified that while the incidence of glaucoma among persons over forty years of age is between two and three percent, it is only .0004 percent among persons under forty. Expert testimony also established that the standard of the ophthalmology profession required an ophthalmologist to give the glaucoma pressure test to any patient whose complaints and symptoms indicated that glaucoma should be suspected. This standard, however, did not afford much protection to the patient under forty years of age. Because the development of glaucoma is accompanied by few noticeable symptoms, the patient is unlikely to complain until his vision has become seriously impaired. Id. at 516-18, 519 P.2d at 982-83.

23. Id. at 519, 519 P.2d at 983.

24. See, e.g., Note, Torts—negligence—physicians and surgeons—a physician's compliance with customary practice does not necessarily insulate him from liability for malpractice, 44 CIN. L. REV. 361, 365-66 (1975) [hereinafter cited as Note, Customary Practice]; Note, Physicians and surgeons—standard of care—medical specialists may be found negligent as a matter of law despite compliance with the customary practice of the specialty, 28 VAND. L. REV. 441, 448-53 (1975).

25. Canterbury v. Spence, 464 F.2d 772, 783 (D.C. Cir. 1972); Sinz v. Owens, 33 Cal.2d 749, 753-54, 205 P.2d 3, 8 (1949); Darling v. Charleston Community Memorial Hosp., 33 Ill.2d 326, 331, 211 N.E.2d 253, 257, aff'd 50 Ill. App.2d 253, 200 N.E.2d 149 (1964), cert. denied, 383 U.S. 946 (1966); Lundahl v. Rockford Memorial Hosp. Ass'n., 93 Ill. App.2d 461, 465, 235 N.E.2d 671, 674 (1968); Viita v. Dolan, 132 Minn. 128, 133, 155 N.W. 1077, 1081 (1916); Tvedt v. Haugen, 70 N.D. 338, 349, 294 N.W. 183, 187 (1940); Morgan v. Sheppard, 188 N.E.2d 808, 816 (Ohio Ct. App. 1963); Incollingo v. Ewing, 444 Pa. 263, 283, 282 A.2d 206, 215 (1971); Hodgson v. Bigelow, 335 Pa. 497, 518, 7 A.2d 338, 348 (1939); Davis v. Kerr, 239 Pa. 351, 355, 86 A. 1007, 1009 (1913).

26. W. Prosser & W. Keeton, supra note 10, §32 at 165.

27. James, Particularizing the standards of conduct in negligence trials, 5 VAND. L. REV. 697, 710 (1952); Morris, Custom and negligence, 42 COLUM. L. REV. 1147, 1149 (1942).

28. Boyce v. Brown, 51 Ariz. 416, 420-21, 77 P.2d 455, 457 (1938); Marchlewski v. Casella, 141 Conn. 377, 380-81, 106 A.2d 466, 467 (1954); Kortus v. Jensen, 195 Neb. 261, 268, 237 N.W.2d 845, 850 (1976); Toth v. Community Hosp., 22 N.Y.2d 255, 262, 239 N.E.2d 368, 372, 292 N.Y.S.2d 440, 447 (1968); Gresham v. Ford, 192 Tenn. 310, 315, 241 S.W.2d 408, 410 (1951); Domina v. Pratt, 111 Vt. 166, 170, 13 A.2d 198, 200 (1940); I. Louisell & H. Williams, Medical malpractice, §8.04 at 200 (1973).

29. Louisiana seems to base its decision on the type of case involved. Guilbeau v. St. Pau Fire & Marine Ins. Co., 325 So.2d 395, 398 (La. Ct. App. 1975), cert. denied 329 So.2d 454 (1976) (physician's compliance with community standard by relying on nurse's count of laparotomy pads will not exonerate); Favalora v. Aetna Cas. & Sur. Co., 144 So.2d 544 (La. Ct. App. 1962) (failure of radiologist to obtain medical history). Other jursidictions hold that the rule requiring the physician to possess and employ only the skill and knowledge ordinarily possessed by physicians is generally subject to the limitations that: (1) due regard be given to the advanced state of the profession at the time of treatment, and (2) the physician is required to exercise the care and judgement of a reasonable person. See Incollingo v. Ewing, 444 Pa. 263, 283, 282 A.2d 206, 213 (1971). See also Moeller v. Hauser, 237 Minn. 368, 375-76, 54 N.W.2d 639, 647-48 (1952).

30. See Keogan v. Holy Family Hosp., 95 Wash.2d 306, 321, 622, P.2d 1246, 1259 (1980).

31. But see Hewitt v. Eisenbart, 36 Neb. 794, 797-98, 55 N.W. 252, 254 (1893) (jury alone may determine the issue of negligence where there is conflicting expert testimony).

32. W. Prosser & W. Keeton, supra note 10, §32 at 165.

33. Id.

34. Morgan v. Sheppard, 188 N.E.2d 808 (Ohio Ct. App. 1963); Note, Customary practice, supra note 24 at 363. Moreover, juries have long been trusted to decide litigation involving complex and technical matter.

35. Incollingo, 444 Pa. at 284, 282 A.2d at 217; Hodgson, 335 Pa. at 505-06, 7 A.2d at 348 Morgan, 188 N.E.2d at 816-17. Moreover, the standard must be that of good medical practice. If the standard of care was that of "average" skill, badly skilled doctors would by definition have to be included; thus, the standard would be too low.

36. 399 S.W.2d 791 (Tex. 1965).

37. Id. at 798 (Smith, J., dissenting). Presumably, such testimony would not be conclusive but would be evidentiary only.

38. 438 S.W.2d 549 (Tex. 1969).

39. Id. at 550.

40. Williams v. Bennett, 610 S.W.2d 144, 146 (Tex. 1980). The issues submitted and approved by the court, while embodying elements of the "locality" rule, nevertheless used as the standard of care that practice that would be employed by a "reasonably prudent physician." Id.

41. 554 S.W.2d 160 (Tex. 1977).

42. 438 S.W.2d 549 (Tex. 1969).

43. 554 S.W.2d at 165.

44. Id. at 164.

45. Hood v. Phillips, 537 S.W.2d 291, 294 (Tex. Civ. App. - Beaumont 1976), aff'd 554 S.W.2d 160 (Tex. 1977).

46. 554 S.W.2d at 165.

47. Id. But see Jackson v. Burnham, 20 Colo. 532, 39 P. 577 (1895) (surgeons must conform to established modes of treatment); Allen v. Voje, 114 Wis. 1, 89 N.W. 924 (1902).

48. 554 S.W.2d at 165.

49. The question of the role of "custom" was recently addressed in Golden Villa Nursing Home, Inc. v. Smith, 675 S.W.2d 343 (Tex. App. - Houston [14th Dist.] 1984, writ ref'd n.r.e.). This case dealt with the negligence of a nursing home that failed to supervise a patient, resulting in his wandering onto the road, injuring himself and the operator of a motorcycle. Suit was brought against the nursing home by both the patient and the cyclist. The plaintiffs contended that the nursing home was negligent in its failure to supervise and control the patient. The trial court rendered judgment for the plaintiffs on the basis of the jury findings. On appeal, the nursing home argued that the care it gave to the patient constituted the same degree of care, skill, and diligence exercised by such homes of the same general type in the same or similar community, and this fact precluded a finding of negligence. The appellate court rejected this contention, holding that while conformity with uniform customs may be considered evidence of proper care, it does not preclude a showing that the custom itself tolerates negligence. In so holding, the court relied upon Air Control Eng'g, Inc., v. Hogan, 477 S.W.2d 941, 946 (Tex. Civ. App. - Dallas 1972, no writ). Other states were declared to have applied this principle to nursing home situations. See, e.g., Stogsdill v. Manor Convalescence Home, Inc., 35 Ill. App.3d 634, 343 N.E.2d 589 (1976).

50. If the "locality" rule is applied.

51. If a "national" rule is applied.

52. But cf. Hood v. Phillips, 554 S.W.2d 160, 168 (Tex. 1977) (Texas Supreme Court did not require exclusion of testimony "that carotid surgery was similar to the removal of a valve from an automobile tire." The court ruled that the testimony was material and relevant to the issue of informed consent. Id.).

53. Questions regarding the standard by which conduct is measured and the role of the expert have ramifications throughout the trial of a malpractice case. For example, medical treatises may be used on direct or cross-examination. Tex. R. Evid. 803(18). If the measuring rule is custom and the witness is only expressing his opinion as to what is "standard" medical practice, then could it not be said that only passages of books

and treatises that tend to support and prove such proposition are relevant? If, on the other hand, the standard of measuring conduct is that of "good" medical care, and the witness is expressing his opinion on this issue, then any statements that tend to support or discredit this proposition would seem material.

54. If the measure of conduct is what is "customary" or "standard," then the teachings of medical schools become irrelevant, unless it can be shown that this bears on what practice was "standard" in the appropriate locality or professional area. Under this test, what is taught at other medical schools also becomes irrelevant. Henderson v. Heyer-Schulte Corp., 600 S.W.2d 844, 848 (Tex. Civ. App. - Houston [1st Dist.] 1980, no writ).

55. Under the "customary" or "standard" rule of care, this becomes critical evidence, and the witness is actually giving an opinion as to what the majority of physicians in a professional community do. If "good" medical practice is the measuring rule, then what other physicians do is relevant, but only evidentiary.

56. While such evidence may not be admissible on direct examination, it may well be appropriate during cross-examination. See, e.g., Bellaire Gen. Hosp. v. Campbell, 510 S.W.2d 94, 98 (Tex. Civ. App. - Houston [14th Dist.] 1974, writ ref'd n.r.e.).

57. *Id.*

58. *Supra* Note 21.

59. The liability of a manufacturer of drugs or medical appliances or equipment may be decided on strict tort liability theories. Airshields, Inc. v. Spears, 590 S.W.2d 574 (Tex. Civ. App. - Waco 1979, writ ref'd n.r.e.).

60. *Id.*

Frank L. Kretzer, Ph.D.
Rekha S. Mehta, B.S.
Donna Goad, M.D.
Helen M. Hittner, M.D.

Whole-eye donations from preterm infants at high risk for the development of retinopathy of prematurity (ROP) are rare and are becoming even more so owing to an increase in their survival rate (infants 750 to 1,000 grams birth weight have a survival rate <75%). Therefore, to probe the pathogenesis of ROP, and to test the possible treatments for ROP, it is desirable to identify animal models whose retinal development completely parallels that of the human retina both morphologically and ontogenetically. Only then can the following concepts be studied under rigorous experimental conditions: vaso-obliteration and endothelial necrosis;[1,2] endothelial proliferation in hyperoxic environments;[3,4] decreased proliferation by slow weaning from oxygen;[5] spindle cell migration through the nerve fiber layer;[6,7] spindle cell induction of ROP;[8,9] prostaglandin enhancement of neovascularization;[10] therapeutic levels of vitamin E to halt vitreal neovascularization;[11,12] cryotherapy to induce regression of neovascularization;[13-17] special stains to document angioblast precursors;[18] and the nature of shunt formation.[19]

METHODS

All animal eyes reported in this chapter were enucleated following ether and Nembutal anesthesia as per the Association for Research in Vision and Ophthalmology Resolution on the Use of Animals in whole globes in a mixture of 2 percent glutaraldehyde and 2 percent paraformaldehyde in cold phosphate buffer (0.135M, pH 7.4) for 1 hour. The globes were then dissected across the pars plana. The posterior hemispheres were fixed in cold, phosphate-buffered 2 percent glutaraldehyde for 12 hours. After a phosphate buffer rinse, a continuous calotte of tissue was isolated in the horizontal meridian from the optic disc to the ora serrata. This calotte was dissected into three equal pieces. The three pieces were fixed in 1 percent osmium tetroxide for 1 hour, washed overnight in phosphate buffer, dehydrated along an acetone gradient (30%, 50%, 70%, 95%, and 100% × 2) at 20 minute intervals, infiltrated overnight with 1:1 acetone:Araldite-Embed, infiltrated 2 hours in 1:4 acetone:Araldite-Embed, embedded in pure Araldite-Embed, and polymerized at 60°C for 24 hours.

Light microscopy involved 0.5-μm-thick sections that were stained with toluidine blue. Continuous montages were constructed from the optic disc to the ora serrata. The developmental stages of the photoreceptors as perceived by light microscopy were confirmed by transmission electron microscopy of thin sections cut from identical regions that were section stained, carbon coated, and examined on a Japan Electron Optics Laboratory 100 CX. Stage I, II, III, and IV photoreceptors were defined by Johnson et al[20,21] and are shown in Chapter 4 (Figs. 4-1, 4-2, 4-3, 4-4, and 4-5) Stage I photoreceptors have nascent inner segments that protrude a short distance beyond the outer limiting membrane. They contain randomly scattered mitochondria, but there is no evidence of outer segment differentiation. Stage II photoreceptors have inner segments that protrude beyond the outer limiting membrane. These inner segments contain some aggregated mitochondria apically and some endoplasmic reticulum supranuclearly. Randomly oriented tubular-membrane profiles are present within the cytoplasm of the balloon-shaped outer segment. Stage III photoreceptors have well formed inner segments bulginig beyond the outer limiting membrane. The inner segments contain densely packed mitochondria. The short outer segments consist of stacked membrane profiles arranged randomly within the cytoplasm. Stage IV photoreceptors have inner segments with a dense mitochondrial ellipsoid. The outer segments contain uniformly stacked disc membranes arranged such that the discs are perpendicular to the long axis of the outer segment.

All segmental montages in this chapter contain six light micrographs taken at the following percentage distance of the total distance from the optic disc to the ora serrata: edge of optic disc and 20 percent of the total distance from the optic disc to the ora serrata, most central piece of calotte; 40 percent and 60 percent, middle piece of calotte; and 80 percent and ora serrata, most peripheral piece of calotte.

DEVELOPMENT OF THE HUMAN RETINA AT 27-WEEKS GESTATIONAL AGE

Figure 8-1 shows the segmental retinal montage from an infant of 27-weeks gestational age, 910 grams birth weight, who survived for 2 hours. The eyes were enucleated and fixed 2 hours post mortem. This montage is characteristic of the most mature retina of infants who are currently at highest risk of developing severe ROP despite continuous vitamin E supplementation from the first hours of life.[22]

Stage IV photoreceptors are restricted to areas adjacent to the optic disc (Fig. 8-1A), Stage III photoreceptors extend radially about 30 percent of the distance from the optic disc to the ora serrata (Fig. 8-1B), and Stage II photoreceptors extend about 20 percent further (Fig. 8-1C). However, 50 percent of the peripheral retina has only Stage I photoreceptors (Figs. 8-1D to 8-1F). Inner retinal vessels are transretinal to Stage III photoreceptors (Fig. 8-1B), tiny inner retinal capillaries interspersed between spindle cells are transretinal to Stage II photoreceptors (Fig. 8-1D). The anterior edge of the migrating apron of spindle cells is transretinal to Stage I photoreceptors (Fig. 8-1D). The anterior edge of the migrating spindle cell apron follows the maturation of the outer plexiform layer[23] (Fig. 8-1D). The vasoformative process of inner retinal vessels occurs by canalization of spindle cells in which solid cords become luminized by the metamorphosis of spindle cells into en-

dothelium.[8,9] Anterior to the peripheral edge of the migrating spindle cell apron, empty cystoid spaces are present within a retina that is still undergoing stratification into the inner and outer nuclear layers (Fig. 8-1E).

In the preterm infant, it has been demonstrated that secretion of interstitial retinol binding protein (IRBP) by photoreceptors is initiated concomitantly with the formation of tubular outer segment discs at Stage II.[20,21] Thus, IRBP within the subretinal space would extend approximately 50 percent of the distance from the optic disc to the ora serrata (Chapter 4, Table 4-8). Since spindle cells are far removed from inner retinal capillaries, only minimal amounts of vitamin E can reach the peripheral spindle cells from these centrally located vessels. In these preterm infants, vitamin E carrier proteins (IRBP) in the hydrophilic subretinal space must play a critical role in the delivery of vitamin E to Müller cells and ultimately to the inner retina. The transretinal Müller cells are assumed to be the most likely critical link between vitamin E carried across the subretinal space by IRBP and spindle cells in the nerve fiber layer. Vitamin E uptake into peripheral retinal membranes is therefore dependent upon retinal maturation (photoreceptor development to Stage II and secretion of IRBP).

Therefore, in the developing retina of the preterm infant less than or equal to 27-weeks gestational age, the following six morphologic relationships are apparent:

1. Cystoid spaces provide the scaffolding through which spindle cells migrate and vessels form.
2. Spindle cells canalize to form inner retinal vessels and migrate peripherally as the outer plexiform layer matures.
3. Spindle cells are predominantly transretinal to Stage I photoreceptors.
4. IRBP secretion parallels Stage II photoreceptor maturation.
5. Innter retinal vessels are transretinal to Stage III and IV photoreceptors.
6. Photoreceptor maturation to Stages III and IV is restricted to the posterior retina.

DEVELOPMENT OF THE PRETERM BABOON RETINA

Figure 8-2 shows the segmental retinal montage from a male baboon of 141-days gestation (term 184 days), 640 grams birth weight, who died at 64 hours of age, while on continuous oxygen administration. At birth, this baboon corresponded chronologically to an

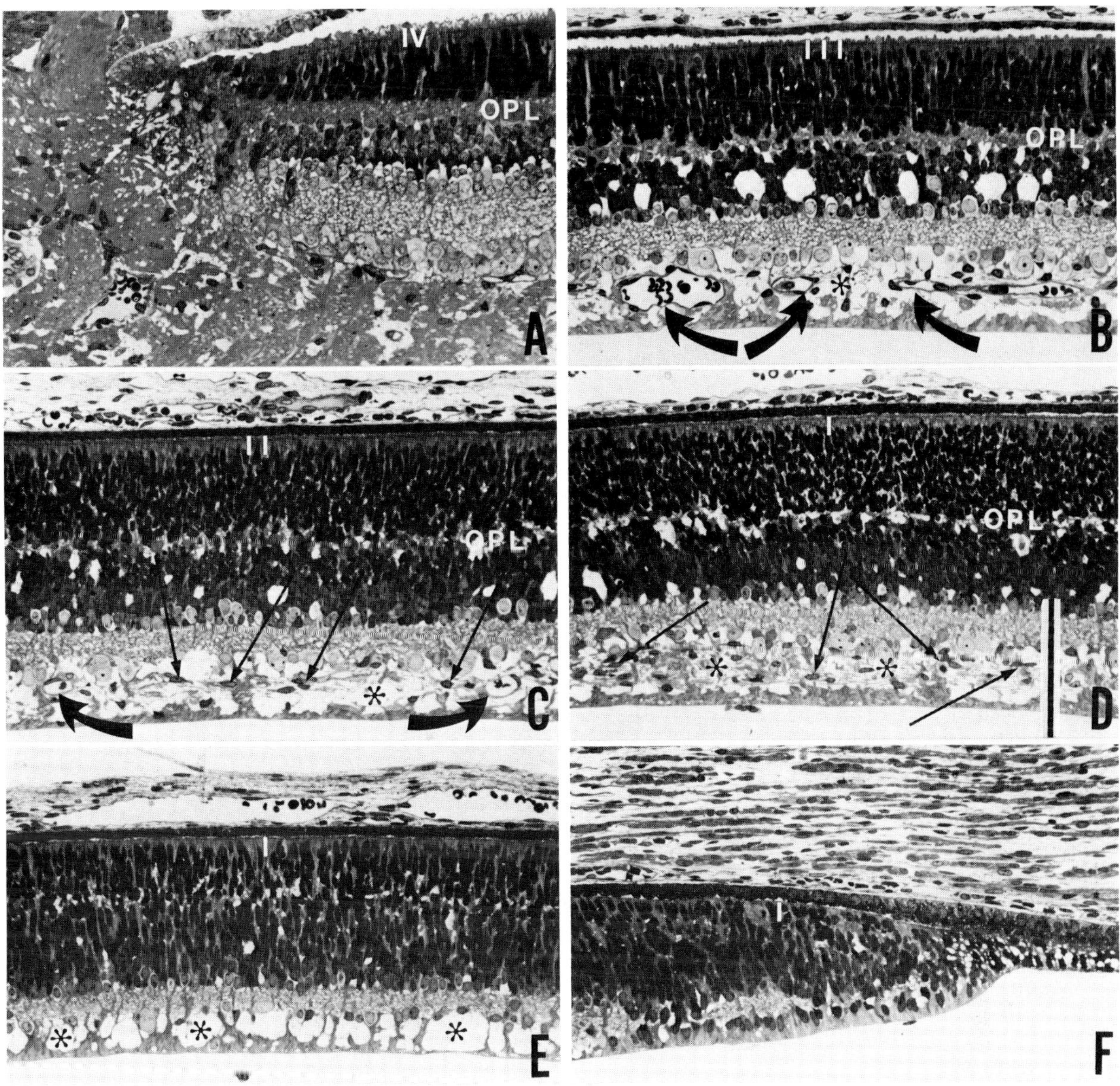

Figure 8-1 Segmental montage of light micrographs (200×) of the retina of a preterm infant of 27-weeks gestational age, 910-grams birth weight, who survived for 2 hours. A, optic disc; B, 20% of the distance from the optic disc to the ora serrata; C, 40% of the distance from the optic disc to the ora serrata; D, 60% of the distance from the optic disc to the ora serrata; E, 80% of the distance from the optic disc to the ora serrata; F, ora serrata. Roman numerals indicate the stage of photoreceptor maturation. (OPL), outer plexiform layer; (*), cystoid spaces; ( ), inner retinal vessels and capillaries; ( ), spindle cells; vertical line in D, anterior edge of migrating spindle cell apron.

infant of 27-weeks gestational age. The baboon eyes, which were enucleated and fixed immediately upon death, were provided by Dr. Rama Bhat, Department of Pediatrics at the University of Illinois College of Medicine at Chicago.

Stage IV photoreceptors extend at least 60 percent of the distance from the optic disc to the ora serrata (Figs. 8-2A to 8-2D), Stage III photoreceptors extend another 20 percent (Fig. 8-2E), and Stage II photorecep-

tors reach the ora serrata (Fig. 8-2F). The nerve fiber layer is compact with no cystoid spaces. Large inner retinal vessels (Figs. 8-2C, 8-2D) and an inner retinal capillary bed (Fig. 8-2E) extend to nearly 80 percent of the distance from the optic disc to the ora serrata. There are no spindle cells among forming capillaries (Fig. 8-2E) nor within the nerve fiber layer adjacent to the ora serrata (Fig. 8-2F). Also, there is no endothelial budding throughout the nerve fiber layer.

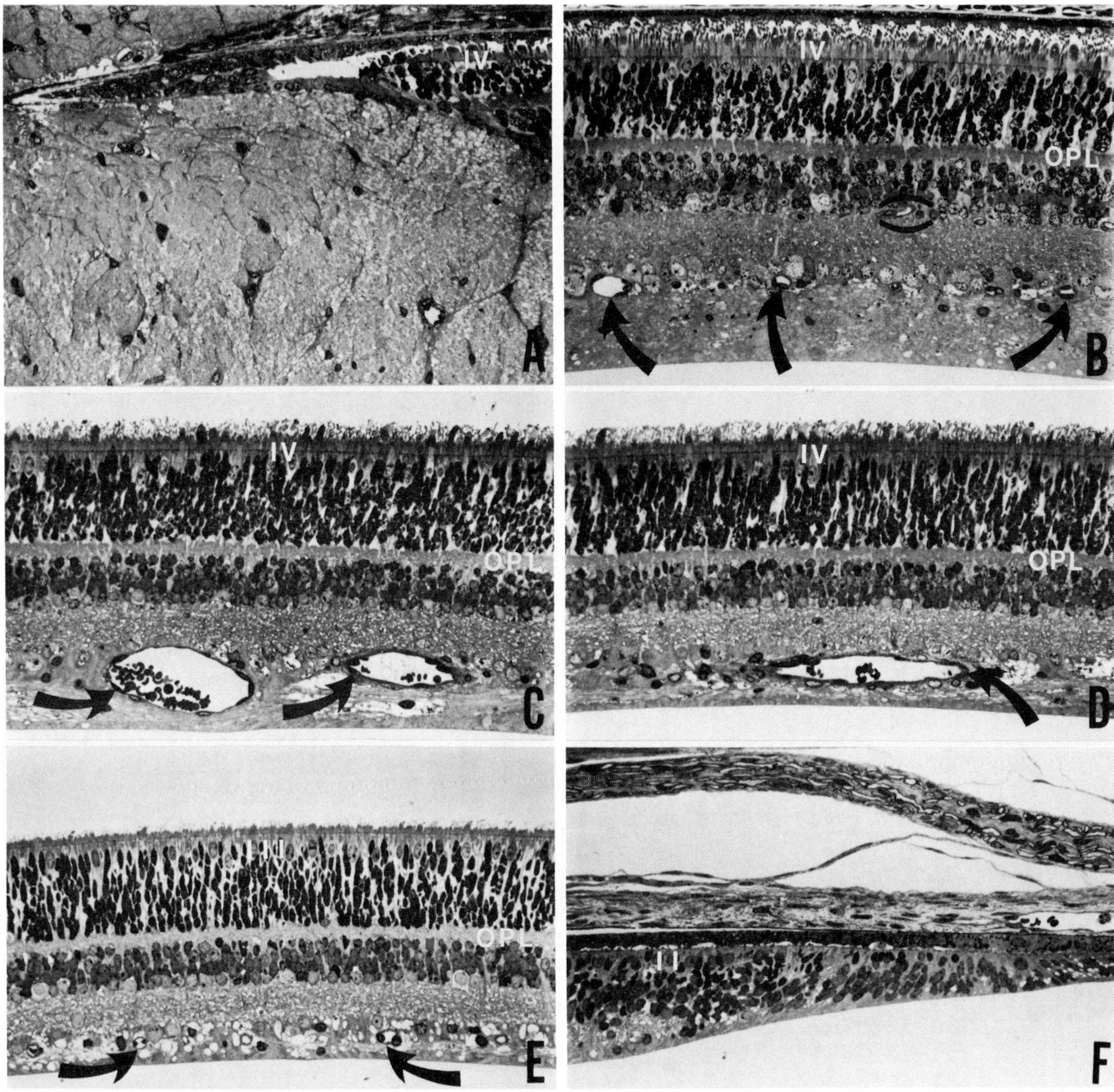

Figure 8-2 Segmental montage of light micrographs (240×) of the retina of a preterm baboon of 141-days gestation (term 184 days), 640-grams birth weight, who died at 64 hours of age while on continuous oxygen administration. A, optic disc; B, 20% of the distance from the optic disc to the ora serrata; C, 40% of the distance from the optic disc to the ora serrata; D, 60% of the distance from the optic disc to the ora serrata; E, 80% of the distance from the optic disc to the ora serrata; F, ora serrata. Roman numerals indicate the stage of photoreceptor maturation. (OPL), outer plexiform layer; (➤), inner retinal vessels and capillaries, (◡), inner retinal vasculature on the inner domain of the inner nuclear layer.

Although IRBP has been shown to be secreted concomitantly with outer segment disc formation in the rat[24,25] and the human,[20,21] IRBP secretion precedes disc formation in the mouse.[26] Therefore, without immunocytochemical studies, it cannot be predicted by photoreceptor maturation alone whether IRBP exists in the subretinal space in the preterm baboon.

There is a second inner retinal vasculature on the inner face of the inner nuclear layer in the retina around the optic disc that is unique to the baboon (Fig. 8-2B). This vasculature is absent in the preterm infant.

Therefore, the developing retina of the preterm baboon is distinctly different from an age-equivalent preterm infant in four ways:

1. There are no cystoid spaces to provide the scaffolding through which vessels form.
2. Where vasoformation is occurring in the most

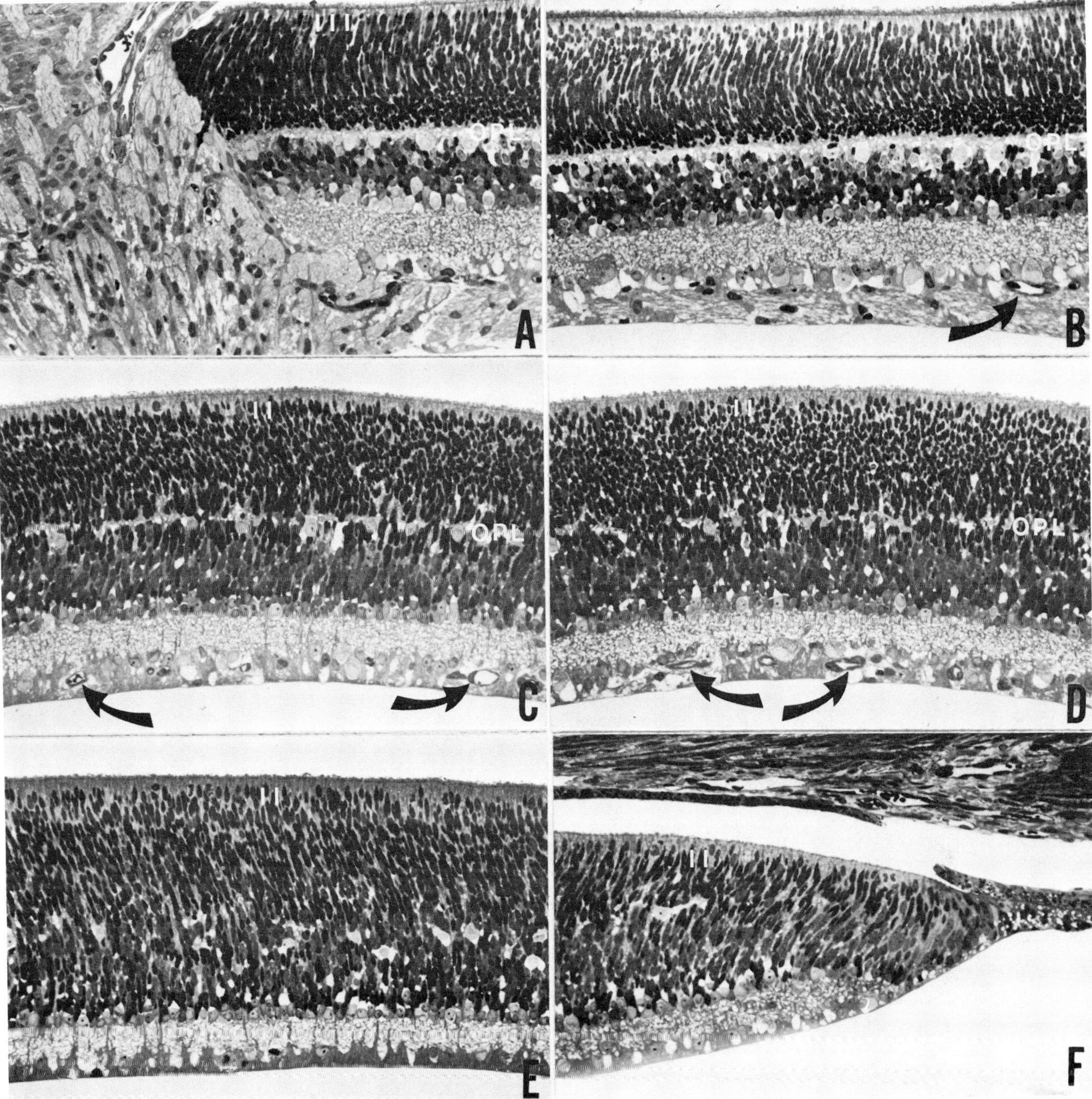

Figure 8-3 Segmental montage of light micrographs (238×) of the retina of a term kitten sacrificed within 4 hours following spontaneous birth. A, optic disc; B, 20% of the distance from the optic disc to the ora serrata; C, 40% of the distance from the optic disc to the ora serrata; D, 60% of the distance from the optic disc to the ora serrata; E, 80% of the distance from the optic disc to the ora serrata; F, ora serrata. Roman numerals indicate the stage of photoreceptor maturation. (OPL), outer plexiform layer; (➤), inner retinal capillaries.

peripheral 20 percent of the baboon retina, there are no spindle cells and no endothelial budding. Therefore, the mechanism of vasoformation is unknown, but certainly different from the preterm infant.

3. Photoreceptor maturation is more advanced. Stage III and IV photoreceptors extend at least 80 percent of the distance from the optic disc to the ora serrata, and Stage II photoreceptors have already reached the ora serrata.

4. Large inner retinal vessels and capillaries are present at least 80 percent of the distance, and a second inner nuclear vascular system is present at least 20 percent of the distance from the optic disc to the ora serrata.

Therefore, even in a close evolution relative to the human, there are drastic morphologic and ontogenetic retinal differences.

DEVELOPMENT OF THE TERM KITTEN RETINA

Figure 8-3 shows the segmental retinal montage characteristic of term kittens (Liberty Laboratories). The term kittens were sacrificed and the eyes enucleated within 4 hours following spontaneous birth.

Stage III photoreceptors extend at least 30 percent of the distance from the optic disc to the ora serrata (Figs. 8-3A and 8-3B), whereas Stage II photoreceptors encroach upon the ora serrata (Figs. 8-3C to 8-3F). The

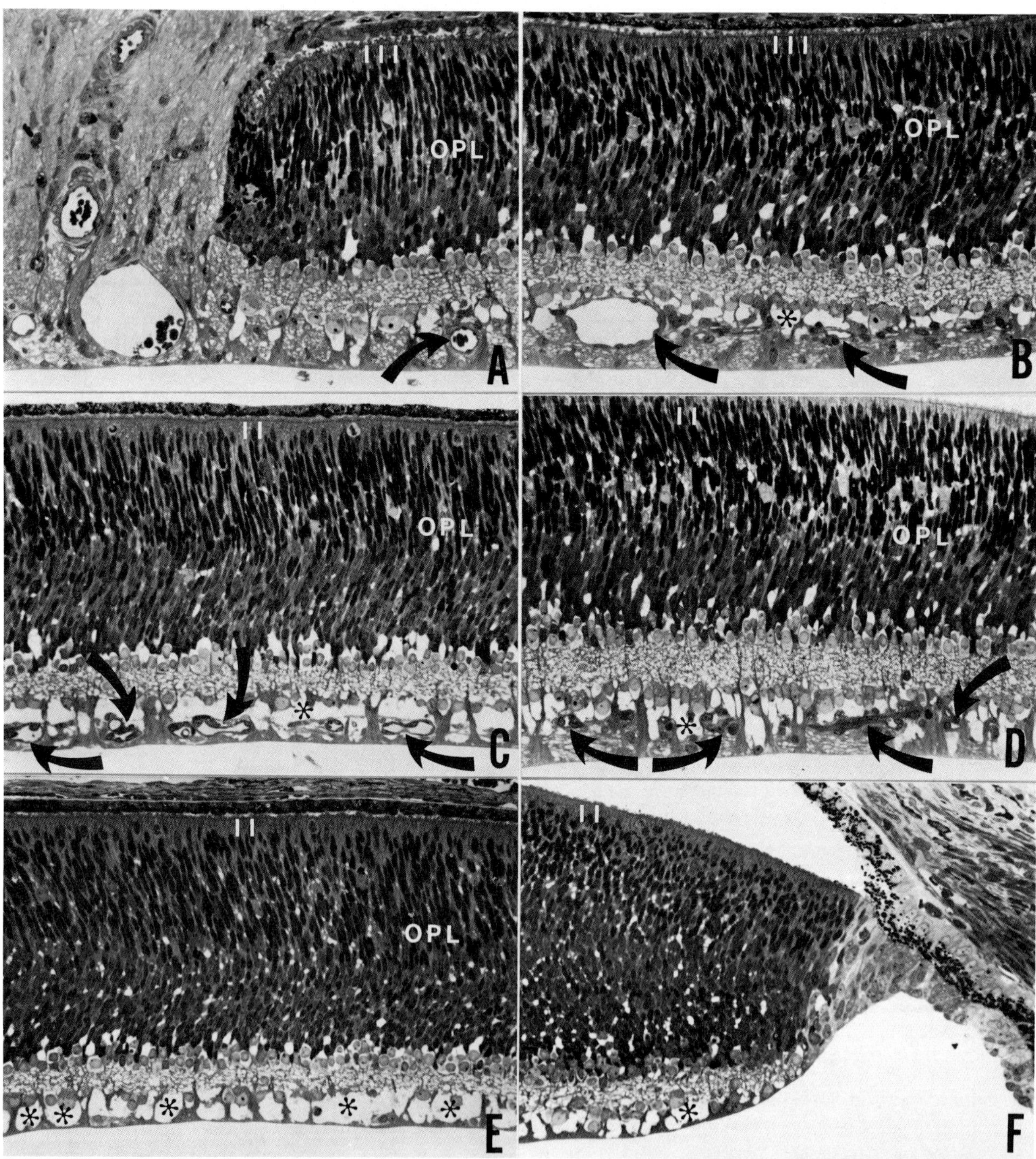

Figure 8-4   Segmental montage of light micrographs (250×) of a term beagle puppy sacrificed immediately following spontaneous birth. A, optic disc; B, 20% of the distance from the optic disc to the ora serrata; C, 40% of the distance from the optic disc to the ora serrata; D, 60% of the distance from the optic disc to the ora serrata; E, 80% of the distance from the optic disc to the ora serrata; F, ora serrata. Roman numerals indicate the stage of photoreceptor maturation. (OPL), outer plexiform layer; (*), cystoid spaces; (➤), inner retinal vessels and capillaries. Endothelial budding is evident in D.

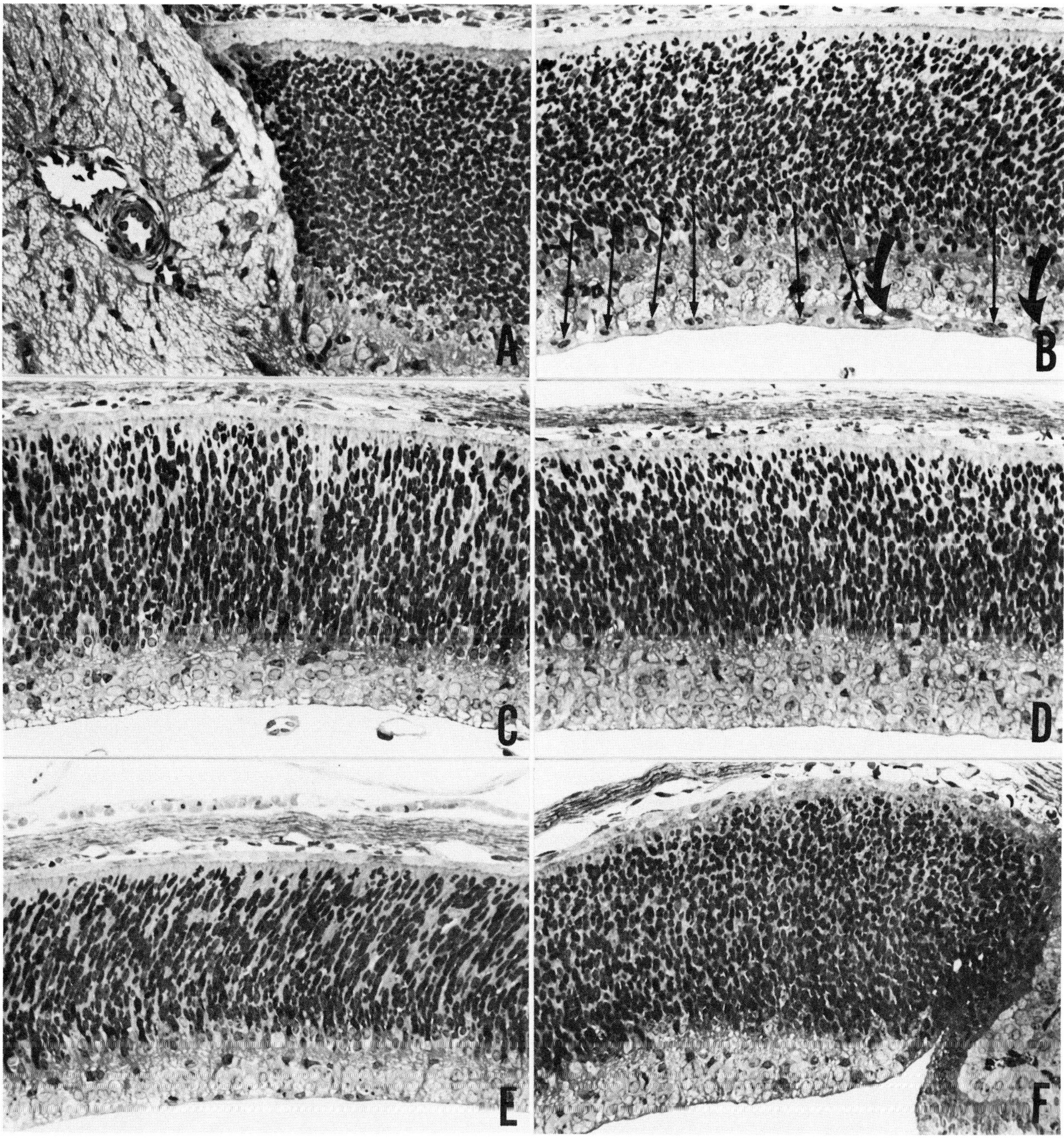

Figure 8-5 Segmental montage of light micrographs (240×) of a term rat (21-days gestation) sacrificed immediately following spontaneous birth. A, optic disc; B, 20% of the distance from the optic disc to the ora serrata; C, 40% of the distance from the optic disc to the ora serrata; D, 60% of the distance from the optic disc to the ora serrata; E, 80% of the distance from the optic disc to the ora serrata; F, ora serrata. Stage I photoreceptors have not developed, and there is no subretinal space between the apical surfaces of the retinal pigment epithelium and the apical surfaces of the neuroblast layer of the nonstratified retina. (↓), spindle cells; (↯), inner retinal capillaries.

nerve fiber layer is compact with no cystoid spaces. Retinal stratification into inner and outer nuclear layers and ontogeny of the outer plexiform layer (Figs. 8-3A to 8-3D) parallels the radial pattern in the preterm infant of 27-weeks gestational age (compare Figs. 8-1 and 8-3). Inner retinal capillaries extend at least 60 to 70 percent of the distance from optic disc to the ora serrata (Figs. 8-3B to 8-3D). However, there are no spindle cells interspersed between the forming capillaries (Figs. 8-3B to 8-3D), and there are no spindle cells within the avascular retina (Figs. 8-3E and 8-3F). Images of endothelial budding are rare immediately after birth into ambient air, but are common features throughout the later post partum period. The kinetics of IRBP secretion from photoreceptors into the subretinal space is undetermined.

Therefore, in the developing term kitten retina, the following five morphologic relationships distinguish it from the preterm infant of 27-weeks gestational age:

1. There are no cystoid spaces.
2. There are no spindle cells.
3. Endothelial budding occurs.
4. Photoreceptor maturation is further developed.
5. Inner retinal capillaries are extensively transretinal to Stage II photoreceptors.

DEVELOPMENT OF THE TERM PUPPY RETINA

Figure 8-4 shows the segmental retinal montage characteristic of term Beagle puppies sacrificed and enucleated immediately following spontaneous birth. The one puppy eye that was studied was provided by Dr. Jan Goddard Feingold, Department of Pediatrics at Baylor College of Medicine.

Like the term kitten, Stage III photoreceptors extend at least 30 percent of the distance from the optic disc to the ora serrata (Figs. 8-4A and 8-4B), and Stage II photoreceptors encroach upon the ora serrata (Figs. 8-4C to 8-4F). Like the preterm infant, cystoid spaces provide the scaffolding (Fig. 8-4) through which the vessels mature. Retinal stratification into inner and outer nuclear layers is barely visible at the light microscopic level, but nuclear differentiation has occurred (Figs. 8-4A to 8-4E). Inner retinal vessels extend at least 60 to 70 percent of the distance from the optic disc to the ora serrata (Figs. 8-4A to 8-4D). Images of endothelial budding are common within the most anterior capillary bed (Fig. 8-4D). The kinetics of IRBP secretion from photoreceptors into the subretinal space is undetermined.

Therefore, in the developing term puppy retina, the following four morphologic relationships distinguish it from the preterm infant of 27-weeks gestational age:

1. There are no spindle cells.
2. Endothelial budding occurs.
3. Stage II photoreceptors encroach on the ora serrata.
4. Inner retinal vessels are extensively transretinal to Stage II photoreceptors.

DEVELOPMENT OF THE TERM RAT RETINA

Figure 8-5 shows the segmental retinal montage from a term rat (Sprague Dawley) that was sacrificed and enucleated immediately following spontaneous birth at 21 days gestation.

In this retina, Stage I photoreceptors have not developed, even around the optic disc (Fig. 8-5A). There is no subretinal space, since junctional complexes still link the apical surfaces of the neural retina with the apical surfaces of the retinal pigment epithelium; this was described in the early human fetus.[27] At term, there is no stratification of the nuclei into outer and inner nuclear layers, and no cystoid spaces exist within the nerve fiber layer (Fig. 8-5). However, spindle cells are canalizing into inner retinal capillaries in the most central 20 percent of the distance from the optic disc to the ora serrata (Fig. 8-5B). Litter mates sacrificed at intervals up to 7 days post partum showed extensive spindle cell migration toward the ora serrata with inner retinal vasoformation through canalization.

Therefore, in the developing rat retina, the following five morphologic relationships are apparent:

1. There are no cystoid spaces through which spindle cells migrate and through which vessels form.
2. Spindle cells canalize to form inner retinal vessels and migrate peripherally, but this migration is not related to the maturation of the outer plexiform layer.
3. Photoreceptor maturation has not occurred at birth.
4. Inner retinal vessels are not spatially restricted to a transretinal location opposite Stage III and IV photoreceptors.
5. Although not demonstrated here, IRBP secretion parallels Stage II photoreceptor maturation.[24,25]

CONCLUSIONS

The preterm infant retina of 27-weeks gestational age establishes five minimal morphologic criteria that animal models should parallel.

1. Spindle cells migrate through cystoid spaces

and form capillaries by canalization.
2. There is no endothelial budding.
3. Inner retinal vessels are transretinal to Stage III and IV photoreceptors.
4. IRBP is secreted by photoreceptors at Stage II maturation, such that the majority of the spindle cell apron is *not* transretinal to IRBP.
5. The ratio of the vascular:avascular retina is approximately 1:1.

Therefore, the retinas of the preterm baboon, the term kitten, the term puppy, and the term rat do not fulfill all of these prerequisites (Table 8-1). The baboon (Fig. 8-2) retinal vasculature and photoreceptor maturation are too advanced. The kitten (Fig. 8-3) and puppy (Fig. 8-4) vascular:avascular retinal ratio approaches that of the preterm infant, but there are no spindle cells, and the dynamic interplay between photoreceptor maturation and inner retinal vasoformation is different; the rat (Fig. 8-5) retina is too immature.

Vitamin E uptake studies in animal models as related to route of administration (oral, intramuscular, slow intravenous infusion, fast intravenous infusion), form (tocopherol or tocopheryl acetate), and vehicle (medium-chain triglycerides, propylene glycol, polysorbates) must fulfill at least two morphologic parameters characteristic of the infant less than or equal to 27-weeks gestational age. The extent of IRBP must be less than or equal to 50 percent of the distance from the optic disc to the ora serrata, and the vascular:avascular retinal ratio must approximate 1:1.

Experimentally, the postnatal rat offers an excellent animal model from which to tissue-culture spindle cells from the retina after 5 days postnatal age. At this age there are significant numbers of spindle cells in the nerve fiber layer.

There are important morphologic variations in the baboon, kitten, puppy, and rat retinas that negate their usefulness as viable animal models in which to study the pathogenesis of ROP. Therefore, whole-eye donations from preterm infants remain the only valid tissue on which to probe the induction of ROP.

ACKNOWLEDGEMENTS

This research was supported by grants from the Retina Research Foundation, United States Public Health Service (USPHS), grant no. AM27685, from the National Institutes of Arthritis, Diabetes, Digestive, and Kidney Diseases of the National Institute of Health (NIH), from Research to Prevent Blindness, from the Cullen Foundation, and from Hoffmann-La Roche. The authors acknowledge the photography of Alexander Kogan and Gilma Miranda; the technical expertise of Evelyn Brown; the secretarial talents of Dorothy Carr; the contributions of Cordell Adams, Richard Fish, M.D., and Chaula Rana, M.D., and Michael Osato, Ph.D. who did the manuscript critique.

REFERENCES

1. Patz A. Current concepts of the effect of oxygen on the developing retina. Cur Eye Res 1984; 3:159–163.
2. Ashton N, Tripathi B, Knight G. Effects of oxygen on the developing retinal vessels of the rabbit. I. Anatomy and development of the retinal vessels of the rabbit. Exp Eye Res 1972; 14:214–220.

TABLE 8–1 Comparison of Morphologic Criteria of Animal Models

Parameters	Preterm Infant	Preterm Baboon	Term Kitten	Term Puppy	Term Rat
Cystoid spaces in nerve fiber layer	+	−	−	+	−
Spindle cells	+	unknown	−		+
Endothelial budding	−	unknown	+	+	−
Retinal stratification into inner and outer nuclear layers	+	+	+	Apparent with Transmission electron microscopy	−
Ratio of vascular:avascular retina	1:1	4:1	3:2	3:2	1:20
Inner retinal vessels follow Stage III and Stage IV photoreceptors	+	unknown	−	−	unknown
IRBP secretion equates with Stage II photoreceptor	+	unknown	unknown	unknown	+
Number of eyes studied	42*	6	8	1	158†

* ≤27-weeks gestational age, surviving ≤4 days
† Surviving up to 7-days post partum

3. Sproul EW, Orlidge A, D'Amore PA. Effects of hyperoxia on the growth and integrity of vascular cells in vitro. Invest Ophthalmol Vis Sci 1985; Suppl 26:284.

4. Graeber JE, Glaser BM. Hyperoxia alters endothelial cell proliferation. Invest Ophthalmol Vis Sci 1985; Suppl 26:284.

5. Phelps DL, Rosenbaum AL. Effects of marginal hypoxemia on recovery from oxygen-induced retinopathy in the kitten model. Pediatrics 1984; 73:1–6.

6. Henkind P, de Oliveira LF. Development of retinal vessels in the rat. Invest Ophthalmol 1967; 6:520–530.

7. Shakib M, de Oliveira LF, Henkind P. Development of retinal vessels. II. Earliest stages of vessel formation. Invest Ophthalmol 1968; 7:689–700.

8. Kretzer FL, Mehta RS, Johnson AT, Hunter DG, Brown ES, Hittner HM. Vitamin E protects against retinopathy of prematurity through action on spindle cells. Nature 1984; 309:793–795.

9. Kretzer FL, McPherson AR, Hittner HM. An interpretation of retinopathy of prematurity in terms of spindle cells: relationship to vitamin E prophylaxis and cryotherapy. Albrecht v Graefes Arch Klin Exp Ophthalmol (in press).

10. Flower RW, Blake DA, Wajer SD, Egner PG, McLeod DS, Pitts SM. Evidence for a role of the prostaglandin cascade in the pathogenesis of oxygen-induced retinopathy in the newborn beagle. Pediatr Res 1981; 15:1293–1302.

11. Phelps DL, Rosenbaum A. The role of tocopherol in oxygen-induced retinopathy: kitten model. Pediatrics 1977; 59:998–1005.

12. Phelps DL, Rosenbaum A. Vitamin E in kitten oxygen-induced retinopathy. II. Blockage of vitreal neovascularization. Arch Ophthalmol 1979; 97:1522–1526.

13. Hindle NW, Leyton J. Prevention of cicatricial retrolental fibroplasia by cryotherapy. Can J Ophthalmol 1978; 13:277–282.

14. Ben-Sira I, Nissenkorn I, Grunwald E, Yassur Y. Treatment of acute retrolental fibroplasia by cryopexy. Br J Ophthalmol 1980; 64:758–762.

15. Hindle NW. Cryotherapy for retinopathy of prematurity to prevent retrolental fibroplasia. Can J Ophthalmol 1982; 17:207–211.

16. Nissenkorn I, Kremer I, Ben-Sira I, Cohen S, Garner A. A clinicopathological case of retinopathy of prematurity (ROP) treated by peripheral cryopexy. Br J. Ophthalmol 1984; 68:36–41.

17. Tasman W. Management of retinopathy of prematurity. Ophthalmology 1985; 92:995–999.

18. Flower RW, McLeod DS, Lutty GA, Goldberg B, Wajer SD. Postnatal retinal development of the puppy. Invest Ophthalmol Vis Sci 1985; 26:957–968.

19. Gole GA, Gannon BJ, Goodger AM. Oxygen-induced retinopathy: the kitten model re-examined. Austral J Ophthalmol 1982; 10:223-232.

20. Johnson AT, Kretzer FL, Hittner HM, Glazebrook PA, Bridges CDB, Lam DMK. Development of the subretinal space in the preterm human eye: ultrastructural and immunocytochemical studies. J Comp Neurol 1985; 233:497–505.

21. Johnson AT, Kretzer FL. Interstitial retinol binding protein in the developing human retina: a proposed explanation for vitamin E suppression of retinopathy of prematurity. In: Bridges CDB, Adler AJ, eds. The interphotoreceptor matrix in health and disease. New York: Alan R. Liss, 1985; 251.

22. Hittner HM, Rudolph AJ, Kretzer FL. Suppression of severe retinopathy of prematurity with vitamin E supplementation: ultrastructural mechanism of clinical efficacy. Ophthalmology 1984; 91:1512–1523.

23. Kretzer FL, Hunter DG, Mehta RS, Brown ES, Blifeld C, Johnson AT, Hittner HM. Spindle cells as vasoformative elements in the developing human retina: vitamin E modulation. In: Coates PW, Kenny AD, Markwald R, eds. Developing and regenerating vertebrate nervous systems. New York: Alan R. Liss, 1983; 199.

24. Gonzalez-Fernandez F, Landers RA, Glazebrook PA, Fong SL, Liou GI, Lam DMK, Bridges CDB. An extracellular retinol-binding glycoprotein in the eyes of mutant rats with retinal dystrophy—development, localization, and biosynthesis. J Cell Biol 1984; 99:2092–2098.

25. Nir I, Cohen D, Papermaster DS. Immunocytochemical localization of opsin in the cell membrane of developing rat retinal photoreceptors. J Cell Biol 1984; 98:1788–1795.

26. Carter-Dawson L, Alvarez RA, Sperling IIG, Bridges CDB. IRBP and retinyl ester in the rod mutant retina. In: Bridges CDB, Adler AJ, eds. The interphotoreceptor matrix in health and disease. New York: Alan R. Liss, 1985; 241.

27. Fisher SK, Linberg KA. Intercellular junctions in the early human embryonic retina. J Ultrastruct Res 1975; 51:69–78.

Efficacy of Vitamin E in Retinopathy of Prematurity

9

Helen M. Hittner, M.D.
Frank L. Kretzer, Ph.D.

A physician without physiology and chemistry flounders along in an aimless fashion, never able to gain any accurate conception of disease, practicing a sort of popgun pharmacy, hitting now the malady and again the patient, he himself not knowing which.

Sir William Osler

OXIDANT-ANTIOXIDANT BALANCE IN THE PRETERM INFANT

In the preterm infant who weighs 1,500 grams or less and is 31-weeks gestational age or less at birth, the oxidant-antioxidant balance is critical, because oxygen-related free radicals potentially damage lipid membranes through auto-oxidation.[1] Since oxygen administration to the very immature infant is a recognized risk factor in the development of ROP,[2-3] prophylactic supplementation with natural antioxidants is a plausible means of suppressing the development of severe ROP. The first natural antioxidant to have undergone the scrutiny of clinical trials in the human preterm infant has been vitamin E.

At birth, the preterm infant is deficient in vitamin E, with plasma levels of 0.4 mg per deciliter owing to a 4:1 placental permeability barrier and low plasma lipid and lipoprotein levels.[4] In addition, there is a decrease in the plasma level if vitamin E is not supplemented in the neonatal period, because there is no adipose storage of the vitamin in the small, premature infant.

An initiating event to the development of ROP is the cluster of oxidative insults to spindle cells, which are the precursors of the inner retinal vasculature (Chapter 4). This cluster of oxidative insults halts normal vasoformation and transforms spindle cells into sites of synthesis and secretion of angiogenic factors.[5-8] This results in retinal and vitreal neovascularization, invasion of myofibroblasts into the vitreous, and in severe cases, retinal detachment.[6-8] Severe ROP can develop when the oxygen challenge exceeds the ability of retinal antioxidants to protect spindle cells.

CRITERIA FOR DEFINITIVE, PROPHYLACTIC CLINICAL TRIALS OF VITAMIN E SUPPLEMENTATION LEADING TO ADEQUATE ANALYSIS AND SUFFICIENT PROTECTION OF SPINDLE CELLS TO SUPPRESS THE DEVELOPMENT OF SEVERE ROP

As a result of the recent understanding of the spindle-cell pathogenesis of ROP, there are 11 criteria that must be fulfilled to establish efficacy or noneffiacy of vitamin E supplementation to suppress the development of severe ROP.

1. The study must evaluate only those infants at high risk of developing ROP. Specifically, infants should weigh 1,500 grams or less at birth.
2. The number of infants enrolled must be adequate to provide a sufficient statistical data base, and the data must be gathered prospectively.
3. The study must be double-masked and randomized to prevent observer bias.
4. Vitamin E must be administered within the first day.
5. Antioxidant protection must be continuous without interruption until the inner retinal vessels reach the temporal ora serrata.
6. There must be a control population whose plasma vitamin E levels are significantly different from the supplemented population, and whose plasma vitamin E levels are unable to provide threshold protection to spindle cells.

7. The treatment dose of vitamin E must be sufficient to provide threshold protection to retinal spindle cells.

8. The form of vitamin E given must be well utilized by the chosen route of administration.

9. An effective and safe initial route of administration of vitamin E must be utilized, since the kinetics of vitamin E uptake into the retinal parenchyma may be tightly linked to initial route of administration.

10. Ophthalmologic examinations must occur with sufficient frequency to determine the most advanced stage of active ROP.

11. A multivariant or variable severity is acceptable, because vitamin E uptake into the retinal parenchyma is dependent on retinal maturation, which is linked to gestational age.

12. A multivariant analysis is mandatory, because vitamin E uptake into the retinal parenchyma is dependent on retinal maturation, which is linked to gestational age.

SEVEN PROPHYLACTIC CLINICAL TRIALS FAILING TO MEET ALL CRITERIA FOR ADEQUATE ANALYSIS AND SUFFICIENT PROTECTION OF SPINDLE CELLS, THAT DO NOT DEMONSTRATE EFFICACY OF VITAMIN E IN SUPPRESSING THE DEVELOPMENT OF SEVERE ROP

1. Puklin, et al.[9,10] The study contained only 20 control and 22 treatment infants, each weighing 1,500 grams or less at birth. The control group was supplemented with intravenous alimentation containing 2.5 IU vitamin E per liter; oral feedings with formula, 16 IU vitamin E per liter, or breast milk, 3 IU vitamin E per liter; and oral vitamin E of 25 IU vitamin E per day for those infants weighing between 1,001 and 1,500 grams at birth; and 50 IU vitamin E per day for those weighing 1,000 grams or less at birth. This resulted in plasma vitamin E levels in the therapeutic range. On the fourteenth day of the study, the control infants had a mean level of 1.11 mg per deciliter, and the vitamin E treatment infants, who received 4 IM doses of 20 mg per kilogram aqueous dl-alpha-tocopherol initially and on days one, two, and seven, had a mean level of 2.23 mg per deciliter. Furthermore, vitamin E supplementation continued only while the infants were on oxygen. A multivariate analy-

sis was not employed; however, there were three infants in the control with intravitreal neovascularization (Stage 3 ROP) and none in the treatment group.

2. Milner, et al.[11] The study contained 133 control and 135 treatment infants, each weighing 1,500 grams or less at birth. By an unstated route of administration, dl-alpha-tocopherol of 25 mg per kilogram per day was administered to the treatment infants. On the seventh day, the plasma vitamin E levels in the control infants attained a mean of 0.87 mg per deciliter, and in the treatment infants, a mean of 2.86 mg per deciliter. However, vitamin E was not continued beyond the age of six weeks, and the ophthalmologic examinations were inadequate to determine the most severe stage of active ROP. Late ophthalmologic examinations determined that five infants in the control group and three in the treatment group had RLF Grades III or IV.

3. Hittner, et al.[12] The 1981 clinical trial was nonmasked, nonrandomized, and noncontrolled. One hundred infants, each weighing 1,500 grams or less at birth, were enrolled with 69 infants surviving for more than ten weeks. Oral dl-alpha-tocopheryl acetate was administered as 100 mg per kilogram daily from the first hours of life. Plasma vitamin E levels on the fourteenth day of life attained a mean of 2.0 mg per deciliter for these infants. They were compared with control infants who had been in the same nursery the previous year. A multivariant significance of p = 0.003 for vitamin E in suppressing the development of severe ROP was obtained.

4. Finer, et al.[13] From May 1981 to September 1982, a nonmasked and nonrandomized clinical trial was performed, which enrolled 44 infants receiving oral dl-alpha-tocopheryl acetate (200 mg per kilogram per day) within the first 12 hours of life and 23 control infants weighing 1,500 grams or less at birth, who survived for more than 8 weeks. Plasma vitamin E levels on the ninth day of life attained a mean of 3.0 mg per deciliter for treatment and 0.7 mg per deciliter for control infants. Four control infants developed RLF, while no treatment infants developed RLF. A multivariant significance of p = 0.0009 for vitamin E in suppressing the development of severe ROP was obtained.

5–7. Johnson, et al.[14-16] Johnson, et al have published three clinical trials. The first study enrolled from February, 1972 to May, 1974; the second from May, 1974 to February, 1976; and the third from January, 1979 to April, 1981. Each targeted a predetermined plasma vitamin E level: 1.5 mg per deciliter, 3.0 mg per deciliter, and 5.0 mg per deciliter respectively. The first two studies were nonmasked and nonrandomized. The number of infants weighing 1,500 grams or less at birth, who survived for more than 1 month, was 33 and 62. The initial parenteral form was dl-alpha-tocopheryl acetate and dl-alpha-tocopherol. The initial route of administration was IM. There was no Stage 3 ROP in the first clinical trial, no statement regarding Stage 3 ROP in the second clinical trial. The trend of the studies is toward vitamin E efficacy.[16]

7. Phelps, et al.[17]   Phelps, et al enrolled 287 infants weighing 1,500 grams or less at birth. Sixty infants died, 31 were not included in the ROP analysis for unknown reasons, and 196 infants completed the trial and were the subject of the final ROP analysis. This large, double-masked, randomized, controlled clinical trial enrolled from December, 1980 through August, 1983. Within the first 24 hours of life and on the second day of life, the trial utilized rapid IV infusion, over 15 to 20 minutes, of aqueous dl-alpha-tocopherol (20 mg per kilogram) as the initial route of administration. Thereafter, a mean plasma vitamin E level of 3.0–3.5 mg per deciliter was targeted by rapid IV administration until the infant no longer required intravenous therapy. The beginning dose for oral supplementation was 100 mg per kilogram per day of dl-alpha-tocopherol. The rapid IV and oral doses were altered according to plasma-tocopherol levels taken twice weekly. IM injections of aqueous dl-alpha-tocopherol were given when the plasma level was recalcitrant to oral doses of 200 mg per kilogram per day. Supplementation was continued until the retinal vessels were mature or the retinopathy was stable at one year of age. However, multiple treatment infants had interrupted therapy. The plasma vitamin E data were expressed as mean weekly levels. For the first week, the mean was 3.5 mg per deciliter for the treated infants. Analysis failed to demonstrate efficacy of vitamin E in suppressing the development of severe ROP. However, ophthalmologic examinations could not be used for multivariant or variable severity analysis. One treatment and one control infant developed Grade V cicatricial RLF.

Summary of these seven clinical trials: In retrospect, the 11 criteria to allow adequate analysis and sufficient protection of spindle cells to suppress the development of severe ROP evolved as the role of spindle cells in the pathogenesis of ROP and the pharmacokinetics of plasma and retinal vitamin E were elucidated. For example, it was impossible to predict, during the planning stages, that rapid IV infusion of vitamin E as an initial route of administration or prolonged pharmacologic elevation of vitamin E plasma levels would result in toxicity. Similarly, the importance of beginning vitamin E within the first day of life, utilizing an effective and safe form and initial route of administration, and the necessity of continuing vitamin E supplementation without interruption until inner retinal vessels reached the temporal ora serrata, could not have been foreseen.

THREE PROPHYLACTIC CLINICAL TRIALS MEETING ALL CRITERIA FOR ADEQUATE ANALYSIS AND SUFFICIENT PROTECTION OF SPINDLE CELLS, THAT DEMONSTRATE EFFICACY OF VITAMIN E IN SUPPRESSING THE DEVELOPMENT OF SEVERE ROP

1. Hittner, et al.[18]   The study enrolled 150 infants (75 control, 75 treatment) weighing 1,500 grams or less at birth, with 101 infants (51 control, 50 treatment) surviving more than 8 weeks. Oral supplementation with dl-alpha-tocopherol began within the first 24 hours of life. The control group was supplemented with 5 mg per kilogram per day; the treatment group, with 100 mg per kilogram per day. This study demonstrated the efficacy of early, initial, oral vitamin E supplementation in suppressing the development of severe ROP (p = 0.012 by multivariate analysis). Details of this study are given in Table 9–1).

2. Finer, et al.[19]   The study enrolled 126 infants (64 control, 62 treatment) weighing 1,500 grams or less at birth, with 97 infants (50 control, 47 treatment) surviving more than 8 weeks. IM supplementation with dl-alpha-tocopheryl acetate began within the first 12 hours of life. The control group was unsupplemented; the treatment group received 50 mg per kilogram on day 1, 20 mg per kilogram on days 2 through 15, and 20 mg per kilogram on days 18, 21, 24, 27, and 30. Following this, 100 mg per kilogram per day of dl-alpha-tocopheryl acetate were administered orally. This study demonstrated the efficacy of early, initial, IM vitamin E supplementation in suppressing the development of severe ROP (p = 0.01 by multivariate analysis). Details of this study are given in Table 9–1.

3. Shaffer, et al.[16]   The study enrolled 424 infants (216 control, 208 treatment) weighing 1,500 grams or less at birth, with 288 infants (147 control, 141 treatment) surviving more than 8 weeks. Primarily slow (4 to 8 hours) intravenous supplementation with dl-alpha-tocopherol began within the first 24 hours of life. The control group

TABLE 9–1   Three Clinical Trials Meeting the Essential Criteria and Demonstrating Efficacy of Vitamin E in Suppressing the Development of Severe ROP

Clinical Parameter	Hittner, et al[18] Control/Treatment	Finer, et al[19] Control/Treatment	SCHAFFER, ET AL[16] Control/Treatment
Infants enrolled ($\leq$1,500 g)	75/75	64/62	194/168
Birth weight of infants enrolled (g)	1,050/1,050	1,203/1,185	1,156/1,162
Infants surviving $\geq$8 weeks	51/50 (+1)*	50/47	147/141
Birth weight of infants surviving			
$\geq$8 weeks (g)	1,113/1,093	1,207/1,197	1,170/1,175
Distribution of these birth weights:			
500–749 g	2/5	--/--	5/2
750–1,000 g	17/15	9/9	22/21
1,001–1,250 g	14/13	15/15	56/56
1,251–1,500 g	18/17	26/23	64/62
Total	51/50	50/47	147/141
Vitamin E:			
Form (dl-alpha)	Alcohol	Acetate	Alcohol
Dosage schedule for 1st week (mg/kg)	5×7/100×7	0×7/(50×1)+(20×6)	0×7/(5–15)×7
Route of administration	oral/oral	--/intramuscular	--/slow intravenous**
Plasma tocopherol level at age one week	1.2	4.6	5.0
ROP Stage $\geq$3 plus in infants surviving			
$\geq$8			
weeks showing distribution according			
to birth weight:			
500–749 g	1/0	--/--	3/0
750–1,000 g	3/0	2/0	2/3
1,001–1,250 g	0/0	1/0	1/0
1,251–1,500 g	1/0	0/0	1/0
Total	5/0	3/07/3	
Multivariate analysis	0.012	0.01	--
Analysis by severity variable	--	--	0.05

* Infant excluded because oral vitamin E therapy was interrupted.[20]

PREDOMINANTLY INITIAL SLOW (4 TO 8 HOURS) INTRAVENOUS, BUT A MINORITY RECEIVED INITIAL INTRAMUSCULAR VITAMIN E.

was unsupplemented; the treatment group received 5–15 mg per kilogram per day to target a plasma vitamin E level of 5.0 mg per deciliter. To maintain this plasma level slow intravenous, intramuscular, and oral supplementation were utilized. This study demonstrated the efficacy of early, initial, slow IV vitamin E supplementation in suppressing the development of severe ROP (p = 0.05 by variable severity analysis). Details of this study are given in Table 9–1.

Summary of these three clinical trials: The total number of infants analyzed in these three double-masked, randomized, controlled clinical trials was 486. It is important to realize that Hittner, et al[18] enrolled infants of smaller birth weight, and thus, had a predictably higher mortality rate and a higher incidence of Stage 3 plus ROP. When evaluating whether prophylactic vitamin E supplementation should be incorporated into routine nursery care, the critical question in evaluating the clinical trials is whether spindle cells were sufficiently protected continuously from the first hours of life until the inner retinal vessels reached the temporal ora serrata.

ANECDOTAL INFORMATION PERCEIVED DURING AND FOLLOWING VITAMIN E CLINICAL TRIALS, EXPLAINED IN TERMS OF THE SPINDLE CELL PATHOGENESIS OF ROP

1. Initiation of vitamin E supplementation must be within the first hours of life. This concept is supported by data of Finer, et al[13] and Hittner, et al.[20] Finer, et al reported a subset of eight infants in which initial oral administration was delayed a mean of 167.5 hours (range = 40–456 hours). Statistically, severe ROP occurred more frequently in these eight infants, as compared to 44 infants in whom initial oral supplementation was started early, at less than 12 hours of life

(p = 0.0008). Hittner, et al documented, as an example, the course of one infant of 29-weeks gestational age, in whom oral vitamin E supplementation was not initiated until the age of 1 month, with development of severe ROP at 8 weeks. This course of development of severe ROP equals that of unsupplemented infants.

These clinical findings correlate with the fact that a cluster of oxidative insults impinges on spindle cells within the first hours of life. Such initial insults trigger a cascade of events that are seen ultrastructurally, by 4 days (96 hours) of life, as extensive gap junction formation between adjacent spindle cells.[5-8] If antioxidant protection occurs after the initial cluster of oxidative insults, spindle cells are already transformed into sites of synthesis and secretion of angiogenic factors. Therefore, antioxidant protection must begin early to yield clinical efficacy.

2. Vitamin E supplementation to the physiological range must be continuous until inner retinal vessels reach the temporal ora serrata.[20] Hittner documented, as an example, the course of one infant of 29-weeks gestational age, in whom oral vitamin E supplementation was interrupted for 10 days within the first month of life, with development of severe ROP at age 8 weeks. This course of development of severe ROP equals that of unsupplemented infants.

This clinical finding correlates with the fact that spindle cells in the hyperoxygenated, peripheral retina can become gap junction linked whenever the retinal oxidant-antioxidant balance is unfavorable. Therefore, vitamin E supplementation must be continuous to be efficacious.

3. Vitamin E supplementation to the physiological range must not be terminated until inner retinal vessels reach the temporal ora serrata, even when oxygen supplementation is no longer required or when only Stages 1 or 2 ROP are observed clinically.[20] Hittner, et al documented, as an example, the course of one infant of 28 weeks gestational age in whom, at the time of discharge from the hospital, oral vitamin E supplementation was halted at 90 days of life. Two weeks later, the infant had developed Stage 3 ROP. This delayed course in the occurrence of severe ROP reflects the vitamin E-induced lag and is equivalent to that of supplemented infants of lower gestational age.

This clinical finding correlates with the fact that spindle cells can be transformed from sites of minimal secretion of angiogenic factors to sites of maximal secretion of angiogenic factors, when the retinal oxidant-antioxidant balance becomes unfavorable owing to premature cessation of vitamin E supplementation. As long as activated spindle cells remain in the peripheral retina, the latent potential for neovascularization persists.

4. With judicious curtailment of oxygen administration, but without vitamin E supplementation, severe ROP can develop in infants of up to 1,500-grams birth weight when sufficient oxidative risk factors are operant. For example, from 1968 to 1971, Johnson, et al[15] reported an incidence of 8 percent Stages 3 and 4 ROP in infants between 1,001- and 1,500-grams birth weight. From 1979 to 1981 utilizing early, initial, slow IV or IM supplementation, severe ROP was present in only three infants whose birth weights were less than 1,000 grams.[16] Hittner, et al[20] reported six infants who received early, initial vitamin E supplementation by oral or IM:oral routes. These infants who developed Stages 3 and 4 ROP had an average birth weight of 790 grams (range 630 to 920 grams).

Vitamin E is transported into the peripheral retina by interstitial retinol binding protein, which is secreted by photoreceptors when they form nascent outer segments.[21] In infants weighing 1,000 grams or less at birth, photoreceptors secreting IRBP extend radially less than 50 percent of the distance from the optic disc to the temporal ora serrata, and spindle cells are far in advance of the IRBP. Thus, a large percentage of the spindle cells is not transretinal to IRBP. These spindle cells cannot be protected through vitamin E supplementation, regardless of the plasma vitamin E level attained with any form of the vitamin by any route of administration. Therefore, clinical failures can be predicted in infants weighing 1,000 grams or less at birth, because vitamin E uptake is closely linked to retinal maturation. In infants weighing 1,000 grams or more at birth, there is a surge of retinal maturation such that a small percentage of spindle cells is not transretinal to IRBP, and vitamin E suppresses the development of severe ROP.[7,8,21,22]

5. In attempting to suppress the development of severe ROP, there is no added efficacy in administering by IM:oral versus the oral, initial route of administration. Hittner, et al[22] demonstrated that gap junction formation between adjacent spindle cells cannot be prevented more effectively by a fast rise in plasma vitamin E.

If retinal development and secretion of IRBP have reached a critical point, retinal uptake of a threshold level of vitamin E occurs when the deficient, preterm plasma vitamin E level is alleviated. Thus, to suppress the development of severe ROP, the oral route alone is sufficient to obtain the maximal effect of vitamin E.

THE CURRENT DILEMMA OF UTILIZING VITAMIN E TO SUPPRESS THE DEVELOPMENT OF SEVERE ROP

Neonatologists are faced with a dilemma regarding the use of vitamin E to suppress the development of severe ROP. Of the ten clinical trials, only three double-masked, randomized, controlled trials enrolled infants at risk (1,500 grams or less birth weight), initiated vitamin E early (at less than 24 hours of life), continued supplementation without interruption until retinal vessels reached the temporal ora serrata, and utilized an effective and safe initial route of administration. These clinical trials documented vitamin E efficacy (486 infants),[16, 18-19]. The critical concept is that antioxidant protection in order to protect spindle cells must reach the periphral, avascular, hyperoxygenated retina as soon as possible following birth.

Although the developing kitten retina is devoid of spindle cells, it is an appropriate model for vitamin E uptake, since the relationship between photoreceptors secreting IRBP and the extent of inner retinal vessels can be equated to that in the developing human retina (Chapter 8). Utilizing this model, Bhat, et al[24] have quantitated retinal levels of vitamin E following initial rapid IV, IM, and oral administration (Fig. 9–1). The rapid IV route produces a biphasic curve of retinal vitamin E. There is an initial, rapid peak reflecting tocopherol within the retinal vessels, but this tocopherol is not transported into the retinal parenchyma. There is a subsequent slow elevation representing tocopherol, which is transported into the retinal parenchyma. ROP is not a disease of retinal, vascular, endothelial necrosis,[5-8] and the presence of tocopherol in centrally located retinal vessels does not favorably influence the oxidant-antioxidant balance in the peripheral retina. By contrast, the IM and oral routes of administration produce a rapid rise in tocopherol within the retinal parenchyma, which protects spindle cells and results in clinical efficacy.

Despite the desirability of utilizing the initial IV route of administration in preterm infants, the uptake of tocopherol into the retinal parenchyma by initial rapid IV route is delayed and by initial slow IV route is unknown. In order to be efficacious, vitamin E as tocopherol must be transported in the plasma, within the hydrophobic core of low-density lipoproteins (LDLP),[25] to sites where transfer of tocopherol occurs to the hydrophobic pocket of the tissue-specific binding protein of the retina, the interstitial retinol binding protein (IRBP).[26]

The rate of transfer of administered tocopherol and tocopheryl acetate to biologically active tocopherol in the hydrophobic core of LDLP may be dependent upon the route of administration, although the precise kinetics are not understood.[27] Following oral administration, the reticuloendothelial system of the duodenal lymphatics readily allows this conversion.[27] The kinetics

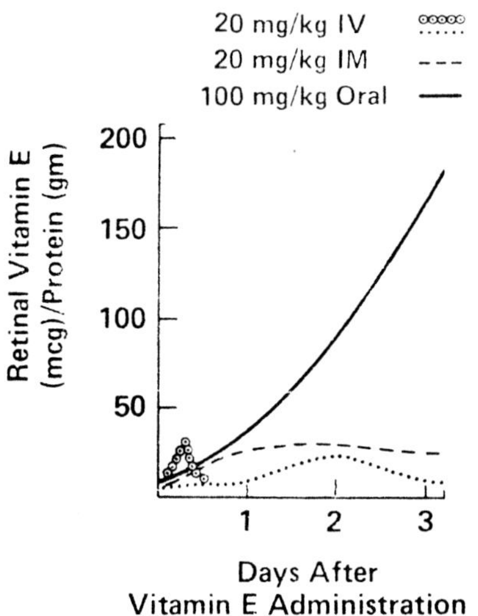

Figure 9–1 Graph demonstrating the retinal vitamin E (tocopherol) levels (μg/gm retinal protein) in the first few days following administration of dl-alpha-tocopherol by the rapid (60 minutes) IV infusion (and), IM ( ), and oral ( ) routes of administration. This graph replots the data of Bhat and Braun[24] in the newborn kitten. They administered 100 mg per kilogram by all three routes of administration; however, these are not the appropriate doses clinically for the preterm infant. Therefore, this graph plots the rapid IV infusion and IM data at 20 mg per kilogram and assumes a linear absorption between 20 and 100 mg per kilogram by the rapid IV infusion and IM routes of administration. This disparity between the parenteral and oral routes reflects the inefficient absorption of tocopherol by the preterm intestine. The curve following rapid IV infusion is biphasic. The initial rapid peak ( ) occurs at 2 hours following administration and represents unbound tocopherol in the plasma of the inner retinal vessels, which provides no antioxidant protection to spindle cells. The second slow elevation ( ) occurs at 2 days following administration and represents tocopherol bound to low-density lipoproteins (LDLP) in the plasma of the inner retinal vessels, and then transported into the retinal parenchyma by interstitial retinol binding protein (IRBP), which provides late antioxidant protection to altered spindle cells after the initial cluster of oxidative insults. The line ( ) below the initial peak that represents tocopherol bound to LDLP in the plasma of the inner retinal vessels and transported into the retinal parenchyma by IRBP, in the first hours following administration, is a hypothetical extrapolation (from the levels between 8 and 24 hours following administration). This explains why initial, rapid IV infusion is nonefficacious in suppressing the development of severe ROP. These replotted lines show that the kinetics of retinal uptake of tocopherol within the critical first 12 hours of life occur equally well following oral and IM administration, but significantly less following rapid IV infusion. The difference between the parenteral and oral routes following this single dose of tocopherol, which becomes greater after 24 hours of life, is not significant as long as continuous threshold protection is provided to spindle cells.

of this transfer of tocopherol or tocopherly acetate by the reticuloendothelial system following IM, slow IV, and rapid IV administration are unknown. The apparently conflicting data regarding intraventricular hemorrhage (decreased incidence—see page 97 versus increased incidence—see page 112) may relate to this transfer. All initial routes of administration (oral, IM, slow IV, and rapid IV) may be efficacious for ROP since the onset of significant clinical disease is delayed by at least 6 weeks. However, initial intravenous routes of administration may not be efficacious for intraventricular hemorrhage since the onset of significant clinical disease is usually within the first few days of life.

INCREASING EXOGENOUS SOURCES OF VITAMIN E

There has been a gradual increase in the amount of exogenous vitamin E given to preterm infants. This trend is reflected in multiple changes. The American Academy of Pediatrics has increased its recommendations for vitamin E supplementation to preterm infants, from nothing in 1966[28] to 5 mg per kilogram per day in 1974[29] to 5 to 25 mg per kilogram per day in 1985[30] Premature formulas, as exemplified by Similac, have increased the content of vitamin E from 5 IU per liter in 1968 to 30 IU per liter in 1985. Breast milk contains large amounts of vitamin E, an average of approximately 10 IU per liter,[31] and the importance of breast feeding preterm infants and milk banks have become widespread in recent years. In the past few years, total parenteral nutrition formulas have substantially increased the content of vitamin E, as dl-alpha-tocopheryl acetate. For example, the multivitamin additive, MVI-Pediatric, has increased its content of vitamin E from 2 IU per vial in 1980 to 7 IU per vial in 1985, with 65 percent of the vial being recommended for infants weighing 1,500 grams or less at birth and 30 percent of the vial for infants weighing 1,000 grams or less at birth.

Thus, the unsupplemented control subjects of the clinical trials of Johnson, et al (1972–1976 and 1979–1981)[14-16], the clinical trials of Hittner, et al (1980–1981)[18,12], and the clinical trials of Phelps, et al (1981–1983)[17] differ from the current experience of Lemons and Maisels (1985).[32] The latter reported that 37 percent of the infants had plasma vitamin E levels above 3.5 mg per deciliter, using 100 mg per kilogram per day of Aquasol E (1985). This contrasts with the experience of Hittner, et al,[12] who found that only 3 percent of their plasma vitamin E levels were above 3.5 mg per deciliter, using the same protocol (1981), (Table 9–2). In the previous year, Hittner, et al[18] found that less than 1 percent of their plasma vitamin E levels were above 3.5 mg per deciliter, utilizing dl-alpha-tocopherol (1980, Table 9–3), and the following year[23] they found that only 7 percent of plasma vitamin E levels were above 3.5 mg per deciliter, utilizing dl-alpha-tocopheryl acetate in medium-chain triglycerides (1982). (Table 9–4). Even when an IM:oral protocol was used, Hittner, et al[23] found that only 17 percent of the plasma vitamin E levels were above 3.5 mg per deciliter (1982) (Table 9–5). These findings emphasize the fact that in order to target mean plasma vitamin E levels in the range of 1.1 to 3.3 mg per deciliter, fixed-dose schedules of vitamin E supplementation to suppress ROP must be modified in each nursery and for each infant by repeated plasma vitamin E determinations. Thus, future clinical trials will

TABLE 9–2 The Distribution of Plasma Tocopherol Levels Measured in Infants with Birth Weights of 500 to 1,500 Grams Who Received Oral dl-alpha-tocopheryl Acetate as Aquasol E in the 1981 Clinical Trial of Hittner, et al.[12]

Tocopherol Level (mg/dl)	Infants Receiving Oral Vitamin E	
	Number of Levels	Percent of Total Number
0.–0.4	50	9.3
0.5–1.4	253	47.1
1.5–2.4	182	33.9
2.5–3.4	38	7.1
3.5–4.4	12	2.2
4.5–5.4	2	0.4
5.5–8.0	0	0.0
>8.0	0	0.0
Total	537	(100 infants)

TABLE 9–3 The Distribution of Plasma Tocopherol Levels Measured in Infants with Birth Weights of 500 to 1,500 Grams Who Received Oral dl-alpha-tocopherol from Hoffmann-LaRoche, Inc. in the 1980 Clinical Trial of Hittner, et al.[18]

Tocopherol Level (mg/dl)	Infants Receiving Oral Vitamin E	
	Number of Levels	Percent of Total Number
0–0.4	156	32.1
0.5–1.4	227	46.7
1.5–2.4	77	15.9
2.5–3.4	23	4.7
3.5–4.4	3	0.6
4.5–5.4	0	0.0
5.5–8.0	0	0.0
>8.0	0	0.0
Total	486	(75 infants)

TABLE 9–4 The Distribution of Plasma Tocopherol Levels Measured in Infants with Birth Weights of 500 to 1,500 Grams Who Received Oral dl-alpha-tocopheryl Acetate in Medium-chain Triglycerides in the 1982 Clinical Trial of Hittner, et al.[23]

Tocopherol Level (mg/dl)	Infants Receiving Oral Vitamin E	
	Number of Levels	Percent of Total Number
0–0.4	69	13.3
0.5–1.4	262	50.7
1.5–2.4	95	18.4
2.5–3.4	53	10.2
3.5–4.4	21	4.1
4.5–5.4	9	1.7
5.5–8.0	5	1.0
>8.0	3	0.6
Total	517	(89 infants)

fail to show efficacy of vitamin E supplementation in suppressing the development of severe ROP, because the increased vitamin E intake of the control infants may have already been sufficient to protect spindle cells; that is, the vitamin E intake of the control infants will be sufficient even when significantly different from that of the treatment infants.

VITAMIN E PRODUCTS, DOSAGE, AND ROUTE OF ADMINISTRATION

1. Tocopherols. Alpha, beta, gamma, and delta forms of tocopherols exist in nature; however, only alpha-tocopherols are vitamin E. Alpha-tocopherol is preferentially absorbed, transported, and retained by tissues.[33]

2. Stereoisomers. The only stereoisomer of vitamin E that is utilized in man as an antioxidant is d-alpha-tocopherol. Owing to expense, a "dl" racemic mixture has been given routinely instead of the pure "d" isomer; however, the "l" isomer is not utilized and may block active receptor sites.[34]

3. Forms. By the oral route of administration, either tocopherol (alcohol form) or tocopheryl acetate (acetate form) can be given, because the acetate is hydrolyzed to the alcohol in the presence of biliary and pancreatic secretions.[35] Both forms have been shown to be efficacious in suppressing the development of severe ROP.[12,18] In the very-low-birth-weight infant, 1,000 grams or less, decreased presence or activity of the

hydrolyzing secretions may be associated with decreased utilization of the acetate forms. This has little clinical significance, however, since there is also decreased retinal utilization of tocopherol in infants weighing 1,000 grams or less at birth. Therefore, while the alcohol may be optimal, stability and lack of any clinical evidence for increased efficacy of tocopherol over tocopheryl acetate has made the acetate the most commonly manufactured form.

When IM vitamin E is administered, either the alcohol or acetate can be used, since IM tocopheryl acetate was efficacious in suppressing the development of severe ROP.[19] Although administration of the alcohol eliminates the need for hydrolysis of the acetate, especially in the most immature infants, there is no evidence for increased efficacy. However, dose schedules for the alcohol and acetate may be different.

Utilization of initial rapid IV infusion of tocopherol has not proven efficacious in suppressing the development of severe ROP.[17] However, in infants too immature or ill to utilize even small quantities of oral vitamin E, initial slow IV infusion of tocopherol may be indicated in the first hours of life to achieve physiological levels. This route of administration may also be clinically useful to maintain physiological levels following early, initial IM injections. Another alternative is the use of a micellar tocopherol, which might circumvent the need for natural plasma carriers (low-density lipoproteins[25]) and rapidly deliver the vitamin to tissue-specific receptor sites. It appears that administering the acetate by the rapid IV route should be avoided.[17]

4. Vehicle. Oral solvents must not cause irritation of the intestinal mucosa; medium-chain triglycerides are

TABLE 9–5 The Distribution of Plasma Tocopherol Levels Measured in Infants with Birth Weights of 500 to 1,500 Grams Who Received IM dl-alpha-tocopherol Plus Oral dl-alpha-tocopheryl Acetate in Medium-chain Triglycerides in the 1982 Clinical Trial of Hittner, et al.[23]

Tocopherol Level (mg/dl)	Infants Receiving IM:Oral Vitamin E	
	Number of Levels	Percent of Total Number
0–0.4	47	10.1
0.5–1.4	102	21.9
1.5–2.4	135	28.9
2.5–3.4	102	21.9
3.5–4.4	53	11.4
4.5–5.4	15	3.2
5.5–8.0	12	2.6
>8.0	0	0.0
Total	466	(79 infants)

ideal.[36] Care must be taken to prevent adding anything to the vitamin that will pose an antigenic challenge.

If appropriate IM products become available, solvents must be aqueous, rather than oil based, for rapid absorption.[37]

If appropriate products become available for slow IV infusion, solvents should be aqueous with minimal levels of emulsifiers.

5. Dosage. In supplementing preterm infants, the dose should achieve, but not exceed adult physiological plasma vitamin E levels, 1.1 to 3.3 mg per deciliter. The dosage must be adjusted to account for all potential sources of vitamin E: oral, breast milk, oral multivitamins, IM, slow IV, parenteral nutrition additives. As a result of poor absorption from the gastrointestinal tract, large mg per kilogram doses given orally produce only minimal plasma elevation, and mg per kilogram doses must be drastically reduced when parenteral routes of administration are utilized. There is a considerable range of plasma vitamin E levels obtained from a single dose by any route of administration, which necessitates frequent determination of plasma vitamin E levels to avoid exceeding the adult physiological plasma vitamin E range. However, it is difficult to exceed this range by the oral route alone.

6. Routes of administration. In the preterm infant, initial oral administration is adequate to suppress the development of severe ROP. If the infant cannot tolerate even small quantities of gavage fluid, then early initial IM administration is the proper alternative and may well be indicated for all infants in order to suppress the development of severe intraventricular hemorrhage.[38,39]

A prospective, randomized, double-masked clinical trial in 226 preterm infants ≤ 32 weeks gestation has demonstrated that IM vitamin E soon after birth protects against periventricular hemorrhage. Among 145 treated inborn babies, there was a decreased incidence of IVH (9.1%) compared with control babies (40.0%) (p<0.0001). Among 81 treated outborn babies, there was also a decreased incidence of IVH (15%) compared with control babies (48%) (p<0.01) (Dr. Malcolm L. Chiswick, personal communication). Early slow IV administration targeting levels below 3.5 mg per deciliter has not been studied prospectively for IVH.

CURRENTLY PROPOSED VITAMIN E DOSE SCHEDULE

1. Vitamin E prophylaxis is unnecessary in infants weighing more than 1,500 grams at birth and who are more than 31-weeks gestational age. These infants are not usually at high risk of developing severe ROP.

2. Begin oral vitamin E supplementation, 100 mg per kilogram per day of tocopherol or tocopheryl acetate in medium-chain triglycerides, to adult physiological levels within the first hours of life. Lower levels of oral supplementation have not been shown to be efficacious in suppressing the development of severe ROP. It is not known whether lower levels of oral supplementation can sufficiently saturate the IRBP carrier system. Certainly, 100 mg per kilogram per day of oral vitamin E administration does not cause toxicity.

3. Maintain physiological supplementation with continuous oral vitamin E until inner retinal vessels reach the ora serrata. Retinal development is halted by initial hyperoxygenation resulting from premature birth, with or without oxygen supplementation. After a variable length of time, the rate of retinal maturation toward the ora serrata proceeds at a rate slower than that in utero. Therefore, the duration of vitamin E supplementation cannot be determined by the simple addition of gestational age at birth and post-partum age. Figure 9–2 proposes guidelines for the minimal duration of vitamin E supplementation at various birth weights and gestational ages. These guidelines cannot be used arbitrarily without careful retinal examinations. Examinations must confirm that the inner retinal vessels have reached the temporal ora serrata, and thus, that all activated spindle cells have disappeared from the peripheral retina.

4. To maintain adult physiological plasma vitamin E levels, utilize 10 mg per kilogram of IM vitamin E (aqueous tocopherol) every third day, in alternate thighs or 3 mg per kilogram of slow IV vitamin E (aqueous tocopherol) every day if the infant is NPO three days or more.

5. Give 3 early IM injections of vitamin E (aqueous tocopherol), on days 1, 2, and 4, of 15 mg per kilogram, 10 mg per kilogram, and 10 mg per kilogram respectively, in alternate thighs, to impede the development of severe intraventricular hemorrhage.

6. Administer vitamin K routinely to prevent a bleeding diathesis.

7. Do not administer oral vitamin E simultaneously with iron.

These recommendations are not absolutes and must be adjusted in accordance with carefully monitored plasma vitamin E levels. They are not intended as legal definitions to establish a standard of care, but are intended to achieve mean target plasma vitamin E levels of approximately 2.5 mg per deciliter to obtain efficacy. Exceeding the 3.5 mg per deciliter plasma vitamin E level as warned by the F.D.A.[40,41] by small increments for short time periods has not been shown to be related to toxicity.

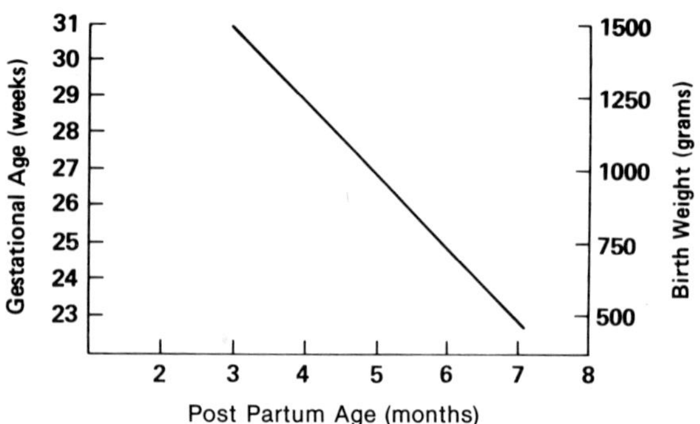

Figure 9–2 Graph demonstrating the relationship between gestational age in weeks (left vertical axis) and birth weight in grams (right vertical axis) and the post-partum ages proposed as guidelines for the minimum duration of continuous vitamin E supplementation. These clinical estimates are not meant to replace careful retinal examinations necessary to document that inner retinal vessels have reached the temporal ora serrata, indicating that there are no activated spindle cells remaining in the retina.

Because the appropriate oral, IM, and slow IV products are not commercially available, the proposed recommendations constitute an ideal protocol that cannot be implemented at the present time. (Fig. 9–3).

Faced with this reality, the practicing neonatologist must decide whether to utilize vitamin E to suppress the development of severe ROP. Then the specialist must decide whether Aquasol E (diluted and given in 4 divided doses with its propylene glycol carrier), or whether the vitamin E solution described in Table 9–6 (given as a single dose in medium-chain triglycerides) should be utilized as an oral supplement. If the decision is made to give early and continuous vitamin E supplementation, and if the nursery does not feed its smallest infants in the first weeks of life, the clinician must utilize MVI-Pediatric by slow IV route for initial vitamin E supplementation. When oral medications are contraindicated, MVI-Pediatric by slow IV route will be required to maintain continuous vitamin E supplementation.

POTENTIAL ANTIOXIDANT PROTECTION FOR INFANTS OF 27-WEEKS GESTATIONAL AGE OR LESS

There are two classes of antioxidants: (1) preventive or primary antioxidants, which reduce the rate of initiation of free radical chains and convert free-radicals to innocuous products; and (2) chain breaking or secondary antioxidants, which trap the chain propagating peroxyl radicals, thereby reducing the length of the auto-oxidation chains (Fig. 9–4).

Vitamin E

Vitamin E is a chain breaking antioxidant whose function is to protect lipid membranes from undesirable auto-oxidation. Since vitamin E is fat-soluble, retinal maturation determines the extent of IRPB present in the subretinal space, to allow threshold levels of vitamin E to be transported to protect spindle cells. Vitamin E is a "panacea" to suppress the development of severe ROP only for those infants of 28-weeks gestational age or more who do not suffer from hypoxia or hypothermia. Endogenous vitamin E levels in the

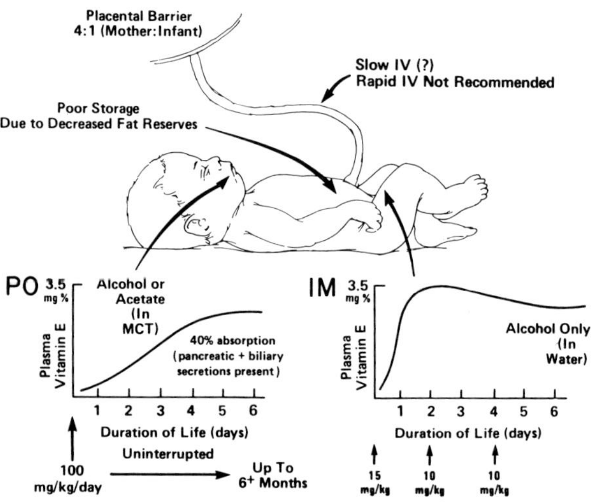

Figure 9–3 Schematic diagram showing the vitamin E status of the deficient preterm infant and the current recommendations for vitamin E supplementation based on the spindle cell pathogenesis of ROP. Graphs summarize the relative relationship between plasma vitamin E (mg/dl) and days of life for initial, oral and IM routes of administration. PO: the slow plasma rise in the first week of life is representative of initial, oral administration of vitamin E in medium-chain triglycerides (MCT) (100 mg per kilogram per day). The 40 percent absorption in the presence of pancreatic and biliary secretions is highly variable and dependent on gestational age. This is the recommended initial route of administration to suppress the development of severe ROP. IM: the rapid, nonpeaking plasma rise in the first week of life is representative of initial, IM administration of vitamin E in water (15, 10, and 10 mg per kilogram on days 1, 2, and 4, respectively, in alternate thighs. This is the recommended initial route of administration to suppress the development of severe intraventricular hemorrhage (IVH). If the infant must be NPO for longer than 3 days, 10 mg per kilogram IM every third day in alternate thighs are recommended. IV: initial slow IV may be efficacious; initial rapid IV is *not* recommended. Oral, IM, and slow IV initial routes of administration are equally efficacious in protecting spindle cells from the initial cluster of oxidative insults. However, initial slow IV has not been shown to suppress the development of severe IVH. The Food and Drug Administration has warned that levels above 3.5 mg per deciliter should be avoided.[40,41]

Selenium

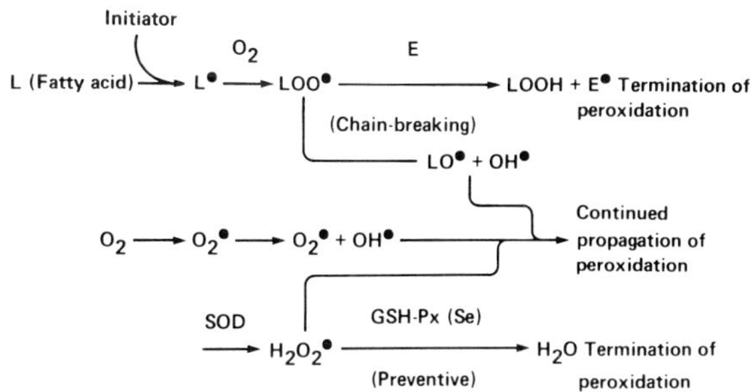

Figure 9–4 Schematic diagram of biochemical pathways involving free radicals. Vitamin E [E] is a chain breaking antioxidant. Selenium, a component of the glutathione peroxidase enzyme system [GSH-Px(Se)], is a preventive antioxidant. SOD = superoxide dismutase. Free radicals = heavy dots.

peripheral retina increase with increasing gestational age (Fig. 9–5).[42] This development parallels the radial distribution of IRBP as photoreceptors mature toward the ora serrata. Exogenous, postnatal vitamin E supplementation produces minimal retinal vitamin E elevation in infants of 27-weeks gestational age or less, but substantial retinal vitamin E elevation in infants of 28-weeks gestational age or more (Fig. 9–5).[42] Parameters of the vitamin E antioxidant system are summarized in Table 9–7.

Selenium is an essential component of the enzyme glutathione peroxidase (four atoms of selenium per mole of enzyme). Glutathione peroxidase catalyzes the reduction of hydrogen peroxide to water, thus preventing peroxidative damage. Preterm infants are deficient in selenium at birth, with plasma levels of 0.06 μg%,[43-47] owing to a 3:2 placental barrier. These levels subsequently decrease in the neonatal period.[44,45,47] There is a wide margin of safety when selenium supplementation is given orally, and toxicity occurs only in endemic areas with unusually high selenium content in the soil.[48] IM preparations can be utilized when the oral route is not appropriate; however, selenium by the slow IV route is known to be rapidly cleared from the plasma.[49]

Glutathione peroxidase is present in human retinal cytosol as early as 20-weeks gestational age, when IRBP is still restricted to a tiny, central region around the optic disc.[21,22] Thus, additional antioxidant protection needed for infants of 27-weeks gestational age or less may be obtained through minimal selenium supplementation. The selenium-dependent glutathione peroxidase [GSH-Px(Se)] antioxidant enzyme system may suppress the development of severe ROP in infants of 27-weeks gestational age or less who do not suffer from hypoxia

TABLE 9–6 **Comparison of Oral Preparations Used in Clinical Studies at Texas Children's Hospital.***

Hoffmann-LaRoche dl-alpha-tocopherol (1980 Study)[18]	Aquasol E dl-alpha-tocopheryl Acetate (1981 Study)[17]	TCH Preparation dl-alpha-tocopheryl Acetate in Medium-Chain Triglycerides (1982 Study)[23]
dl-alpha-tocopherol	dl alpha tocopheryl acetate	dl-alpha-tocopheryl acetate (26.8 g)†
Polysorbate 80	Polysorbate 80	Polysorbate 80 (2.8 g=2.6 ml)
Propylene glycol	Propylene glycol	MCT Oil (60 g=63.6 ml)‡
Distilled water	Distilled water	Distilled water (90 ml)
	Sorbitol	
	Oil of Anise	
	Sodium saccharin	
	Imitation butterscotch flavor	
Osmolality: 3,000 mOsm	Osmolality: 3,000 mOsm	Osmolality: 150 mOsm
pH: 6.5	pH: 5.7	pH: 5.4

* Aquasol E is the only commercially available oral preparation.
† Hoffmann-LaRoche investigational drug containing 500 IU vitamin E/g compounded with gelatin and 3% silicon dioxide, 0.2% sorbic acid and 0.1% sodium benzoate. Prepared as above emulsion contains 100 IU/1.5 ml with a total volume of 201 ml. It is stable for at least 6 weeks if refrigerated and protected from light.
‡ Medium-chain triglycerides.

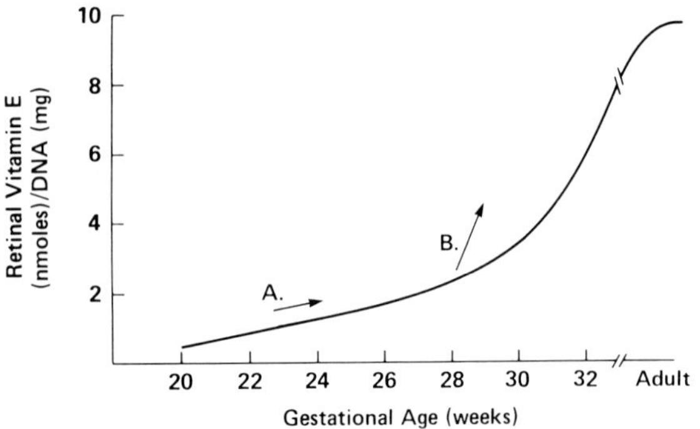

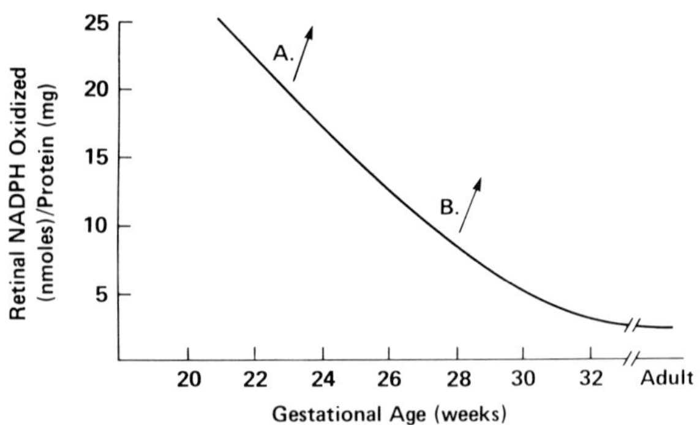

Figure 9–5 Graph summarizing the relationship of peripheral, avascular retinal vitamin E levels (nmoles/mg retinal DNA) to gestational age (weeks) of preterm infants, and to adults. Endogenous retinal vitamin E levels increase as a function of gestational age (n = 6) and are high in adults (n = 8). These preliminary data are courtesy of JC Nielsen and RE Anderson.[42] Endogenous retinal vitamin E levels are lowest in infants currently at greatest risk for developing severe ROP. This antioxidant system is of secondary importance as compared to the selenium-dependent glutathione peroxidase antioxidant enzyme system (Fig. 9–6 and Table 9–7) in infants of 27-weeks gestational age or less who are at highest risk in the current ROP epidemic (Fig. 9–7). The clinical relevance in preventing the development of severe ROP of the vitamin E antioxidant system increases as retinal development occurs. The rise in endogenous vitamin E levels lags behind, but parallels, the appearance of the retinal vitamin E carrier protein (IRBP), which is secreted by photoreceptors when they first form outer segment discs. Line A is an example of an infant of 27-weeks gestational age or less who received IM and oral vitamin E supplementation. There is no significant increase in retinal levels of vitamin E above the baseline. This explains why supplementation is nonefficacious despite adequate plasma vitamin E levels. In these infants, IRBP is restricted to a central domain such that the majority of the spindle cells are not transretinal to a source of antioxidant protection. In contrast, line B is an example of an infant of 28-weeks gestational age or more who received IM and oral vitamin E supplementation. There is a substantial increase in retinal levels of vitamin E above the baseline. This explains why supplementation is efficacious, as anticipated, with adequate plasma vitamin E levels. In these infants, IRBP encroaches on the ora serrata, and the majority of the spindle cells are transretinal to a source of antioxidant protection. These data explain the clinical "break point" of 27 weeks, relating to the efficacy for vitamin E supplementation in protecting the preterm retina from the development of severe ROP.

Figure 9–6 Graph summarizing the relationship of retinal selenium-dependent glutathione peroxidase (expressed as retinal NADPH oxidized in nmoles/mg retinal protein) to gestational age (weeks) of preterm infants and to adults. Endogenous, retinal, selenium-dependent glutathione peroxidase [GSH-Px(Se)] levels decrease as a function of gestational age (n = 20) and are low in adults (n = 2). These preliminary data are courtesy of Dr. Helen W. Lane. Endogenous retinal GSH-Px(Se) levels are highest in infants currently at greatest risk for developing severe ROP. This antioxidant system is of primary importance as compared to the vitamin E system (Fig. 9–5 and Table 9–7) in infants of 27-weeks gestational age or less who are at highest risk in the current ROP epidemic (Fig. 9–7). The clinical relevance in preventing the development of severe ROP of the GSH-Px(Se) antioxidant system decreases as retinal development occurs. Selenium is water soluble, and thus, no carrier protein is required. This makes selenium retinal uptake independent of gestational age and retinal maturation. Line A is an example of an infant of 27-weeks gestational age or less who received slow IV infusion of selenium supplementation. There is a substantial increase in retinal levels of GSH-Px(Se) above the baseline. This explains why selenium supplementation is potentially efficacious in providing antioxidant protection to spindle cells for those smallest infants in whom vitamin E uptake is morphologically impossible. Line B is an example of an infant of 28-weeks gestational age or more who received slow IV infusion of selenium supplementation. There is a substantial increase in retinal levels of GSH-Px(Se) above the baseline. This explains why selenium supplementation is potentially efficacious in these larger infants. However, the vitamin E antioxidant system is already adequate in these infants if they receive oral, IM, or slow IV vitamin E supplementation. Additional selenium supplementation is not mandatory to provide antioxidant protection to spindle cells.

or hypothermia. Endogenous retinal GSH-Px(Se) levels decrease with increasing gestational age (Dr. Helen W. Lane, personal communication) (Fig. 9–6). Exogenous prenatal or postnatal selenium supplementation can produce substantial retinal GSH-Px(Se) elevation in infants of all gestational ages (Dr. Helen W. Lane, personal communication) (Fig. 9–6). Parameters of the GSH-Px(Se) antioxidant enzyme system are summarized in Table 9–7.

An Antioxidant "Cocktail"

In the retina, the anaerobic GSH-Px(Se) antioxidant enzyme system is decreasing, while the aerobic vitamin E antioxidant system is increasing as a function of gestational age. This transition anticipates the change from the low oxygen tension in utero to the high oxygen tension of ambient air or oxygen supplementation following birth. Vitamin E supplementation has diminished efficacy in very-low-birth-weight infants. Selenium supplementation may be efficacious in these infants but should only be necessary until photoreceptors begin secreting IRBP. As retinal maturation occurs slowly postnatally, vitamin E supplementation alone will be sufficient and should continue until inner retinal vessels reach the ora serrata. Thus, the concept of an antioxidant "cocktail" designed for infants of specific gestational ages must evolve. For infants weighing 1,000 grams or less at birth, who are currently at highest risk of develop-

TABLE 9–7   Comparison of the Vitamin E and Selenium-Dependent Glutathione Peroxidase Antioxidant Systems

Parameter	Vitamin E System	Selenium-Dependent Glutathione Peroxidase System
Deficiency in preterm infants	Yes	Yes
Active form	d-alpha-tocopherol	l–selenium
Predominant type of metabolism protected	Aerobic metabolism	Anaerobic metabolism
Solubility	Fat soluble	Water soluble
Required carrier protein	Low-density lipoprotein (LDLP) in plasma and interstitial retinol binding protein (IRBP) in subretinal space because of fat solubility	No carrier required because of water solubility
Endogenous retinal levels as a function of gestational age	Increases with gestational age (retinal maturation) (Fig. 9–5)	Decreases with gestational age (retinal maturation) (Fig. 9–6)
Potential for infant post-partum supplementation	Gestational-age (retinal maturation) dependent because of IRBP requirement: infants >1,000 g birth weight will benefit most	Gestational-age (retinal maturation) independent because no carrier required: infants ≤1,000 g birth weight will benefit most
Potential efficacy related to initial route of administration	Oral, IM and slow IV are efficacious and safe in preventing the development of severe ROP	Unknown
Dosage and form	Dependent on route of administration because of carrier requirement	Independent of route of administration because of no carrier requirement
Comparison of plasma and retinal levels	Dependent on route of administration because initial IV levels may reflect inactive tocopherol within plasma and within inner retinal vessels in first hours. Initial oral and IM levels reflect only active tocopherol within plasma (LDLP) and within retinal parenchyma (IRBP) (Fig. 9–1)	Independent of route of administration because of no carrier requirement
Maternal: infant placental barrier	4:1 plasma vitamin E ratio	3:2 plasma selenium ratio
Potential for maternal pre-partum supplementation	Not feasible because of placental barrier	Feasible because of placental equilibrium

ing severe ROP, such a ''cocktail'' would be weighted primarily toward selenium initially. With increasing postnatal age, the ''cocktail'' would gradually change and be weighted primarily toward vitamin E.

THE FUTURE CHALLENGE

Historically, nursery practices have altered the retinal oxidant antioxidant balance and, in turn, have changed the number of infants who are at risk of developing severe ROP (Fig. 9–7). Following the introduction of oxygen into intensive care nurseries, Terry reported the first case of RLF in 1942.[50] An epidemic of RLF ensued, until the association between ROP and oxygen administration was suggested by the observations of Campbell in 1951.[2] The epidemic ended and the controversy that surrounded the identification of this risk factor was resolved through the multicenter results of Kinsey, et al in 1956.[3] The original epidemic of ROP primarily involved infants who weighed more than 1,000 grams at birth; the survival rate for infants weighing between 750 and 1,000 grams at birth was then less than 8 percent. Severe ROP developed in these large infants because the few spindle cells in the small peripheral retina were maximally activated in an uncontrolled oxygen environment. With judicious curtailment of oxygen, the infants who remained at risk were primarily in the 1,500-gram or less group.

Following the higher survival rate of low-birth-weight infants, as a result of technological advances and the concomitant increase in ROP, the association between ROP and antioxidant deficiency were suggested by Johnson, et al in 1974,[14] and substantiated by Hittner, et al in 1981,[18] Finer, et al in 1982,[19] and Schaffer, et al in 1986.[16] Vitamin E has been recognized as an essential nutrient for the preterm infant. It is necessary to recognize vitamin E as an essential antioxidant for the preterm infant, especially effective in infants weighing 1,000 grams or more at birth. Then early and continuous vita-

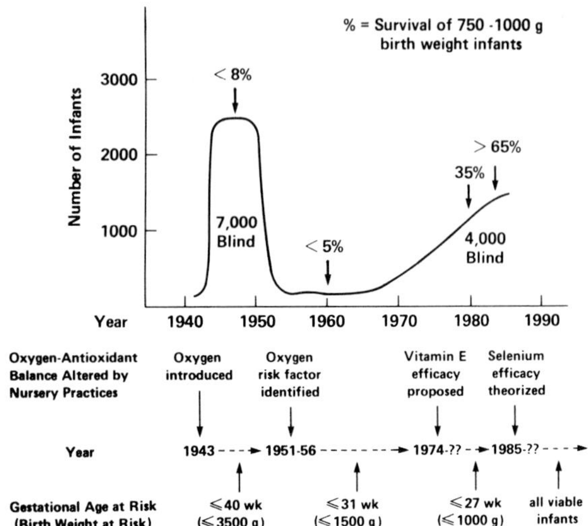

Figure 9–7 Historical review of oxygen-antioxidant balance as it relates to both the gestational ages (birth weights) of infants at risk for ROP and to the number of totally blind infants in the U.S.A. The percentage of surviving infants who weighed between 750 and 1,000 grams at birth are given at four critical years (%). The first epidemic occurred between 1943 and 1952 (7,000 blind infants). The current epidemic (since 1970) has blinded 4,000 infants to date. These two epidemics are shown in relation to alterations in nursery practices and to gestational ages (birth weights) of infants at risk for developing severe ROP. In the early 1940s, oxygen was introduced, and in 1942, the first case of ROP was reported. At that time, all infants of 40-weeks gestational age or less, weighing 3,500 grams or less at birth, were at risk for ROP. In 1951, oxygen was suggested as a primary ROP risk factor. Thus, the first epidemic ended. In 1956, oxygen was established conclusively as a primary ROP risk factor. From that time, with judicious curtailment of oxygen administration, only infants of 31-weeks gestational age or less, weighing 1,500 grams or less at birth, were at risk for developing severe ROP. In 1974, efficacy was reproposed for physiological supplementation of the fat-soluble antioxidant, vitamin E. With appropriate vitamin E administration, only infants of 27-weeks gestational age or less, weighing 1,000 grams or less at birth, are at risk for developing severe ROP. In 1985, efficacy was theorized for the physiological supplementation of the water-soluble component of the glutathione peroxidase antioxidant enzyme, selenium. In the future, with appropriate selenium administration, all viable infants who do not sustain intrauterine or postpartum hypoxia or hypothermia may be protected from severe ROP, which develops secondary to postnatal, oxygen-related ROP risk factors. Thus, the second epidemic may end.

min E supplementation (slow IV, IM and oral vitamin E), combined with the increasing baseline of plasma vitamin E levels in premature infants—owing to breast milk, supplemented formulas, multivitamins, and slow, parenteral nutrition—can reduce the birth weight of those infants who remain primarily at risk of developing severe ROP, from 1,500 grams or less to 1,000 grams or less. It should be realized that even given the availability and utilization of early and continuous vitamin E supplementation, the magnitude of the current epidemic will not be substantially affected. This is owing to the fact that the great majority of the infants who are developing severe ROP weigh 1,000 grams or less at birth, since the

survival rate of those weighing between 750 and 1,000 grams at birth exceeds 65 percent. Severe ROP develops in these infants because the large peripheral retina contains huge numbers of spindle cells that are in an unfavorable oxidant-antioxidant balance, even with judicious oxygen curtailment and early, continuous vitamin E supplementation. The current epidemic will end only after spindle cells are protected by antioxidants whose retinal uptake is not gestational age dependent.

REFERENCES

1. Slater TF, Riley PA. Free-radical damage in retrolental fibroplasia. Lancet 1970; 2:467.
2. Campbell K. Intensive oxygen therapy as a possible cause of retrolental fibroplasia: a clinical approach. Med J Aust 1951; 2:48–50.
3. Kinsey VE. Retrolental fibroplasia: cooperative study of retrolental fibroplasia and the use of oxygen. Arch Ophthalmol 1956; 56:481–543.
4. Farrell PM. Vitamin E deficiency in preterm infants. J Pediatr 1979; 95:869–872.
5. Kretzer FL, Mehta RS, Johnson AT, Hunter DG, Brown ES, Hittner HM. Vitamin E protects against retinopathy of prematurity through action on spindle cells. Nature 1984; 309:793–795.
6. Hittner HM, Kretzer FL. Retinopathy of prematurity: a new look at pathogenesis, prevention, and treatment. In: Chiswick ML, ed. Recent advances in perinatal medicine. London: Churchill Livingston, 1985; 2:145–163.
7. Kretzer FL, Hittner HM. Initiating events in the development of retinopathy of prematurity. In: Silverman WA, Flynn JT, eds. Retinopathy of prematurity. Boston: Blackwell Scientific Publication, 1986; 121–152.
8. Kretzer FL, McPherson AR, Rudolph AJ, Hittner HM. Pathogenic mechanism of retinopathy of prematurity; a controversial explanation for the efficacy of oral and intramuscular vitamin E supplementation and cryotherapy. Bull N Y Acad Med 1985; 61:883–900.
9. Puklin JE, Simon RM, Ehrenkranz RA. Influence on retrolental fibroplasia of intramuscular vitamin E administration during respiratory distress syndrome. Ophthalmology 1982; 89:96–102.
10. Ehrenkranz RA, Puklin JE. Letters to the editor: RLF and vitamin E. Ophthalmology 1982; 89:988–989.
11. Milner RA, Bell E, Blanchette V, Ling E, Watts JL, Zipursky A. Vitamin E supplement in under 1,500 gram neonates. Retinopathy of Prematurity Conference. Ross Laboratories, December 4–6, 1981; 703–716.
12. Hittner HM, Godio LB, Speer ME, Rudolph AJ, Taylor MM, Blifeld C, Kretzer FL. Retrolental fibroplasia: further clinical evidence and ultrastructural support for efficacy of vitamin E in the preterm infant. Pediatrics 1983; 71:423–432.
13. Finer NN, Schindler RF, Peters KL, Grant GD. Vitamin E and retrolental fibroplasia: improved visual outcome with early vitamin E. Ophthalmology 1983; 90:428–434.
14. Johnson L, Schaffer D, Boggs TR. The premature infant, vitamin E deficiency and retrolental fibroplasia. Am J Clin Nutr 1974; 27:1158–1173.
15. Johnson L, Schaffer D, Quinn G, Goldstein D, Mathis MJ, Otis C, Boggs TR. Vitamin E supplementation and the retinopathy of prematurity. Ann N Y Acad Sci 1982; 393:473–494.
16. Schaffer DL, Johnson L, Quinn GE, et al. Vitamin E and retinopathy of prematurity: the ophthalmologist's perspective. In: Flynn JT, Phelps DL, eds. Birth defects original article series: retinopathy of prematurity: update 1985. New York: Alan R. Liss, 1986. In press.
17. Phelps DL, Rosenbaum A, Isenberg SJ, Leake RD, Dorey F. Effect of IV tocopherol (vit E) on retinopathy of prematurity. Pediatr Res 1985; 19:357A.

18. Hittner HM, Godio LB, Rudolph AJ, Adams JM, Garcia-Prats JA, Friedman Z, Kautz JA, Monaco WA. Retrolental fibroplasia: efficacy of vitamin E in a double-blind clinical study of preterm infants. N Eng J Med 1981; 305:1365–1371.

19. Finer NN, Grant G, Schindler RF, Hill GB, Peters KL. Effect of intramuscular vitamin E on frequency and severity of retrolental fibroplasia: a controlled trial. Lancet 1982; 1:1087–1091.

20. Hittner HM, Rudolph AJ, Kretzer FL. Suppression of severe retinopathy of prematurity with vitamin E supplementation: ultrastructural mechanism of clinical efficacy. Ophthalmology 1984; 91:1512–1523.

21. Johnson AT, Kretzer FL, Hittner HM, Glazebrook PA, Bridges CDB, Lam DML. Development of the subretinal space in the preterm human eye: ultrastructural and immunocytochemical studies. J Compar Neurol 1984; 233:497–505.

22. Johnson AT, Kretzer FL. Interstitial retinol binding protein in the developing human retina: a proposed explanation for vitamin E suppression of retinopathy of prematurity. In: Bridges CDB, Adler AJ, eds. The interphotoreceptor matrix in health and disease. New York: Alan R. Liss, 1985; 251–277.

23. Hittner HM, Speer ME, Rudolph AJ, Blifeld C, Chadda P, Holbein MEB, Godio LB, Kretzer FL. Retrolental fibroplasia and vitamin E in the preterm infant: comparison of oral versus intramuscular:oral administration. Pediatrics 1984; 73:238–249.

24. Bhat R, Braun RJ. Retinal and tissue vitamin E kinetics in the newborn kitten following vitamin E administration. Pediatr Res 1984; 18:149A.

25. Thellman C, Shireman RB. Major route of vitamin E transport into cells: low density lipoprotein receptor pathway. Fed Proc 1984; 43:691A.

26. Fong SL, Liou GI, Landers RA, et al. Characterization, localization, and biosynthesis of an interstitial retinol-binding glycoprotein in the human eye. J Neurochem 1984; 42:1667–1676.

27. Gallo-Torres HE. Transport and metabolism. In: Machlin LJ, ed. Vitamin E: a comprehensive treatise. New York: Marcel Dekker. 1980: 193–267.

28. Committee on Nutrition: Nutritional needs of low-birth-weight infants. Pediatrics 1977; 60:519–530.

29. Committee on Nutrition: Vitamin and mineral supplement needs in normal children in the United States. Pediatrics 1980; 66:1015–1021.

30. Committee on Nutrition: Nutritional needs of low-birth-weight infants. Pediatrics 1985; 75:976–986.

31. Lammi-Keefe CJ, Jensen RG. Fat-soluble vitamins in human breast milk. Nutrition Rev 1984; 42:365–371.

32. Lemons JA, Maisels MJ. Commentary: Vitamin E—How much is too much? Pediatrics 1985; 76:625–627.

33. Machlin LJ. Vitamin E. In: Machlin LJ, ed. Handbook of vitamins: nutritional, biochemical and clinical aspects. New York: Marcel Dekker, 1984; 99–145.

34. Horwitt MK, Elliott WH, Kanjananggulpan P, Fitch CD. Serum concentrations of alpha-tocopherol after ingestion of various vitamin E preparations. Am J Clin Nutr 1984; 40:240–245.

35. Bell EF, Brown EJ, Milner R, Sinclair JC, Zipursky A. Vitamin E absorption in small premature infants. Pediatrics 1979; 63:830–832.

36. Williams ML, Oski FA. Vitamin E status of infants fed formula containing medium chain triglycerides. J Pediatr 1980; 96:70–72.

37. Pantoja A, Ukrainski C, Belenky D, Grinberg A, Hulac P, Mathis J. Vitamin E (VE) kinetics in infants < 1500 grams: intramuscular (IM) vs. oral administration. Pediatr Res 1984; 18:157A.

38. Chiswick ML, Johnson M. Woodhall C, Gowland M, Davies J, Toner N, Sims DG. Protective effect of vitamin E (dl-alpha-tocopherol) against intraventricular haemorrhage in premature babies. Br Med J 1983; 287:81–84.

39. Speer ME, Blifeld C, Rudolph AJ, Chadda P, Holbein MEB, Hittner HB. Intraventricular hemorrhage and vitamin E in the very low birth weight infant: evidence for efficacy of early intramuscular administration. Pediatrics 1984; 74:1107–1112.

40. Sobel S, Gueriguian J, Troendle G, Nevius E. Correspondence: vitamin E in retrolental fibroplasia. N Engl J Med 1982; 306:867.

41. Hittner HM, Kretzer FL, Rudolph AJ, Holbein MEB, Troendle G, Sobel S. Correspondence: vitamin E in retrolental fibroplasia. N Engl J Med 1983; 309:669–670.

42. Nielson J, Anderson R. Vitamin E levels in preterm infant retinas. Presentation at Baylor College of Medicine, 22nd Annual Ophthalmology Alumni Association Meeting. June 8, 1985.

43. Rhead WJ, Cary EE, Allaway WH, Saltzstein SL, Schrauzer GN. The vitamin E and selenium status of infants and the sudden infant death syndrome. Bioinorg Chem 1972; 1:289–294.

44. Gross S. Hemolytic anemia in premature infants: relationship to vitamin E, selenium, glutathione peroxidase, and erythrocyte lipids. Semin Hematol 1976; 13:187–199.

45. Lombeck I, Kasparek K, Harbisch HD, Feinendegen LE, Bremer HJ. The selenium state of healthy children. I. serum selenium concentration at different ages; activity of glutathione peroxidase of erythrocytes at different ages; selenium content of food of infants. Eur J Pediatr 1977; 125:81–88.

46. Rudolph N. Wong SL. Selenium and glutathione peroxidase activity in maternal and cord plasma and red cells. Pediat Res 1978; 12:789–792.

47. Verlinden M, van Sprundel M, Van der Auwera JC, Eylinbosch WJ. The selenium status of Belgian population groups. Biol Trac Elem Res 1983; 5:103–113.

48. Yang G, Wang S, Zhou R, Sun S. Endemic selenium intoxication of humans in China. Am J Clin Nutr 1983; 37:872–881.

49. Van Rij AM, McKenzie JM, Thomson CD, Robinson MF. Selenium supplementation in total parenteral nutrition. J Parenteral Enteral Nutr 1981; 5:120–124.

50. Terry TL. Extreme prematurity and fibroblastic overgrowth of persistent vascular sheath behind each crystalline lens. I. Preliminary report. Am J Ophthalmol 1942; 25:203–204.

Baruch A. Brody, Ph.D.

THE ETHICAL AND LEGAL BACKGROUND FOR OUR EXAMINATION OF THE VITAMIN E STUDY

The fundamental ethical problem in all human experimentation is really very simple. On the one hand, tremendous benefits result from human experimentation. The advances in medical knowledge and the resulting improvement in patient care mandates, not merely permits, the required medical experimentation. On the other hand, there are always risks involved in experimentation, and it is wrong, in any case, to use people as subjects to help advance knowledge without ensuring that they participate knowingly. The ethical problem is then how to balance the legitimate moral concerns that mandate and challenge the legitimacy of experimentation upon human subjects.

The crucial sections[1] of the Code of Federal Regulations strike this balance with two major requirements for legitimate research involving human subjects. *a* The risks to the subject are minimized, and are reasonable in relation to the anticipated benefits to the subjects and the importance of the expected resulting knowledge. *b* Informed consent is obtained from the subjects or their legally authorized representative. Such informed consent eliminates the problem of using people without their permission. Requirement *a* does not eliminate risk to the subject, but it at least attempts to minimize it and to make the risk worthwhile. Similar provisions are found in the World Medical Association's Declaration of Helsinki[2] and most other recent codes governing experimentation upon human subjects.

Not all cases of human experimentation are alike. Some are complicated by additional factors that require careful moral consideration. We are concerned here with studies evaluating the efficacy of oral vitamin E in prevent

ing the development of retrolental fibroplasia (RLF), involving at least two such complicating factors. First, the human subjects were preterm infants incapable of making any decisions concerning their care. Moreover, the parents, the infants' legally authorized representatives, were often just coming to grips with the problem of having small preterm infants and might have had tremendous difficulties in making any intelligent decisions. Second, the investigators were also involved in providing professional care to the patients. This might give rise to a conflict of interest, because there might be cases in which the research needs would conflict with the best interests of their patients.

The first complication has, after many years of delay, finally been addressed in recent additions to the Code of Federal Regulations.[3] As soon as it involves anything more than minimal risk, research on children is restricted to cases in which the research subjects, or others with the condition are expected to benefit. If it is only others with the condition who are expected to benefit. If it is only others with the condition who are expected to benefit, the research is allowable only if the risk is a minor increment over normal minimal risk. Parents and/or guardians may not volunteer children to be placed at substantial risk.

The second complication has not really been addressed in the federal regulations. It was, however, addressed in the World Medical Association's Declaration of Helsinki, in which the following crucial passage occurs:

> The doctor can combine medical research with professional care, the objective being the acquisition of new medical knowledge, only to the extent that medical research is justified by its potential diagnostic or therapeutic value for the patient.

This claim, as it stands, seems too strong, for it rules out all clinical research that does not directly benefit the subject himself, even if the subject is exposed to no more than normal risk. To avoid the conflict of interest between the physician as care provider and the physician as experimentor, particularly in research involving infants, it seems fair to say that doctors treating infants can combine research with professional care only with the parents' consent and only if an outside institutional review board agrees, either that the risks are minimal, or that the risks are justified by the potential diagnostic or therapeutic value to the patient. This is a slight strengthening of the new federal regulation governing research for infants, since I am ruling out lesser increments of risk, when the patients are minors who will not directly benefit. This strengthening of the regulation seems a just way of dealing with the conflict of interest problem posed by clinical research involving infants.

A third complication requires very careful consideration. This is the moral question of using control groups in randomized clinical trials. A randomized clinical trial, such as the research with which we shall be concerned, involves the following factors: *a* the treatment group receives the therapy being tested, while the control group being treated in otherwise the same fashion does not. *b* individual subjects are assigned randomly to the treatment or the control group. *c* where feasible, neither the investigator nor the subject knows until the conclusion of the study who is in which group; such studies are called double-blind studies. Many commentators have expressed moral doubts about one or another aspect of double-blind randomized clinical trials. Some[4] claim that randomization introduces dehumanization; others[5] claim that randomization cannot be effectively explained to the patient. These are not, to my mind, the crucial issues. We need to consider whether the randomized clinical trial might not be imposing illegitimate risks upon the control group.

We rarely conduct a randomized clinical trial without some background indications of the safety and efficacy of the treatment being studied. In some cases, we have indications that two or more competing forms of treatment have advantages and disadvantages, but no indication of which is more favorable. Each group in the proposed study gets one of these treatments, and each patient, or guardian, consents, in an informed fashion, to random inclusion in the study to determine the best form of treatment. These cases involve no problems either with the control group or with the experimental group; to my mind, the scientific benefits to the consenting patient outweigh the alleged dehumanization of randomization.

In other cases, we have background knowledge indicating that a proposed treatment produces some bene-fits and some risks, but we have no clear indication of their respective weights. The treatment group gets the benefits but runs the risks, whereas the control group foregoes the benefits and avoids the risks. As long as each patient, or guardian, consents in an informed fashion to random inclusion in the study, there is still no problem.

But there is a third situation, in which our background knowledge indicates a form of treatment is advantageous, but conclusive statistical proof of its advantage is not yet available. This can arise before or in the middle of a study, if it is not a double-blind study, or if the partial results are independently analyzed. Can we justifiably continue to withhold the treatment from the control group, thereby imposing this risk upon them? In particular, can we do this in a randomized clinical study involving infants? Can we do this if the treatment could avoid mortality or serious morbidity, e.g., blindness?

These questions are not explicitly addressed in the federal regulations, and they are, I suspect, often neglected by institutional review boards. We are used to double-blind clinical studies as the paradigm of good scientific medicine, and we usually think of the risks to the treatment group and not to the control group, so the neglect of these questions is not surprising. To be sure, some ethicists have commented on them, but I see little evidence of sufficient awareness of the problem. The Code of Helsinki[2] is satisfied with the following claim:

> In any medical study, every patient—including those in a control group, if any—should be assured of the best proven diagnostic and therapeutic method.

Since the method is not "proven" until the study is completed, the Code of Helsinki would presumably allow double-blind, randomized clinical trials even in the cases we are now considering. But I have my severe doubts, for two reasons.

First, I doubt that any parent or guardian of a patient, if he were truly informed, would consent in such a case to randomization. Suppose we were to tell him or her the following: our background information indicates, but does not yet conclusively prove, that this new form of treatment will substantially improve your child's chance of avoiding death or serious illness. It also fails to indicate any serious risks. Still, we have not yet completely proven the case. Would you allow us, then, to randomly enter your child into the treatment group or the control group, so that we can complete our study and prove or disprove the current indication? In so doing, you could be taking a 50 percent risk; that is, it is likely that your child's chances of dying or becoming seriously ill would be substantially increased. Suppose they understood all of this. Who would, being informed, consent to randomization? Wouldn't all insist upon their children receiving the treatment? Wouldn't you?

Robert Levine[5] suggested that we ask subjects to accept the scientific community's standard of proof, and not to draw any conclusions about what they want based on what the background information indicates. This is supposed to be a way to obtain informed consent. But why should subjects accept those standards? An appropriate standard of proof for scientific acceptance is certainly different from an appropriate standard of proof for a patient desiring treatment. Similarly, Robert Veatch[6] suggested that we ask consent to provide incomplete information, that we ask consent to withhold the indications. But why in the world should subjects agree to that? Would you? I submit, then, that in the cases under consideration, randomized clinical trials cannot be justified, because we cannot obtain appropriate informed consent.

There is a second difficulty with randomized clinical trials when the subjects are children. In the cases we are describing, control group members are at a considerable risk of not getting the probably beneficial therapy and their participation as controls is unlikely to be of benefit to them. In such cases, the latest federal regulations[3] would not allow such research, and our earlier analysis certainly supported those regulations. Even if the children's parents consented—and even if we could convince ourselves that they understood what they were consenting to—their consent would not meet the regulations' requirements.

I conclude, therefore, that the following principles must guide us in evaluating the research on the efficacy of oral vitamin E in preventing RLF in low-birth-weight preterm infants:

1. Research involving children requires the informed consent of their parents or legal guardians.
2. Clinical research involving children, particularly if the investigators are also the treating physicians, requires either that there be no more than minimal risk to the patients participating, or that the risks be outweighed by direct benefits to the patients.
3. As a result of the first two conditions, children cannot be randomly assigned to control groups

once the background knowledge or early study results indicate—even though they do not prove—that there are substantial benefits and few risks to receiving the treatments scheduled for the treatment group.

One cannot, of course, specify the weight of evidence sufficient to stop the randomized clinical study. The best one can say is that the evidence is sufficiently strong to lead most knowledgeable parents to demand the treatment, and to refuse to allow participation in the control group.

THE HISTORIC AND SCIENTIFIC BACKGROUND FOR OUR EXAMINATION OF THE VITAMIN E STUDY

The understanding and treatment of RLF is a fascinating study in scientific advances that create problems resulting in further advances, further problems, and so forth. Terry first identified RLF as a separate condition in the 1940s[7], shortly after it became technologically feasible to deliver high dose oxygen to premature neonates. Even though most low-birth-weight neonates, who most often needed the oxygen, did not survive in those early years, many larger neonates receiving oxygen did, and the incidence of RLF increased. It is estimated that this condition caused 7,000 cases of blindness in the late 1940s and early 1950s. In 1951, Campbell[8] first suggested that intensive oxygen therapy was important in RLF development. A cooperative study headed by V. Everett Kinsey[9] confirmed this suggestion, and oxygen administration was drastically curtailed in the United States. In 1960, however, Avery and Oppenheimer[10] published a study showing that this curtailment of oxygen administration resulted in greater mortality from respiratory distress syndrome. When others confirmed this study, the pendulum swung back to a more liberal use of oxygen. But even with this return, a careful titration of oxygen doses to minimize the concentration was recommended. Despite this careful titration, increased oxygen usage, combined with a much higher survival rate of the very-low-birth-weight neonate, has resulted in an increased incidence of RLF since the mid 1960s. Associated with this were lawsuits charging excessive use of oxygen; so, the issue of RLF became emotionally charged for many neonatologists.

Ironically, as early as 1949,[11] one report suggested that vitamin E supplementation might minimize RLF development; this report was apparently neglected as interest focused on oxygen levels. Lois Johnson's group at the Pennsylvania Hospital first refocused attention on the possible role of vitamin E[12]. In a first trial (1972–1974) and a second trial (1974–1976), they noted important improvements subsequent to prophylactic use of vitamin E. The first study showed a reduction in both incidence and severity, with the differences being significant at P 0.02; since there were no severe cases (Grade III or worse), this was only a study of low grade retinopathy. The second study showed the same trend, but the differences between the groups did not reach the same level of statistical significance. Johnson and associates had been encouraged to carry on further studies by Phelps's and Rosenbaum's[13] work with kittens, which indicated a great usefulness of vitamin E. Apparently, Johnson's group is currently carrying on a large scale randomized clinical study.

Two randomized clinical trials were conducted between 1978 and 1981. Finer and associates[14] tested the effect of intramuscular vitamin E on the frequency and severity of RLF. They simultaneously conducted a second, more confusing, experiment involving oral vitamin E. The crucial finding of the first and more important study was that while the frequencies of active RLF in the treatment and the control groups at discharge were not significantly different, vitamin E did significantly reduce the severity of RLF at a follow-up examination after discharge.

The other randomized, double-blind clinical trial was carried out by Hittner and colleagues at Baylor College of Medicine. Published in 1981,[15] their first study covered neonates who weighed less than 1,500 grams at birth, required supplemental oxygen, and were born between November 1979 and December 1980. This study showed a significant reduction in severe (Grade III or greater) disease in the treatment group receiving oral vitamin E, but no noteworthy reduction in the total incidence of the disease. More importantly, a multivariate analysis showed a significant ability of vitamin E to reduce RLF severity.

In 1981, Hittner and colleagues conducted a second study.[16] All infants who weighed less than 1,500 grams and who received supplementary oxygen received oral vitamin E. The control group was the historical control group for the 1980 study; no randomized control group was used in 1981 because of the 1980 trial's positive results. This decision is at the heart of our critical discussion in the third section of this chapter. Moreover, unlike the 1980 study, the univariate analysis in the 1981 study showed no important reduction in any Grade RLF. However, the more significant multivariate analysis showed

a marked reduction in RLF severity in the treatment group.

While Hittner conducted her clinical studies, a colleague, Frank L. Kretzer[17] carefully studied whole eyes donated by parents of deceased neonates from the control and the treatment groups. He found a new approach to RLF etiology that explained *a* why vitamin E therapy must be initiated at birth, *b* why it only decreases severity but not total incidence, and *c* why it does not help in infants less than 27 weeks of age.

Not all agreed with these findings. A Yale group, headed by Puklin and Ehrenkranz[18] reported in 1982 that vitamin E supplementation did not result in any further reduced incidence of active RLF over the incidence seen with standard neonatal care, which included daily oral vitamin E supplementation. Commentators[19] immediately pointed out that the normal vitamin E supplementation for the control group made that group equivalent to Hittner's treatment group—and made the Yale study irrelevant. A more crucial development was an article by Phelps[20] in the September 1982 issue of *Pediatrics*. She agreed that there is some strength to the claim that vitamin E reduces RLF severity. Her more crucial point, however, was that we need larger samples before we can conclude that there are no safety risks in the use of vitamin E prophylactically. Phelps did not argue that the risks were actually present; the argument was simply that they could not be ruled out, given the sample sizes in the studies carried out. Rosenbaum,[21] Phelps's colleague at Los Angeles, endorsed that view in an important editorial in the *Journal of Pediatrics Ophthalmology and Strabismus*. I quote the crucial argument:

> An estimated 37,000 infants weighing less than 1.5 kg are born annually in the United States. Of these, 22,000 will survive. Demographic analysis by Dr. Dale Phelps has suggested that of these 22,000, 500 will be blind from retrolental fibroplasia, and an additional 1,500 will have significant visual problems due to the disease. The remaining 20,000 infants will not get retrolental fibroplasia, but could be exposed to any proposed treatment such as vitamin E. It is, therefore, essential that efficacy be clearly established and potential side effects elucidated before administering an annual pharmacologic dose of this vitamin to 20,000 infants who would not actually be developing the disease.

Moreover, Rosenbaum announced that two large double-blind, carefully controlled trials are in progress at the Children's Hospital in Philadelphia and the University of California Medical Center in Los Angeles. This announcement also raises a crucial question in our discussion of ethics. Are these studies morally legitimate, given Hittner's argument, or is the Los Angeles group correct in arguing that morality demands these studies?

Where, then, does our story stand? Two major clinical groups are making dramatically opposed ethical claims. Hittner and her Baylor colleagues argue that further double-blind, randomized clinical trials cannot be carried out in light of the data currently available. The Los Angeles group argues, to the contrary, that large-scale trials of this type are morally required. In the final section of this chapter, we will look at this debate from the perspective of the moral and legal structure developed in the first section of the chapter.

THE ETHICS OF RANDOMIZED PATIENT INCLUSION IN A FURTHER VITAMIN E STUDY

We are now ready to consider the two crucial moral issues: *a* did Dr. Hittner and her group correctly claim, in January, 1981, that the data from the first part of their study made it morally impermissible to randomly place more patients in a control group, the goal being to continue a randomized clinical trial testing the efficacy of vitamin E in diminishing RLF severity? *b* is the Los Angeles group right in insisting that further randomized clinical trials are permissible and, in fact, required before the administration of vitamin E becomes standard practice? Obviously, only one group can be right in its claims.

It seems evident to me, in light of the moral and legal backdrop constructed in section one, that Dr. Hittner's group is correct. There are several different ways to argue this claim. The first is simply to apply our third principle in section one to this case: this indicates that Dr. Hittner is correct. Or we can go back to the first principle, informed consent, and argue that it is highly unlikely that any properly informed parent would agree to his child's random inclusion in future studies, rather than simply receiving vitamin E. Alternatively, we can go back to the second principle, or even the slightly weaker principle embodied in the recent additions to the Code of Federal Regulations, and show that either one rules out the study, even if the parents consent.

Principle three holds that children cannot be randomly assigned into control groups once the background knowledge or the early study results indicate—even though they do not prove—that there are substantial

benefits and few risks to receiving the treatment scheduled for the treatment group. Was that condition satisfied at Baylor on January 1, 1981? I submit that it was. The first Baylor study revealed a statistically significant reduction in RLF severity, whether the analysis was univariate or multivariate. (To be sure, the second study did not show a significant result by univariate analysis, but it did by multivariate analysis. So the situation continued unaltered even after the second study.) Clearly, then, the early results indicated with sufficient strength—they were statistically significant—that there were substantial benefits to be had from the treatment scheduled for the treatment group. What about the risks from that treatment? Phelps discussed three possible risks: mortality, necrotizing enterocolitis, and central nervous system (CNS) hemorrhage. She observed that the mortality rates were similar for the control group and the treatment group, that there were no data on necrotizing enterocolitis, and that the Hittner study showed no significant problem with CNS hemorrhage. Her point was simply that there were insufficient figures to rule out these possible side effects. There are no present indications of these risks, so the data at least indicate, although they do not prove, that there are few risks. So according to principle three, Hittner and her group were right.

Let's now look at the likelihood of getting informed parental consent to random assignment of the infants to the study groups. Suppose the parents understand all of the following: your child is very small and requires supplementary oxygen to support breathing. Unfortunately, about 9 percent of such children who survive (2,000 of 22,000 annually) develop severe problems with their eyesight. We are concerned about that. Studies indicate that giving the affected children extra vitamin E from birth helps them see better. Everyone agrees the studies show this; some say they actually prove this, but others say the studies just indicate that vitamin E improves sight. There is, of course, the possibility that vitamin E might cause some harm, but we have not yet detected any. Unfortunately, we have not studied enough cases to rule out the possibility of harm. *a* would you prefer to have your child receive vitamin E, along with its likely although not certain benefit of increasing the chances of seeing well? Remember, there might be some as yet undetected risks. *b* would you prefer to have your child not receive vitamin E, and so avoid those undetected but possible risks? If you choose this option, your child will forego the likely benefit of being helped to avoid eyesight problems. *c* will you permit us to randomly assign your child either to receive or not to receive the vitamin E, so that our study can settle all these questions? In doing so, the benefits and risks to your child will depend upon the group to which your child is randomly assigned.

All of this, I submit, *must* be told parents to obtain their informed consent to random assignment. Further, I submit that once these ramifications are understood, few parents will choose other than the first option. Thus principle one, informed consent, probably entails that a randomized trial could not have been carried out after January 1, 1981. It would be interesting to know exactly what those who are still running randomized clinical trials said to the parents who agreed to enroll their children in them.

Finally, we look at principle two and the even weaker principle embodied in the amended Code of Federal Regulations. Both permitted enrolling a child in a randomized trial, as opposed to giving him vitamin E, if the risks of doing so were minimal. But since doing so means a 50 percent chance of decreasing the probability of avoiding severe RLF, which is not a minimal risk, enrolling a child in the randomized study cannot be justified on that basis. Both principles also permit enrolling the child in a randomized trial, as opposed to giving him vitamin E, if the risks are more than minimal, but the benefits to the patient outweigh the risks. The risks of enrolling the child, as opposed to giving him vitamin E, are serious, and the benefits to the patient—the mere possibility of avoiding the currenty unknown and undetected side effects—are obviously much less significant. Therefore, enrolling the child, as opposed to giving him vitamin E, cannot be justified on that basis.

Finally, the amended Code of Federal Regulation would allow, but I would oppose, enrolling a child in a randomized study, versus giving him vitamin E, if the risks are only slightly more than minimal, and the knowledge to be obtained is vitally important to understanding the patient's disorder or condition. Again, I cannot see how the risk of foregoing the probable prophylactic benefit of vitamin E can be described as only a minor increase over minimal risks.

For all these reasons, I conclude that Dr. Hittner and her group correctly stopped randomized clinical trials in January, 1981. Here is a classic conflict of interest between society's interest in obtaining knowledge and the patient's right to the best care available. Lacking some special further arguments, I conclude that the Baylor group made the right choice.

One final point. From the perspective of scientific medicine, these conclusions are no cause for rejoicing.

The history of medicine reminds us of the value of repeated studies in finally establishing the soundness of a clinical practice. We pay a price in not continuing the vitamin E random studies; the heart of our argument is, however, that the patients pay the price if we do continue, and that must be our first concern.

REFERENCES

1. Code of Federal Regulations: Basic HHS Policy for Protection of Human Subjects 45 CFR 46.
2. Levine RJ. Ethics and Regulation of Clinical Research. Baltimore: Urban and Schwarzenberg, 1981; 287–289.
3. Subpart D of 45 CFR 46, printed in Federal Register. March 8, 1983; 48(46):9818.
4. Fried C. Medical Experimentation: Personal Integrity and Social Policy. New York: American Elsevier, 1974; 50.
5. Levine RJ, Lebacqz K. Some ethical considerations in clinical trials. Clinical Pharmacology and Therapeutics 1979; 25: 728–741.
6. Veatch R. Longitudinal studies, sequential design and grant renewals: what to do with preliminary data. IRB 1979; 1(4):1–3.
7. Terry TL. Extreme prematurity and fibroplastic overgrowth of persistent vascular sheath behind each crystalline lens. Am J Ophthalmol 1942; 25:203–204.
8. Campbell K. Intensive oxygen therapy as a possible cause of retrolental fibroplasia: a clinical approach. Med J Aust 1951; 2:48–50.
9. Kinsey VE. Retrolental fibroplasia: cooperative study of retrolental fibroplasia and the use of oxygen. Arch Ophthalmol 1956; 56:481–543.
10. Avery ME, Oppenheimer EH. Recent increase in mortality from hyaline membrane disease. Journal of Pediatrics 1960; 57: 553–559.
11. Owens WC, Owens EU. Retrolental fibroplasia in premature infants. II. Studies on the prophylaxis of the disease: the use of alpha tocopheryl acetate. Am J Ophthalmol 1949; 32: 1631–1637.
12. Johnson L, Schaffer D, Quinn G, et al. Vitamin E supplementation and the retinopathy of prematurity. NY Acad Sci 1982; 393:473–495.
13. Phelps DL, Rosenbaum A. Vitamin E protection in experimental retrolental fibroplasia in kittens. Clin Res 1976; 24:194A.
14. Finer N, Schindler RF, Peters KL, et al. Vitamin E and retrolental fibroplasia. Improved visual outcome with early vitamin E. Ophthalmology 1983; 90:428–435.
15. Hittner HM, Godio LB, Rudolph AJ. Retrolental fibroplasia: efficacy of vitamin E in a double-blind clinical study of preterm infants. N Engl J Med 1981; 305:1365–1371.
16. Hittner HM, Godio LB, Speer ME. Retrolental fibroplasia: further clinical evidence and ultrastructural support for efficacy of vitamin E in the preterm infant. Pediatrics 1983; 71:423–432.
17. Kretzer FL, Mehta RS, Johnson AT, Hunter DG, Brown ES, Hittner HM. Vitamin E protects against retinopathy of prematurity through action on spindle cells. Nature 1984; 309:793–795.
18. Puklin JE, Simon RM, Ehrenkranz RA. Influence on fibroplasia of intramuscular vitamin E administration during respiratory distress syndrome. Ophthalmology 1982; 89:96–103.
19. Gellis S. More on retrolental fibroplasia and effect of vitamin E. Pediatric Notes 1982; 6(13):49.
20. Phelps DL. Vitamin E and retrolental fibroplasia in 1982. Pediatrics 1982; 70:420–425.
21. Rosenbaum A. Vitamin E and RLF. J Pediatr Ophthalmol Strabis 1982; 19(4):5.

Toxicity of Vitamin E in Preterm Infants

11

Helen M. Hittner, M.D.
Frank L. Kretzer, Ph.D.

UNORTHODOX APPROACH TO CLINICAL TRIALS

Since the suggestive evidence presented by Johnson, et al in 1974, that vitamin E supplementation in the preterm infant could suppress the development of severe ROP,[1] numerous centers have attempted to confirm this efficacy. None of these clinical trials had systematic Phase I, II, and III studies. Phase I studies should determine absorption and elimination, safe dosage range, preferred route of administration, and toxicity. Phase II studies should be initial clinical trials involving a limited number of patients for a specific indication. Phase III studies are, then, extensive clinical trials involving large numbers of patients, performed only if Phase I and II studies demonstrate reasonable safety and effectiveness.

Unfortunately, the clinical trials in preterm infants, assessing vitamin E efficacy to prevent severe ROP and determining toxicity, have been done by targeting variable plasma vitamin E levels, utilizing multiple routes of administration, and employing different forms of vitamin E in various vehicles. Because of this unorthodox approach to Phase II clinical trials, multiple toxicities have been reported due to dosage, route of administration, and product composition.

TOXICITY RELATED TO DOSAGE

From 1979 to 1981, Johnson, et al[2] conducted a randomized, double-masked, controlled clinical trial utilizing primarily initial slow (4 to 8 hours) IV infusion of dl-alpha-tocopherol (Ephynal, Hoffmann-LaRoche, Nutley, New Jersey) targeting a plasma vitamin E level of 5.0 mg per deciliter (Fig. 11-1). This protocol was justified by two observations. First, Phelps and Rosenbaum[3] had utilized IM injections of dl-alpha-tocopheryl acetate in the kitten. They proposed that regression of intravitreal neovascularization could be induced by pharmacological doses that produced mean plasma vitamin E levels of 10.2 mg per deciliter. Second, Johnson, et al[4] showed a significantly improved visual outcome in ten infants when vitamin E therapy aimed at plasma levels of 5.0 mg per deciliter was started after severe acute ROP had developed.

With the prolonged mean plasma plateaus maintained at 5 mg per deciliter,[2] there was a significant increase in the incidence of confirmed sepsis in babies receiving the study medication for more than 1 week, and in the incidence of documented necrotizing enterocolitis in babies receiving the study medication for more than 2 weeks. Johnson, et al felt that the sustained high plasma levels of vitamin E probably exerted their effect in the microbes (predominance of streptococcal species lacking catalase), as well as in the neutrophils (decrease in overall bactericidal capacity of the polymorphonuclear cells).

An FDA review of this data base revealed that "in the vitamin E-treated group, the incidence of sepsis and necrotizing enterocolitis was increased. This occurred primarily in infants under 1,500-grams birth weight, in whom peak blood levels averaged approximately 8 mg per deciliter."[5] Since Hittner, et al[6] established vitamin E efficacy using 100 mg per kilogram per day of oral dl-alpha-tocopherol at 1.2 mg per deciliter, pharmacological therapy is not needed to saturate interstitial retinal binding protein to a critical level. This occurs at lower nontoxic plasma vitamin E levels that result in adequate protection of spindle cells from the initial cluster of oxidative insults, which ultimately may result in the development of severe ROP.

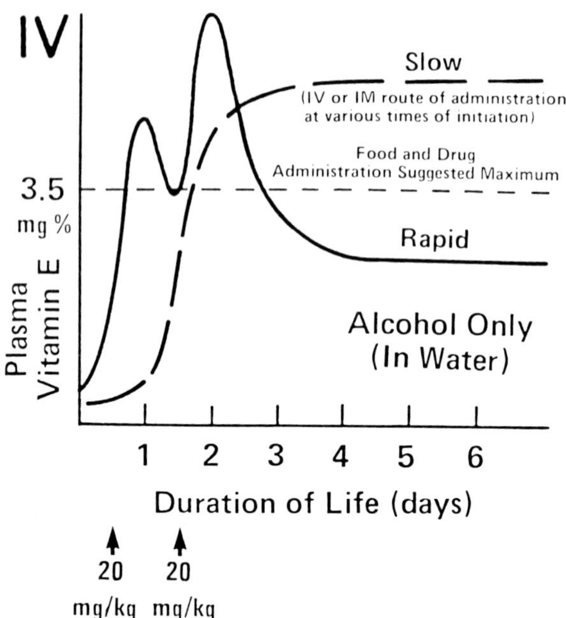

Figure 11–1 Graph demonstrates the mean plasma vitamin E levels produced by initial slow (four to eight hours) (— —) and initial rapid (15–20 minutes) (———) intravenous administration. The high plasma plateau (5 mg per deciliter) was obtained by initial slow IV vitamin E in a subset of the infants reported by Johnson, et al.[2] The prolonged pharmacological level of vitamin E was associated with sepsis and necrotizing enterocolitis in some of the infants enrolled in the study. Early high plasma peaks could have been obtained by initial rapid IV vitamin E of 20 mg per kilogram on days one, two and sometimes three in a subset of the infants reported by Phelps, et al.[7] The transient pharmacological level of vitamin E was associated with intraventricular and early retinal hemorrhages in some of the infants enrolled in the study. The Food and Drug Administration suggested 3.5 mg per deciliter (– – –) as a maximum.[5] Both Johnson, et al[2] and Phelps, et al[7] utilized Ephynal (Hoffmann-LaRoche, Nutley, New Jersey), which is dl-alpha-tocopherol in water.

TOXICITY RELATED TO ROUTE OF ADMINISTRATION

From 1981 to 1983, Phelps, et al[7] conducted a randomized, double-masked, controlled clinical trial utilizing initial rapid (15 to 20 minutes) IV infusion of dl-alpha-tocopherol (Ephynal, Hoffmann-LaRoche, Nutley, New Jersey) targeting a plasma vitamin E level of 3.0 to 3.5 mg per deciliter, (Fig. 11-1). The actual treatment dose schedule was initial rapid IV infusion of 20 mg per kilogram on days one and two and sometimes three, with subsequent doses adjusted according to plasma tocopherol levels performed twice weekly. When an infant no longer required IV therapy, the oral dose of dl-alpha-tocopherol was 100 mg per kilogram per day. These doses were also adjusted according to plasma tocopherol levels performed twice weekly.

The treatment group's mean plasma vitamin E level for the first week of life was 3.5 mg per deciliter. However, in infants weighing 1,000 grams or less at birth, 10 of 42 infants in the treatment group suffered severe intraventricular hemorrhages (IVH Grades 3 and 4) after receiving initial rapid IV infusion of vitamin E, compared to two of 43 infants in the control group. Thirty-five percent of babies with clinical signs of IVH had early retinal hemorrhage, compared to only 5 percent of babies without clinical signs of IVH with early retinal hemorrhage. Twenty-five percent of babies who had maximum plasma vitamin E levels of 7 mg per deciliter or more had early retinal hemorrhage, compared to only 7 percent of babies who had maximum plasma vitamin E levels of 1.5 mg per deciliter or less with early retinal hemorrhage.[8]

Myers, et al[9] described the pharmacokinetics of rapid (60 minutes) IV infusion of 10 mg per kilogram of dl-alpha-tocopherol in six preterm infants with a mean birth weight of 920 grams. Thirty minutes after infusion, the mean plasma vitamin E level was 8.8 mg per deciliter (range of 6.6 to 10.6 mg per deciliter). This rapidly declined, and 24 hours after infusion, the mean plasma level was 2.8 mg per deciliter (range of 1.9 to 4.4 mg per deciliter). Although Phelps, et al[7] expressed plasma vitamin E levels in terms of weekly means, it can be deduced from the data of Myers, et al that twice the dose given three times as fast could produce, in a subset of very-low-birth-weight infants, daily peaks of at least 17.6 mg per deciliter 30 minutes after infusion. Such transient peaks could induce the reported intraventricular and early retinal hemorrhages.[8]

Helson[10] reported a decrease in factors II, VII, IX, and X in one child with neuroblastoma receiving 2,300 mg per m² per day of dl-alpha-tocopherol for 4 or more days, with plateau plasma vitamin E levels of 12.5 mg per deciliter. He found that when the ratio between vitamin E and vitamin K exceeded 400:1, these four vitamin K-dependent clotting factors became abnormal. Corrigan and Marcus[11] found a decrease in the same four vitamin K-dependent clotting factors in one adult with hyperlipoproteinemia who was treated with warfarin and self-administered 800 IU of vitamin E per day. They felt that the mechanism was a direct interference of vitamin E with vitamin K. Although vitamin K is routinely given to the preterm infant as a single 0.5 to 1.0 mg dose, the vitamin E-related toxicity of intraventricular and early retinal hemorrhages may be linked to transient high plasma vitamin E peaks competing with vitamin K-dependent clotting factors. Such high plasma peaks of vitamin E can only be achieved by rapid IV infusion or extremely high doses of slow IV infusion.

Thus, Johnson, et al[2] did not find a similar increase in IVH, despite the prolonged plasma plateaus of 5 mg per deciliter.

TOXICITY RELATED TO PRODUCT COMPOSITION

The primary considerations in formulating vitamin E products are types of tocopherols, stereoisomers, forms, and vehicles. Alpha-tocopherols are the only products that are vitamin E. The only natural antioxidant is d-alpha-tocopherol.

Purified d-alpha-tocopherols (natural vitamin E) are expensive to produce, but no toxicity results from administering dl-alpha-tocopherols. However, the "l" stereoisomer is absorbed and may decrease potency by competing for active binding sites.

Vitamin E is usually administered as a free alcohol or an acetate. Since the alcohol forms are more expensive, the acetate forms are frequently produced. This has little significance when the oral and IM routes of administration are employed, because hydrolysis and binding to appropriate plasma binding proteins (low-density lipoproteins) within the gastrointestinal tract and muscle are not rate limiting. However, the use of acetate forms may have great significance when the rapid IV route of administration is employed, because hydrolysis and binding to appropriate plasma binding proteins by the reticuloendothelial system delays utilization and may stress the preterm liver and spleen.

The vehicles (propylene glycol, Emulphor El-100, polysorbate 80, polysorbate 20, sesame seed oil) have been the primary cause of toxicity related to vitamin E administration in preterm infants.

Aquasol E

From 1981 to 1982, Finer, et al [12] utilized oral dl-alpha-tocopheryl acetate (Aquasol E, USV Pharmaceuticals, now Armour Pharmaceuticals, Tarrytown, New York, Chapter 9, Table 3) at 200 mg per kilogram per day in an effort to improve vitamin E efficacy in preventing the development of severe ROP. Aquasol E (at 100 mg per kilogram per day) produced plasma vitamin E levels that approached 2.0 mg per deciliter at 1 week of life. Finer, et al felt that these levels should be elevated to produce plasma vitamin E levels similar to those infants who received IM vitamin E in their previous studies. Aquasol E was diluted 1:2 and given 50 mg per kilogram every 6 hours, which resulted in mean plasma

vitamin E levels of 2.6 mg per deciliter by the seventh day of treatment. However, using this protocol, Finer, et al found an increased incidence of necrotizing enterocolitis [treatment, 20 of 114 (17.5%); control, 4 of 105 (3.8%)].

Lambert, et al[13] studied oral Aquasol E in 22 preterm infants with a mean birth weight of 1,140 grams at 50, 100, and 200 mg per kilogram per day, undiluted and undivided, and by the seventh day of treatment obtained mean plasma vitamin E levels of 0.96 mg per deciliter, 1.96 mg per deciliter, and 2.18 mg per deciliter. They concluded that there was no advantage in administering vitamin E in oral doses greater than 100 mg per kilogram per day in preterm infants. Thus, oral administration of vitamin E alone cannot produce mean plasma vitamin E levels that approach 3.5 mg per deciliter; however, with increasing dosage, the vehicle can introduce toxicity. This may be due to hyperosmolarity and/or toxicity of propylene glycol,[12] or it may be due to hydrogen binding properties of propylene glycol, which cause significant dehydration at concentrations greater than 50 percent.[2] This toxicity can be circumvented by the administration of dl-alpha-tocopheryl acetate, with medium-chain triglycerides as a vehicle (Chapter 9, Table 3).

E-Ferol-IM, E-Vicotrat, Ephynal

In 1983 and 1984, E-Ferol-IM (O'Neal, Jones & Feldman Pharmaceuticals, Maryland Heights, Missouri, Table 11-1) was available in the United States for IM injections in preterm infants to prevent the development of severe ROP. Pantoja, et al[14] demonstrated lack of absorption of this product, whose vehicle was sesame seed oil.

Schroder, et al[15] reported on three infants who received in the anterior thighs 21 IM injections of E-Vicotrat (Heyl, Berlin, Federal Republic of Germany, Table 11-1) of 30 mg per day. The infants developed hard, woody ossifications at the sites of injection, which after some months became smooth without visible muscle atrophy or contractures. Schroder, et al do not report plasma vitamin E levels for this product whose carrier is polysorbate 80.

Smith, et al[16] reported on two infants who received in the anterior thighs 22 and 10 IM injections respectively of Ephynal (Hoffmann-LaRoche, Basel Switzerland, Table 11-2) of 25 mg per kilogram per day, with the development of hard, woody ossification at the sites of injection by 2 months of age. They do not report plasma

TABLE 11–1 Comparison of E-Ferol -IM (O'Neal, Jones and Feldman) with E-Vicotrat® (Hedl) per ml Solution

Eferol®-IM		E-*Vicotrat®*	
Component	*Amount*	*Component*	*Amount*
dl-alpha-tocopheryl acetate	200.00 mg	dl-alpha-tocopheryl acetate	50.000 mg
Benzyl alcohol	20.00 mg	methyl-4-hydroxybenzoate	0.476 mg
		propyl-4-hydroxybenzoate	0.204 mg
Sesame Seed Oil U.S.P. qs	1.00 mg	polysorbate 80	128.400 mg

vitamin E levels for this product, whose carrier is Emulphor El-100. However, Finer, et al[17] and Chiswick, et al[18] demonstrated good absorption of vitamin E utilizing this product, with production of plasma vitamin E levels at their desired target levels. Table 11-2 compares the content of IM/IV Ephynal (Hoffmann-LaRoche, Basel, Switzerland) with that of IM/IV Ephynal (Hoffmann-LaRoche, Nutley, New Jersey). The latter is optimal for IM or IV use, since only it contains dl-alpha-tocopherol.

The toxicity of these IM injections is transient and minimal in comparison to the toxicities associated with IV administration of vitamin E (sepsis, necrotizing enterocolitis, intraventricular hemorrhage, and hepatic necrosis). Thus, the risk:benefit ratio of IM vitamin E may be warranted, especially in infants of 1,000 grams or less at birth, who are at highest risk for ROP and IVH.

The localized inflammation associated with IM injections can be minimized by limiting the number of injections, decreasing the volume (dosage) at each injection site, and alternating thighs. The use of Ephynal (Hoffmann-LaRoche: Nutley, New Jersey) for three initial IM injections on days one, two, and four of 15 mg per kilogram, 10 mg per kilogram, and 10 mg per kilogram respectively, and for subsequent IM injections every third day of 10 mg per kilogram, when an infant cannot tolerate even small gavage feedings, does not result in local calcifications but does produce mean plasma vitamin E levels in the adult physiological range (1.1 to 3.3 mg per deciliter).[19]

E-Ferol-IV and MVI-Pediatric

From November 1983 to April 1984, E-Ferol-IV (O'Neal, Jones & Feldman Pharmaceuticals, Maryland Heights, Missouri, Table 11-3) was marketed in the United States as a high-potency vitamin E, with the recommendation that 25 to 50 mg be added to slow IV infusion solutions. In their brochure,[20] the clinical indication was "to help assure adequate daily intake of vitamin E." However, the clinical pharmacology stated that "substantial doses of vitamin E will reduce the severity of retrolental fibroplasia in neonatals." The references cited were Johnson, et al[1] (1974, IM dl-alpha-tocopherol), Hittner, et al[6] (1981, oral dl-alpha-tocopherol), and Finer, et al[17] (1982, IM dl-alpha-tocopheryl acetate). Many

TABLE 11–2 Comparison of Ephynal® (IM/IV) (Hoffmann-LaRoche, Basel, Switzerland) with Ephynal® (IM/IV) (Hoffmann-LaRoche, Nutley, New Jersey) per ml Water

Ephynal® (IM/IV) (*Basel, Switzerland*)		*Ephynal®* (IM/IV) (*Nutley, New Jersey*)	
Component	*Amount*	*Component*	*Amount*
dl-alpha-tocopheryl acetate	50.00 mg	dl-alpha-tocopherol	55.00 mg
	50.00 IU		60.50 IU
Emulphor El-100	41.60 mg	Emulphor El-620	105.00 mg
Phenol crystaline	5.00 mg		
Glycerine	50.00 mg		
		Benzyl alcohol	0.01 ml
		Propylene glycol	0.10 ml
		Ethyl alcohol (200 proof)	0.10 ml
		Sodium acetate trihydrate	0.30 mg
		Glacial acetic acid	2.50 mg
		Sodium chloride	9.00 mg
		Disodium edetate	0.10 mg

**TABLE 11–3   Comparison of E-Ferol-IV   (O'Neal, Jones and Feldman)
with MVI   Pediatric (Armour Pharmaceuticals, formerly
USV Pharmaceuticals) per ml Sterile Water**

E-Ferol-IV		MVI Pediatric	
Component	Amount	Component	Amount
dl-alpha-tocopheryl acetate	25.00 mg	dl-alpha-tocopheryl acetate	1.40 mg
polysorbate 80	97.00 mg	polysorbate 80	10.00 mg
polysorbate 20	11.00 mg	polysorbate 20	0.16 mg
		butylated hydroxytoluene	11.60 μg
		butylated hydroxyanisol	2.80 μg

* If formulated according to U.S.P. standards on a volume-to-volume basis.

neonatologists had been anxiously awaiting the marketing of an IV preparation of vitamin E endorsed by these researchers. Use of the product was widespread, with at least 38 documented deaths. This tragic saga of vitamin E toxicity has been chronicled in the FDA's Regulation of the Marketing of Unapproved New Drugs: The Case of E-Ferol Vitamin E Aqueous Solution, which was a report on a hearing before a U.S. House of Representatives subcommittee on government operations. This episode has redefined the role of the FDA in monitoring the marketing of unapproved new drugs.

E-Ferol-IV contains dl-alpha-tocopheryl acetate, with polysorbates 80 and 20 as vehicles. The pathology reports documented a sequence of distinctive hepatic lesions that were dose related. The cumulative dose varied from 350 to 4,290 units, which were administered for periods ranging from 6 to 44 days.[21] A precise etiologic relationship between the clinical syndrome[22] and the therapy has not been established; however, Bhat, et al[23] induced ultrastructural hepatic lesions and physiological cessation of cellular bile acid uptake and secretion in rabbits, utilizing polysorbates 80 and 20 alone.

The components of E-Ferol-IV are similar to MVI-Pediatric (USV Pharmaceuticals, now Armour Pharmaceuticals, Tarrytown, New York, Table 11-3), although the ratio of vitamin E to polysorbates 80 and 20 per ml product are vastly different (Table 11-3). Since MVI-Pediatric, a multivitamin product, is being added to slow IV infusion solutions, there is a potential danger of reaching cumulative toxic levels and producing distinctive hepatic lesions similar to E-Ferol-IV, especially in infants of 1,000 grams or less at birth. Furthermore, toxic plasma vitamin E levels can be approached when MVI-Pediatric is used in combination with oral or IM supplementation to prevent the development of severe ROP. This has warranted a change in the package insert of MVI-Pediatric, such that the daily dose in infants weighing 1,000 grams or less is not to exceed 30 percent of a single vial.

REFERENCES

1. Johnson L, Schaffer D, Boggs TR. The premature infant, vitamin E deficiency and retrolental fibroplasia. Am J Clin Nutr 1974; 27:1158-1173.
2. Johnson L, Bowen FW, Abbasi S, et al. Relationship of prolonged pharmacologic serum levels of vitamin E to incidence of sepsis and necrotizing enterocolitis in infants with birth weight 1,500 grams or less. Pediatrics 1985; 75:619–638.
3. Phelps DL, Rosenbaum A. Vitamin E in kitten oxygen-induced retinopathy. II. Blockage of vitreal neovascularization. Arch Ophthalmol 1979; 97:1522-1526.
4. Johnson L, Schaffer D, Quinn G, Goldstein D, Mathis MJ, Otis C, Boggs TR. Vitamin E supplementation and the retinopathy of prematurity. Ann N Y Acad Sci 1982; 393:473-494.
5. Sobel S, Gueriguian J, Troendle G, Nevius E. Correspondence: vitamin E in retrolental fibroplasia. N Engl J Med 1982; 306:867.
6. Hittner HM, Godio LB, Rudolph AJ, Adams JM, Garcia-Prats JA, Friedman Z, Kautz JA, Monaco WA. Retrolental fibroplasia: efficacy of vitamin E in a double-blind clinical study of preterm infants. N Eng J Med 1981; 305:1365-1371.
7. Phelps DL, Rosenbaum A, Isenberg SJ, Leake RD, Dorey F. Effect of IV tocopherol (vit E) on retinopathy of prematurity. Pediatr Res 1985; 19:357A.
8. Rosenbaum AL, Phelps DL, Isenberg SJ, Leake RD, Dorey F. Retinal hemorrhage in retinopathy of prematurity associated with tocopherol treatment. Ophthalmology 1985; 92:1012–1014.
9. Myers PR, Quissell BJ, Peterson PG. Pharmacology of intravenous vitamin E in the very-low-birth-weight (VLBW) newborn. Pediatr Res 1984; 18:157A.
10. Helson L. The effect of intravenous vitamin E and menadiol sodium diphosphate on vitamin K dependent clotting factors. Thrombosis Res 1984; 35:11-18.
11. Corrigan JJ, Marcus FI. Coagulopathy associated with vitamin E ingestion. JAMA 1974; 230:1300-1301.
12. Finer NN, Peters KL, Hayek Z, Merkel CL. Vitamin E and necrotizing enterocolitis. Pediatrics 1984; 73:387-393.
13. Lambert GH, Papp LA, Paton JB. Megadoses of vitamin E in oxygen-dependent premature newborn infants. J Perinatol 1985; 5:44-47.
14. Pantoja A, Ukrainski C, Belenky D, Grinberg A, Hulac P, Mathis J. Vitamin E (VE) kinetics in infants < 1,500 grams: intramuscular (IM) vs. oral administration. Pediatr Res 1984; 18:157A.

15. Schroder H, Schulz M, Aeissen K. Muscular calcification following injection of vitamin E in newborn infants. Eur J Pediatr 1984; 142:145-146.

16. Smith IJ, Buchanan MFG, Goss I, Congdon PJ. Correspondence: vitamin E in retrolental fibroplasia. N Engl J Med 1983; 309:669.

17. Finer NN, Grant G, Schindler RF, Hill GB, Peters KL. Effect of intramuscular vitamin E on frequency and severity of retrolental fibrplasia: a controlled trial. Lancet 1982; 1:1087-1091.

18. Chiswick ML, Johnson M, Woodhall C, Gowland M, Davies J, Toner N, Sims DG. Protective effect of vitamin E (dl-alpha-tocopherol) against intraventricular hemorrhage in premature babies. Br Med J 1983; 287:81-84.

19. Hittner HM, Rudolph AJ. Retinopathy of prematurity. In: Nelson NM, ed. Current therapy in neonatal-perinatal medicine 1985-1986. Toronto: B.C. Decker, 1985; 295-299.

20. FDA's regulation of the marketing of unapproved new drugs: the case of E-Ferol vitamin E aqueous solution. Hearing before a subcommittee of the Committee on Government Operations, House of Representatives, Ninety-eighth Congress, May 4, 1984, 39:238 0. Washington: U.S. Government Printing Office, 1984; 6-7.

21. Bove KE, Bodenstein CJ, Saldivar VA, Balistreri WF, Haas JE. A distinctive hepatic lesion is present in premature infants given intravenous vitamin E/polysorbates. Lab Invest 1985; 52:10A.

22. Lorch V, Murphy MD, Hoersten LR, Harris E, Fitzgerald J, Sinha SN. Unusual syndrome among premature infants: association with a new intravenous vitamin E product. Pediatrics 1985; 75:598-602.

23. Bhat R, Jiang JX, Walsh JM, Mortensen ML, Vidyasagar D, Evans MA. Effect of vitamin E and polysorbate on bile acid transport in newborn rabbit hepatocytes. Pediatr Res 1985; 19:213A.

Intensive Care of the Low-Birth-Weight Infant

12

James M. Adams, M.D.

It is perhaps paradoxical that in an era of advanced medical specialization, neonatal intensive care has risen to unprecedented levels of sophistication and cost, witnessed striking reductions in mortality, and yet remained such a little-known endeavor outside the realm of the perinatologist. At the core of the rapid growth of this field remains the same public health problem that prompted its inception—the low-birth-weight infant. The medical profession, the health care provider, and the medical consumer are only now beginning to place in perspective the importance of diseases of the perinatal period and have yet to fully realize the impact of low birth weight as a public health problem.

It is now possible to deliver to the critically ill neonate virtually all modes of cardiopulmonary support and monitoring available to older children and adults. Moreover, such care can be implemented with expectation of substantially better results than those obtained from currently accepted therapy of many malignancies, cardiovascular diseases, and chronic progressive diseases of adulthood. Such results, however, require substantial monetary resources, large number of support personnel and equipment, and techniques that can be difficult to make cost effective. The low-birth-weight baby requires specialized hospital care for weeks to months; the cyclic, acute-chronic nature of his course places unique pressures upon his family and caretakers. Constant re-evaluation of techniques and results is required, and each new therapeutic step is accompanied by the need to grapple with complex ethical dilemmas.

It seems, therefore, most important to disseminate a better understanding of what can be accomplished by applications of neonatal intensive care—as well as what realistically cannot. Failure to accurately appraise these issues places both the medical profession and the medical consumer at risk of unjustified pessimism or unrealistic expectations in approaching the low-birth-weight infant.

THE DEVELOPMENT OF NEONATAL INTENSIVE CARE

The 1960s witnessed progressive development of neonatal intensive care. Previously, mortality in babies who weighed less than 1,500 grams exceeded 70 percent[1], and morbidity was concentrated among survivors who weighed more. The clinical application of research data regarding thermal physiology and metabolic disturbances produced important reductions in mortality.

Hypoglycemia was recognized as an important cause of morbidity, and neonatalogists appreciated that anticipating the condition could, in many instances, lead to prevention. Glucose-containing intravascular fluids became a cornerstone of care for seriously ill neonates. Medical care of all forms of acute neonatal disease became increasingly organized into special neonatal intensive care units. Vigorous research activity into pulmonary physiology and hyaline membrane disease (HMD) produced a wealth of new information and understanding. Techniques of mechanical ventilation, initially introduced in a few neonatal centers, were applied with increasing frequency. The use of electronic monitoring, indwelling catheters, and blood gas analysis increased. By the end of the decade, several aspects of this organized approach to care were accompanied by a substantial reduction in neonatal mortality.[2] Unfortunately, such impact was much more pronounced in babies weighing over 1,000 grams than in those less mature.

Two notable features dominated the care of the critically ill neonate in the 1970s. The first was the increased emphasis placed on the maternal-fetal unit and perinatal, rather than just neonatal, care. The second was a large-scale therapeutic attack on HMD. Data from several centers in North America suggested that at least 5 percent of live births could require neonatal intensive care, and that nearly two thirds of pregnancies resulting in a distressed neonate could be anticipated prior to birth.[3] It was noted that maternal diabetes, preeclampsia, infections, and multiple gestations were particularly prone to result in a low-birth-weight or otherwise compromised infant. This introduced the concept of the high-risk pregnancy and resulted in widespread development of regional centers specializing in the care of the high-risk mother and her distressed neonate. Along with this regional organization, techniques for transporting mothers and critically ill babies were refined and more widely applied. In many areas of the United States and Canada, perinatal facilities were elaborately organized into primary, secondary, and tertiary institutions. Data documenting improved survival of low-birth-weight infants delivered and cared for in tertiary care centers accumulated in the medical literature.[4]

At the same time, perinatologists mounted a massive attack on HMD, from the standpoints of treatment in the nursery and more vigorous attempts at prevention. Obstetrical attempts to avoid premature delivery were emphasized; earlier observations[5] that antepartum corticosteroid administration could induce fetal lung maturity and reduce the risk of HMD underwent more extensive trials and clinical application. A reduction of "preventable" forms of HMD was realized in many perinatal centers.

Neonatologists, meanwhile, developed increasingly refined—and invasive—techniques of physiological and laboratory monitoring. A wealth of data was accumulated regarding physiologic and metabolic derangements in premature infants. Many babies underwent mechanical ventilation for HMD; many neonatologists became highly adept at such techniques. By the end of the decade, gratifying reductions in deaths related to this disease had been realized.[6]

Such care was not without complications, however. Among ventilated babies, pneumothorax was frequent, and bronchopulmonary dysplasia was recognized as a new clinical entity.[7] Intracranial hemorrhage was recognized as a major cause of death and morbidity, and retinopathy of prematurity (ROP) once again became increasingly prevalent in high-risk centers. Both were largely diseases of babies of less than 34-weeks gestation, or 1,500 grams, and both stimulated intense research into the respective pathophysiological mechanisms. Survival became virtually the rule among large premature and term babies. Death and morbidity had been pushed back into the lowest-birth-weight categories; many of these very small survivors had serious residual effects, however.

By the early 1980s, neonatologists possessed a large body of data and perhaps the most realistic perceptions regarding the care of critically ill neonates. A select group of entities accounts for most of the mortality and morbidity in the first month of life (Table 12–1). Most occur among low-birth-weight babies, and most in each category occur among the lowest-birth-weight groups. Depending on regional, socioeconomic, and ethnic influences, approximately 7.5 percent of all live-born infants can be expected to weigh less than 2,500 grams,[8] the majority being truly premature. Although low-birth-weight infants represented only 15 percent of the inborn population at the University of Colorado Health Sciences Center from 1974 to 1980, they accounted for 87 percent of deaths.[9] During the past decade, most perinatal centers have produced steady improvements in survival among low-birth-weight infants (Table 12–2). Mortality of the younger gestational age babies has fallen to nearly half that previously seen. Indeed, in a regional perinatal facility, any live-born baby of 25-weeks gestation or greater has at least a 50 percent chance of survival.

Survival per se, however, can no longer be considered a sensitive indicator of the results of perinatal care. The quality and cost of survival is of ever increasing concern to those involved in caring for low-birth-weight infants. Follow-up data from babies born from 1974 to 1977 demonstrated a neurodevelopmental handicap rate of up to 49 percent[10] in less than 800-gram babies. More recent data on such small infants, however, demonstrates a reduction to as low as 11 to 19 percent[11,12] in central nervous system handicaps among survivors. The cost of such care is now as high as that of any medical care in North America. Phibbs and associates, in 1981, reported the average cost of care for less than 1,500-gram infants requiring mechanical ventilation and surgery to be $25,496.00.[13] Johnson and associates estimated that the cost of hospital care for the low-birth-weight infant was

TABLE 12-1 Causes of Death*

Entity	Percent of Infants
Pulmonary	38 [pneumothorax (16)]
Congenital anomalies	26
Infection	18
Asphyxia	8
Intraventricular hemorrhage	5
Necrotizing enterocolitis	4
Others	1

* Texas Children's Hospital, Neonatal Intensive Care Unit

TABLE 12-2 Mortality in Low-Birth-Weight Infants*

1976

Weight(ing)	Admitted	Died	Mortality
500 – 750	9	7	78%
751–1,000	27	12	44%
1,001–1,250	31	12	39%
1,251–1,500	35	12	34%
1,501–2,000	90	10	11%
2,001–2,500	103	11	11%
Total	295	64	Average 36%

1983

Weight(ing)	Admitted	Died	Mortality
500 – 750	35	18	51%
751–1,000	34	5	15%
1,001–1,250	57	2	4%
1,251–1,500	38	2	5%
1,501–2,000	82	8	9%
2,001–2,500	44	2	5%
Total	290	37	Average 15%

* Texas Children's Hospital, Neonatal Intensive Care Unit

reduced by $901.00 per each additional day spent in utero between 27 and 33 weeks.[14] Even the most sophisticated nursery care is clearly much less efficient than the uterine environment.

MAJOR CLINICAL PROBLEMS IN LOW-BIRTH-WEIGHT INFANTS

Hyaline Membrane Disease

As we have seen, the low-birth-weight baby is particularly predisposed to certain entities that influence survival and potential quality of life. Despite perinatologists' intensive efforts to reduce the prevalence of HMD, it remains a major clinical problem. Its incidence rises progressively with decreasing gestational age, occurring in 10 to 15 percent of all low-birth-weight infants. Despite a decline in incidence and mortality, HMD still accounts for approximately 10 percent of total infant deaths in the United States.[15] HMD is associated with increased risk of death and intracranial hemorrhage, as well as markedly accelerated hospital costs.

Intraventricular Cerebral Hemorrhage

Since the early 1970s, neonatologists have increasingly appreciated that intraventricular cerebral hemorrhage (IVH) is a major cause of death and neurologic morbidity in low-birth-weight babies (Table 12–2). IVH occurs in approximately 43 percent of babies weighing less than 1,500 grams[16] and is relatively infrequent in those larger. Follow-up suggested a high incidence of neurological residuals in babies who have large hemorrhages.[17] Concern about such morbidity prompted much research into the physiology of IVH.

Present information suggests that relative immaturity or loss of autoregulation of cerebral blood flow might be common in small premature infants. This results in a pressure passive cerebral circulation most vulnerable to episodes of ischemia or hyperemia.

Infections

The specter of infection stalks the newborn infant. Congenital or early-onset infections occur in two to three infants per 1,000 live births. The risk increases in the face of maternal infection, unexplained fever, or prolonged (over 24 hours) rupture of maternal membranes. Low-birth-weight infants have a three- to tenfold greater risk of infection, depending on severity of illness and gestational age.[18] Chronic hospitalization, nutritional state, and the need for intubation and indwelling catheters make the small infant in the neonatal ICU an especially vulnerable host. During the average hospital stay, infection or the suspicion thereof accounts for significant numbers of procedures, as well as much laboratory work and administration of medications. Despite some impact of antibiotics on outcome, mortality rates for major categories of neonatal infections are still in the 14 to 40 percent range. Clearly, as long

TABLE 12–3 Intraventricular Hemorrhage

1981			
Weight(ing)	*Admitted*	*Died*	*Mortality*
500 – 750	14	10	71%
751–1,000	64	40	63%
1,001–1,250	32	14	44%
1,251–1,500	36	6	17%
Total	146	70	Average 49%
1983			
Weight(ing)	*Admitted*	*Died*	*Mortality*
500 – 750	34	17	50%
751–1,000	34	12	35%
1,001–1,250	57	12	21%
1,251–1,500	38	5	13%
Total	163	46	Average 30%

* Texas Children's Hospital, Neonatal Intensive Care Unit

as significant numbers of premature infants require prolonged hospital care, infection will continue as a major factor in the outcome.

Retinopathy of Prematurity

The markedly increased survival rates of very-low-birth-weight infants in recent years again brought clinicians to confront the problem of retinopathy of prematurity (ROP). Present data suggest that severe ROP is recognized in at least 7 percent of babies weighing less than 1,500 grams, with a sharp increase in incidence in those smaller than 1,000 grams.[19] This disorder increases as gestational age decreass, as does its severity. Indeed by far the dominant risk factor is very low birth weight. It has become increasingly clear that ROP is not a disease of oxygen excess in these small babies, but rather a multifaceted disorder in which oxygen administration is but one factor—or in some cases not a factor at all. Remember that the survival and function of a small premature infant in room air in the extrauterine development requires arterial oxygen tensions two- to threefold higher than those encountered by the immature retina in utero. Since the small premature baby is a displaced fetus, ROP represents only one of many circumstances in which, to survive, he must make certain physiological compromises.

This is a particularly frustrating disorder when—after the baby's long hospitalization, during which all available forms of sophisticated and costly care were utilized—the disorder produces severe visual impairment in the neurologically intact survivor. Fortunately, however, some recent developments described in this volume make the visual prognosis for the very-low-birth-weight baby considerably brighter. Recent research into the interaction of vitamin E and the developing retina provides a promising new tool for preventing ROP or ameliorating its severity. At the same time, retinal surgical procedures, though requiring further study of long-term effectiveness, offer a therapeutic approach for those already involved with this disorder. All physicians involved in the care of low-birth-weight infants can anticipate some intensive dialogue regarding this aspect of newborn care, as well as re-examination of the medicolegal ramifications of ROP.

SURGICAL CARE OF LOW-BIRTH-WEIGHT INFANTS

During the past decade, surgical procedures for premature infants have been commonplace, particularly involving insertion of TPN catheters, ligation of patent ductus arteriosus, and laparotomy for intra-abdominal bowel repair. A large experience has accumulated and defined areas requiring special consideration in the care of these small patients. Except for surgical management of necrotizing enterocolitis, intraoperative mortality for most of these procedures approaches zero. In the absence of special precautions, however, morbidity can be significant.

Thermal Environment

Clinical application of the basic principles of thermal physiology in the neonate, learned in the 1950s and

1960s, has become a cornerstone of acute care of the neonate. Well before the advent of mechanical ventilation and organized neonatal intensive care, control of the thermal environment led to significant reductions in mortality in critically ill neonates.[20]

This particularly applies to the surgical situation. The main goal is to maintain normal body temperatures and to simultaneously minimize oxygen consumption and metabolic rate. Metabolic responses to cold stress include increased oxygen consumption, increased catecholamine secretion, increased levels of free fatty acids, and greater risk of hypoglycemia—all undesirable in small prematures. Frank hypothermia decreases oxyhemaglobin dissociation, can raise pulmonary vascular resistance, and can be accompanied by apnea during rewarming.

Such metabolic derangements can be avoided by transporting the infant to the operating room in a controlled thermal environment and by warming and preparing the room in advance. It is the practice in many centers to perform neonatal surgery under servo-controlled radiant warmers, but it must be remembered that surgical drapes interfere with the delivery of radiant heat. A small premature should also be placed on a thermal conducting pad, whose temperature can be varied as needed during the procedure. Obviously, maintaining a normal core temperature during surgery does not guarantee a minimal metabolic rate, but a low core temperature indicates without doubt that the infant's thermal defenses have been overwhelmed and the metabolic consequences have already taken place.

Fluid Levels

Close monitoring of fluid administration is essential to avoiding the hazards of inadvertent hypervolemia, hyperglycemia, or hypo-osmolality. Clearly, small prematures fasted or deprived of a glucose supply can soon become hypoglycemic. Physiological solutions infused during surgery, therefore, should include 5 percent glucose. Higher concentrations should be avoided, because should rapid fluid administration become necessary, significant hyperglycemia could occur. Fluid may be administered using a neonatal infusion pump or hand syringe, but accurate record keeping is the best preventive measure.

Much time can be saved and cold exposure reduced by performing procedures such as intubation, placement of a good intravenous line, and manipulation of fluids and pumps in the neonatal unit before moving to the operating room. But then careful attention must be paid to avoid airway displacement and vascular access when moving or positioning the infant.

Pulmonary Function

Intraoperative ventilatory management of these small infants requires a somewhat different approach than for the older patient. Many of these babies still have some impaired pulmonary function at the time of surgery and require supplemental oxygen. The need to control inspired oxygen concentration and to measure therapy adequacy is of major concern, perhaps requiring blood-gas analysis during the procedure. Transcutaneous oxygen monitoring of these patients is becoming increasingly common in the operating room.

Finally, many of these babies have immature control of breathing mechanisms, and apnea is a common clinical problem. Increasingly, we have recognized that surgery and anesthesia seem to be among many factors that can disturb stability of control of breathing. Even among older, gestationally maturing prematures, surgical procedures can be followed by episodes of apnea that persist for several days. These can occur in babies who have previously had control of breathing problems, or in those who have had no apnea. Therefore, it is prudent to cautiously wean these patients off postoperative ventilatory support, and to extubate them only after a demonstrated period of sustained controlled breathing. It is not unusual for some of these babies to require several days of supplementary ventilatory support.

Surgery in Intensive Care Unit

The hazards and difficulties of transport to and from the operating room are frequently greater than those of the surgical procedure itself. Many surgical procedures involving small babies can be safely and effectively performed in the neonatal intensive care unit, thus avoiding transport-related morbidity. In addition to insertion of TPN catheters and urologic drainage procedures, we have now performed more than 50 patent ductus ateriosus ligations in the neonatal intensive care unit at Texas Children's Hospital. In a few selected cases, exploratory laparotomy and bowel resection have been possible in very ill, unstable infants. Others report similar experiences.[21] Such an approach might be helpful in the developing surgical management of infants with ROP. These patients frequently still require mechanical ventilation and are relatively small at the time of their initial procedures, so that subsequently they might require a series of examinations and further procedures. If the role of surgery expands in managing this entity, it will be the task of neonatologists, anesthesiologists, and ophthalmologists to work together to improve the total care of these patients, and to reduce the cumbersome nature of delivering that care.

REFERENCES

1. Gordon RR. Neonatal and "perinatal" mortality rates by birth weight. Br Med J 1977; 2:1202–1204.
2. Kleinman JC, Kovar MG, Feldman JJ, Young CA. A comparison of 1960 and 1973–1974 early neonatal mortality in selected states. Am J Epidemiol 1978; 108:454–469.
3. Committee on Perinatal Health: toward improving the outcome of pregnancy: recommendations for the regional development of maternal and perinatal health services. The National Foundation March of Dimes, White Plains, New York, 1976; 26.
4. Harris TR, Isaman J, Giles HR. Improved neonatal survival through maternal transport. Obstet Gynecol 1978; 52:294–300.
5. Liggins GC, Howie RN. A controlled trial of antepartum glucocorticoid treatment for prevention of the respiratory distress syndrome in premature infants. Pediatrics 1972; 50:515–525.
6. Tooley WH. Hyaline membrane disease, telling it like it was. Am Rev Respin Dis 1977; 115(6):19–28.
7. Northway WH, Rosan RC, Porter DY. Pulmonary disease following respirator therapy of hyaline membrane disease. N Engl J Med 1967; 276:357–368.
8. Characteristics of Births, United States 1973–1975; Series 21, No 30. National Center for Health Statistics, U.S. Department of Health, Education and Welfare.
9. Koops BL, Morgan LJ, Battaglia FC. Neonatal mortality risk in relation to birth weight and gestational age: Update. J Pediatr 1982; 101:969–976.
10. Britton BS, Fitzhardinge PM, Asby S. Is intensive care justified for infants weighing less than 801 g at birth? J Pediatr 1981; 99:937–943.
11. Hirata T, Epcar JT, Walsh A, Mednick J, Harris M, McGinis MS, Sehring S, Papedo G. Survival and outcome of infants 501 to 750 g: a six year experience. J Pediatr 1983; 102:741–748.
12. Bennett FC, Robinson NM, Sells CJ. Growth and development of infants weighing less than 800 g at birth. Pediatrics 1983; 71:319–323.
13. Phibbs CS, Williams RL, Phibbs RH. Newborn risk factors and costs of neonatal intensive care. Pediatrics 1981; 68:313–321.
14. Johnson DE, Munson DP, Thompson TR. Effect of antenatal administration of betamethasone on hospital costs and survival of premature infants. Pediatrics 1981; 68:633–637.
15. Wegman ME. Annual summary of vital statistics—1982. Pediatrics 1983; 72:755–765.
16. Papile L, Burstein R, Koffler H. Incidence and evaluation of subependymal and intraventricular hemorrhage: a study of infants with birth weights less than 1500 g. J Pediatr 1978; 92:529–534.
17. Papile L, Munsick-Bruno G, Schaefer A. Relationship of cerebral intraventricular hemorrhage and early childhood neurologic handicaps. J Pediatr 1983; 103:273–277.
18. Goldmann DA, Durbin WA, Freeman J. Nosocomial infections in a neonatal intensive-care unit. J Infect Dis 1981; 144:449–459.
19. Lucey JF, Dangman B. A reexamination of the role of oxygen in retrolental fibroplasia. Pediatrics 1984; 73:82–96.
20. Silverman WA, Fertig JW, Berger AP. The influence of the thermal environment upon the survival of newly born premature infants. Pediatrics 1985; 22:876–886.
21. Eggert LD, Jung AJ, McGough EC, Ruttenberg HD. Surgical treatent of patent ductus arteriosus in preterm infants: four-year experience with ligation in the intensive care unit. Pediatr Cardiol 1982; 2:15–18.

Anesthetic Considerations in Surgery for Retinopathy of Prematurity

13

H. Hollis Oxspring, M.D., Ph.D.
Vincent Whitehead, M.D.

In the past few years, there has been increasing interest in the special problems of anesthesia for the preterm infant.[1,2,3] Indeed, owing to the relatively recent establishment and accessibility of comprehensive neonatal care units, increasing numbers of preterm infants survive the early difficulties associated with their prematurity and can require surgery. The anatomic, physiologic and pharmacologic peculiarities of the pediatric patient are well known but often not fully appreciated. Although these characteristics are dramatic in the infant and neonate, they are accentuated, because of immature organ systems, in the preterm child. In planning an anesthetic for a preterm child presented for elective surgery in the first few months of life, an understanding of the newborn physiology and preterm pathophysiology is essential.

A complete discussion of the type, extent, and impact of these differences on the perianesthetic management of these patients is beyond the scope of this chapter. Our remarks, rather, are tailored to considerations pertaining to ophthalmic procedures on patients who have retinopathy of prematurity (ROP). Such patients are typically preterm infants from 2 to 8 months old at the time of surgery. Virtually all have histories of respiratory problems requiring oxygen therapy. Many have evidence of bronchopulmonary dysplasia, and some have histories of problems such as intraventricular hemorrhage and sepsis. Many take multiple medications. The consequences and significance of their status, from the anesthesiologist's point of view, are presented in what follows. We conclude by relating our experience with these patients over the past six years.

ANATOMIC CONSIDERATIONS

The anatomic and proportional differences of the neonate have clinical import to the anesthesiologist. The increased surface-area-to-weight ratio, the relative body composition, and the anatomy of the airway are most important.

With the increased surface-area-to-weight ratio comes the implication of greater ventilatory, fluid, and caloric requirements. It also makes thermoregulation more challenging.

Total body water and extracellular fluid volume are increased on a percent-body-weight basis in the infant, as compared to the adult; this volume is even more substantial in the preterm child. It influences the uptake and distribution of anesthetics and has important implications for fluid management. Although, in general, fluid replacement is not as challenging in ophthalmic surgery as in more invasive surgery, which leads to dramatic third-space translocation of fluid, care must still be taken to ensure that adequate maintenance fluids are given.

The anatomy of the infant's upper airway makes him an obligate nose breather. Nasal obstruction from any cause, including a nasogastric tube, can dictate the use of an oral airway.

The cephalad placement of the vocal cords with anterior caudad slope can make intubation difficult. A straight blade with the light source near the tip is optimal for direct vision. The narrowest portion of the larynx is at the cricoid cartilage. It is important to select a proper tube size that provides for a small air leak to avoid postoperative subglottic edema.

The newborn's trachea is short, 4 to 5 centimeters, and the endotracheal tube should extend 1 to 1.5 centimeters past the cords before fixation. Both main bronchi rise at an angle of about 55 degrees, so that each is equally likely to be entered by an excessively long tube. Head movements, as can occur in ophthalmic surgery, place the infant at high risk of accidental extubation or endobronchial intubation. Of course, proper placement must be continuously confirmed by auscultation and observation.

PHYSIOLOGICAL CONSIDERATIONS

Thermoregulation

Because of an increased surface-area-to-weight ratio in the infant, heat loss from radiation, evaporation, convection, and conduction is proportionately increased. The immediate consequence of hypothermia is increased oxygen consumption. Thermogenesis through fat metabolism, with a resultant increase in free fatty acids, can result in metabolic acidosis. Also, hypothermia increases the likelihood of apneic spells. To avoid these potential hazards, the following steps should be considered: *a* transport the infant in a heated module, *b* increase the operating room temperature, *c* use warmed solutions for prepping and infusion, *d* humidify and warm inspired gases, and *e* use heating blankets and radiant warmers when necessary. It is important that temperature be accurately monitored, and that timely therapeutic measures be undertaken to restore and maintain normothermia.

Respiration

Because their nervous systems are still developing, the preterm infant, as well as the preterm and term neonate, might not manifest fine control of respiratory functions. Seemingly inappropriate reactions to metabolic or environmental stimuli are often observed. For example, hypoxia decreases ventilation in the preterm infant.[4] The expected response of sustained hyperventilation develops more slowly in the preterm than in the term neonate.[5] Also, hypercarbia provides decreased ventilatory stimulation to the neonate and can be a respiratory depressant to the preterm child.[6] Preterm infants exhibit a higher incidence of periodic breathing—

that is, regular ventilation with pauses lasting up to six seconds—than do term infants. However, apneic spells lasting longer and accompanied by bradycardia are not uncommon. These spells can accompany minor changes, such as elevated environmental temperature, or can be associated with pathological states, such as intraventricular hemorrhage.

In addition to the increased immaturity of respiratory control, the ventilatory patterns of preterm infants differ from full-term infants, because of decreased lung compliance, increased chest-wall compliance, increased dead space to tidal-volume ratios, and different inspiratory to expiratory ratios. The neonate's oxygen consumption and carbon dioxide production, on a weight basis, is approximately twice that of an adult. Although tidal volume on a weight basis is about the same, increased alveolar ventilation from an increased respiratory rate compensates.

Infants are almost exclusively diaphragmatic breathers. The neonatal diaphragm contains relatively few high-oxidative muscle fibers and is thus susceptible to early fatigue. Intercostal muscle tone allows easy rib-cage excursion on inspiration and decreased chest wall recoil on expiration.

The anesthesiologist must appreciate the impact of anesthetic drugs and muscle relaxants on the mechanics of ventilation. Functional residual capacity can be precariously close to closing volumes; anesthetics can decrease muscle tone, further reducing this capacity.[7] Anesthetics also affect ventilatory control mechanisms; even minor depression from residual anesthetics, combined with immature control of ventilation, can easily lead to postoperative hypoventilation. Recent evidence suggests that the preterm infant with a preanesthetic history of apnea is at especially high risk of unexplained apnea during recovery from anesthesia.[3]

Many infants presented for ophthalmic procedures related to their ROP have residual lung disease. Fortunately, the lungs continue to develop through early childhood, so that their residual lung disease can become less severe with growth. However, those who survive respiratory distress syndrome, but require prolonged positive pressure ventilation at increased inspired oxygen concentration, could develop bronchopulmonary dysplasia and might not have normal blood gases even after one year. These infants frequently manifest decreased pulmonary compliance, an exacerbated ventilation-perfusion mismatch, and tachypnea. They are also prone to an increased incidence of lower respiratory tract infections. Optimal management can require controlled ventilation, with continuous positive airway pressure maintained postoperatively until the infant is awake and ready for extubation.

Cardiovascular System

Preterm infants have a relatively higher cardiac output and lower peripheral vascular resistance than do term infants. In general, blood pressure in the neonate increases with postnatal age and weight. Cardiac output in infants is primarily heart rate dependent because of the relatively noncompliant nature of the young myocardium. The limited ability to increase cardiac output in response to a volume load makes meticulous fluid management a necessity.

Bradycardia is common, and its cause is not always readily apparent, but it is judicious to consider hypoxia responsible until proven otherwise. The management, in order of preference, follows:

1. Verify adequate ventilation by auscultation and observation.
2. Increase the inspired oxygen concentration.
3. Decrease the anesthetic agent.
4. Eliminate possible mechanical or reflex causes, including surgical stimulation.
5. Administer an anticholinergic agent in a vagolytic dosage.
6. Administer a fluid challenge to correct possible hypovolemia.
7. Consider the use of a beta-1 agonist.

Most of the potent anesthetic agents are cardiodepressants. It must be appreciated that the infant has particularly limited ability to compensate for hypotension in the perioperative period, as baroreceptor and other reflexes can be altered. Also, since adequate tissue oxygen delivery is the ultimate goal, consideration must be given to other factors that vary with gestational and postnatal age as well as iatrogenic etiologies, e.g., the quantitative and qualitative aspects of the hematocrit.

Renal Function

In general, the child attains good renal function by the second postnatal month. However, the consequences of renal immaturity include a low glomerular filtration rate and a decreased capacity to excrete a water or sodium load. Moreover, the rapid postnatal increase in glomerular filtration rate in the term infant can be attenuated in the preterm neonate. The ability to control sodium balance is also decreased[8]; although sodium and water must be supplied, excess sodium can lead to edema, if water is available for extracellular fluid volume expansion, and can lead to hypernatremia if insufficient water is available.

In addition to the mandate for meticulous fluid management to prevent both fluid underloading and fluid overloading, decreased renal function has other important implications for the anesthesiologist. For example, the effects of anesthetics dependent on renal clearance for elimination will be prolonged.

Gastrointestinal Tract

Because of poor nutrition or concomitant gastrointestinal disorders, many infants coming to surgery are being fed by peripheral or central veins, or have a nasogastric tube in place. The anesthesiologist should recognize the potential complications in such circumstances. Nasogastric tubes can interfere with obligate nose breathing and can make masking or intubation more difficult or hazardous. Total parenteral nutrition is often associated with electrolyte imbalance, minor mineral deficiencies, and sepsis. To prevent contamination, it is desirable to avoid use of the central line. However, if it must be used, a determined effort must be made to keep it sterile.

Infants receiving total parenteral nutrition are also at risk of hyperglycemia or hypoglycemia perioperatively. Because of stress, the infant will likely be in a catabolic rather than an anabolic state, with insulin antagonism and increased adrenergic activity that can lead to perioperative hyperglycemia or even hyperosmolar coma. Conversely, hypoglycemia can develop if insulin secretion has been stimulated by a glucose load that suddenly stops. If the infant has a concentrated glucose infusion, discontinue it and substitute an infusion of low dextrose concentration. Monitoring the blood glucose levels in such situations is imperative.

Hepatic Function

The main concern with the liver is its role in biotransformation and drug metabolism by the various systems in the endoplasmic reticulum. Hepatic immaturity can result in prolonged activity of many drugs. Also, the immature liver is especially susceptible to damage from the stress of hypoxia or hypotension.

PHARMACOLOGIC CONSIDERATIONS

Inhalational Anesthetics

Uptake and elimination of inhalational anesthetics in the neonate are accelerated. The time constant is decreased, since functional residual capacity is smaller and alveolar ventilation is larger than in the older child or adult. Also, since both cardiac output and ventilation are increased relative to body mass, alveolar gas tension approaches inspired tension more rapidly. This convergence is also enhanced by the relatively increased percentage of total body mass occupied by tissue belonging to the vessel-rich group.

The volatile anesthetics have a dose-dependent myocardial depressant effect and can increase ventilation-perfusion abnormalities. The more rapid uptake of inhaled anesthetics makes the neonate susceptible to rapid change in anesthetic depth, with attendant deleterious cardiovascular changes. The neonate is especially at risk of suffering profound hypotension if hypovolemia is concomitant. It is, therefore, imperative to decrease this risk by frequent monitoring.

Muscle Relaxants

Neonates have immature neuromuscular transmission and decreased neuromuscular reserve; their muscle mass is also more than proportionately reduced compared to that of the adult, implying an increased sensitivity to muscle relaxants. However, a relatively increased volume of distribution, because of an increased total body-water-to-weight ratio, should tend to minimize this sensitivity.

There seems to be a wide dose-response relationship with nondepolarizing muscle relaxants. It seems prudent to start with a dose considerably smaller than that usually recommended, with subsequent titration depending on tolerance and desired effect. It is advisable to reverse the relaxant effects, even if the interval since the last dose has been long and the effects have apparently dissipated. These patients' limited reserves make the postoperative potentiation from possible respiratory acidosis a substantial risk. If there is any doubt about the patients' ventilatory reserve, they should be artificially ventilated postoperatively. Also, consider other common causes of potentiation, e.g.,

hypothermia, electrolyte and mineral imbalances, and other drugs, especially antibiotics and furosemide.

The high dose of succinylcholine required for neuromuscular blockade probably reflects the relatively large extracellular fluid volume of these infants, with the resultant large volume of distribution for this highly ionized agent. Pretreatment with nondepolarizing muscle relaxants is not required. However, pretreatment with a muscarinic blocking agent is desired, to prevent or to attenuate the bradycardia and cardiac arrhythmias frequently experienced as a result of the administration of succinylcholine alone.

Narcotics

The necessary narcotic dosage for adequate analgesia in the preterm infant is less, because reduced plasma volume and a low plasma protein concentration result in a higher serum concentration of the drug. Also, the immaturity of metabolic pathways and excretory organs prolongs the effects of the parent compound and active metabolites.

Anesthesia Induction Technique

Perioperative care is provided through the coordinated efforts of neonatology/pediatric, ophthalmology, and anesthetic teams. Most patients are either long-term inpatients or are admitted at least one day prior to surgery, to give adequate time for preoperative assessment and therapy.

Procedures are scheduled, as much as possible, as first cases. Any infant from a neonatal intensive care or an intermediate-care unit is accompanied by a neonatal transport team composed of a neonatal fellow and, if necessary, pediatric nursing personnel. The infant arrives in a transport incubator with an intravenous infusion connected through a continuous infusion pump, continuous electrocardiographic monitoring, and with resuscitation equipment and drugs available. A portable respirator and additional monitoring systems for continuous assessment of vital functions are also available.

This transport arrangement fosters informal conferences among the neonatologist, surgeon, and anesthesiologist, often producing important information that refines the intraoperative and postoperative plans. Such information could rarely be extracted only by chart review.

Before the infant arrives, the operating room is preheated to 28 to 30°C, and the anesthetic equipment, drugs, and monitors are checked and ready. Once all is in order, the patient is taken to the operating room and transferred under full monitoring to the operating table, where the level of support previously required is maintained. During preoxygenation, a precordial stethoscope is applied, adequate venous access is verified, and if not present, a T-connector to minimize dead space is added to the tubing. With another anesthesiologist and often the neonatologist present or immediately available, together with the surgical team and operating-room personnel, the anesthetist begins awake intubation and/or induction.

The anesthetic agents chosen vary with the anesthesiologist and the infant's status but are usually one of the following general anesthetic combinations, used with controlled or assisted ventilation via a Jackson Rees system:

1. Halothane or isoflurane and oxygen, with or without nitrous oxide.
2. Narcotic and oxygen, with or without nitrous oxide, with nondepolarizing muscle relaxants.
3. Ketamine and oxygen, with or without narcotics, or nitrous oxide, or muscle relaxants.

Each infant is intubated, with or without muscle relaxants, and has electrocardiographic and temperature monitoring. Depending on various factors, the blood pressure can be monitored by cuff, with or without the aid of a Doppler flow detector, or by invasive means. Also, inspired gases can be humidified and warmed. Other monitoring aids, such as nerve stimulators and transcutaneous oxygen analyzers, as well as routine laboratory analysis, are available.

At the conclusion of the procedure, and in view of the preoperative and intraoperative history and experience, the patient's postoperative needs are assessed and the postoperative plans formulated. Transport to the recovery room entails at least the level of monitoring and support required preoperatively. Subsequent therapeutic, transport, and level of care modalities, required postoperatively, are reassessed or confirmed during recovery room observation. This is the joint effort of the neonatologist, surgeon, and anesthesiologist.

RESULTS

We studied, retrospectively, 71 preterm ROP patients less than 2 years old, who were presented for 216 ophthalmic procedures under general anesthesia from January 1978 to January 1984. Their birth weights were 460 to 2,414 grams, with a mean of 975 grams and a standard deviation of 312 grams. The mean and standard deviation of gestational ages were 27.8 weeks and 2.4 weeks, respectively. Postnatal age at the time of procedure varied from 3 to 628 days, with a mean of 148 days and a standard deviation of 96 days. Weights at the time of first procedure varied from 1,100 to 5,300 grams, with a mean of 2,778 grams and a standard deviation of 1,175 grams. Relative frequency distributions for birth weight, gestational age, weight at time of first procedure, and postnatal age at time of procedure are given in Tables 13–1 to 13–4, respectively.

TABLE 13–1 Relative Frequency Distribution of Birth Weights

Birth Weight (in g)	Percent
< 500	4.2
500 to 1,000	60.5
1,000 to 1,500	32.5
1,500 to 2,000	1.4
> 2,000	1.4

TABLE 13–2 Relative Frequency Distribution of Gestational Age

Gestational Age (weeks)	Percent
< 24	2.8
24 to 26	24.0
26 to 28	46.5
28 to 30	16.9
30 to 32	4.2
32 to 34	4.2
> 34	1.4

TABLE 13–3 Relative Frequency Distribution of Weight at Time of First Surgery

Weight (in g)	Percent
< 1,500	11.9
1,500 to 2,000	21.4
2,000 to 2,500	19.0
2,500 to 3,000	9.5
3,000 to 3,500	16.6
3,500 to 4,000	4.7
> 4,000	16.6

TABLE 13–4 Relative Frequency Distribution of Postnatal Age at Time of Procedure

Age (weeks)	Percent
< 8	2
8 to 16	44
16 to 24	31
24 to 32	9
32 to 40	6
40 to 48	3
48 to 56	3
> 56	2

Review of a representative chart sample revealed a 13 percent incidence of postoperative apnea. Nine percent experienced apnea with bradycardia and flaccidity. However these infants responded satisfactorily to mechanical stimulation and required only prolonged observation. Four percent experienced multiple, prolonged apneic episodes requiring either artificial ventilation with bag and mask or intubation and mechanical ventilation. The oldest in this latter group had a postnatal age of 16 weeks.

Other complications included an instance of mucus plugging of the endotracheal tube intraoperatively, unresponsive to suctioning and requiring reintubation; rare instances of suspected perioperative fluid overloading, requiring diuretic therapy; and one episode of intraoperative ventricular tachycardia, with successful resuscitation and no apparent long-term sequelae.

Young infants presented for ophthalmic procedures related to their ROP often have a very precarious history, suffering multiple disease states and requiring intensive medical and surgical therapy. Increasing knowledge and availability of therapy for these infants' difficulties promises increased survival rates. To maximize the infant's potential for a healthy, productive life, it is important to identify and minimize potential risks and to evaluate the risk-benefit of early surgical intervention in ROP.

REFERENCES

1. Steward DJ. Preterm infants are more prone to complications following minor surgery than are term infants. Anesthesiology 1982; 56:304–306.
2. Gregory GA, Steward DJ. Life-threatening perioperative apnea in the ex-"premi." Anesthesiology 1983; 59:495–498.
3. Liu LMP, Cote CJ, Goudsorsouzian NG, Ryan JF, Firestone S, Dedrick DF, Liu PL, Todres ID. Life-threatening apnea in infants recovering from anesthesia. Anesthesiology 1983; 59:506–510.
4. Schulte FJ. Apnea. Clin Perinatol 1977; 4:65–76.
5. Rigatto H. Ventilatory response to hypoxia. Semin Perinatol 1977; 1:357–362.
6. Rigatto H. Ventilatory response to hypercapnia. Semin Perinatol 1977; 1:363–367.
7. Muller NL, Bryan AC. Chest wall mechanics and respiratory muscles in infants. Pediatr Clin North Am 1979; 26(3):503–516.
8. Greenberg AJ, McNamara H, McCrory WW. Renal tubular response to aldosterone in normal infants and children with adrenal disorders. Clin Endrocrinol Metab 1967; 27:1197–1202.

Treatment of Acute Retinopathy of Prematurity with Cryotherapy: The Beilinson Experience

Isaac Ben-Sira, M.D.

Ilana Nissenkorn, M.D.

By early detection of active retrolental fibroplasia (RLF) and treatment when indicated, the ophthalmologist can make a contribution to the protection of vision in premature infants who still develop this disease occasionally.

Arnall Patz, M.D.[1]

Acute retinopathy of prematurity (ROP) and active stages of retrolental fibroplasia (RLF) are the terms we use in this chapter; these as well as descriptions of the various disease stages are in accord with the new international classification of ROP[2]. Cryotherapy, as used herein, refers to applications of cold lesions only to the avascular areas of the retina.

The purpose of this review is to present our personal approach to the treatment of acute ROP. Over the past 8 years, Ilana Nissenkorn personally examined and followed up over 1,500 preterm infants, many having various degrees of ROP. During these years, Isaac Ben-Sira performed cryotreatment on some 100 eyes having ROP. All of these babies are still being followed.

The vast majority of ROP cases were referred from the neonatal intensive care unit (NICU) at the Beilinson Medical Center (S. Reisner, M.B., Ch.B.), a tertiary ICU. Statistics on admissions and survival rates of various birth-weight groups from this NICU are found in Tables 14-1 to 14-5 and discussed in the data base section.

WORKING HYPOTHESIS

ROP is a retinovascular disease seen at the border between the vascularized and avascularized retina of the premature baby. The more posterior the disease, the younger the preterm, and the greater amount of involved retinal avascular tissue, the more serious is the disease.

The natural history and the evolution of events at the border between vascularized and avascularized retina is usually toward resolution with vascularization of the avascular retina or, rarely, progression to cicatrization by contraction of fibrovascular elements with various degrees of destruction of normal ocular architecture.

Cryotherapy on avascular retina stops active ROP[3] immediately upon application, possibly by destroying cells, perhaps spindle cells[4], in the avascular maturing retina. Cryoapplication on avascular retina does not interfere with contraction or cicatrization of the existing fibrovascular tissue. Since cicatrization, which is proportional to the amount of fibrovascular tissue, appears rather early in the disease (usually in the middle of Stage 3) it is suggested that cryotherapy on avascular retina will be effective in preventing severe cicatrization. However, this is true only when cryotherapy is applied

TABLE 14-1 Six Years Experience with Retinopathy of Prematurity* General Data Base

Data	Birth Weight (g)		
	< 1,500	> 1,500	Total
Admissions (N)	568	601	1,169
Survivors (N)	401	541	942
Survivors (%)	70.6	90.0	80.6†
Cases of acute ROP (N)	133	42	175
Cases of acute ROP (%)	32.9	7.7	18.5†
Cases of cicatricial RLF Grade III or greater (N)	0	0	0
Cases of blindness (N)	0	0	0

* In Beilinson NICU 1977-1982
† Averages

TABLE 14-2   Survival and ROP Related to Birth Weight*

| | Birth Weight (g) | | | | | | |
Data	<750	751-1,000	1,001-1,250	1,251-1,500	1,501-2,000	2,001-2,500	Total
Admissions (N)	46	123	188	211	432	169	1,169
Survivors (N)	9	64	142	186	394	147	942
Survivors (%)	19.5	52.0	75.5	88.1	91.2	87.0	80.6†
Cases of acute ROP (N)	3	43	50	37	40	2	175
Cases of acute ROP (%)	33.3	67.2	35.2	19.8	10.1	1.4	18.5†

* Beilinson NICU 1977-1982
† Average

TABLE 14–3   Acute ROP and Treatment by Cryotherapy

Data	1977	1978	1979	1980	1981	1982	Total
Survivors (N)	139	170	155	156	162	160	942
Survivors with acute ROP (N)	16	32	26	27	36	37	175
Survivors with acute ROP (%)	11.5	18.8	16.7	17.3	22.2	23.7	18.5†
Survivors treated by cryotherapy (N)	4	9	4	9	5	8	39
Survivors treated by cryotherapy out of acute ROP (%)	25.0	28.7	15.3	33.3	13.9	21.0	22.4†
Survivors treated by cryotherapy out of total survivors (%)	2.8	5.2	2.6	5.7	3.0	5.0	4.1†

† Average

TABLE 14–4   Acute ROP and Cryotherapy in Relation to Birth Weight*

| | Birth Weight (g) | | | |
Data	<1,000	1,001-1,500	1,501-2,500	Total
Survivors (N)	73	328	541	942
Survivors with acute ROP (N)	46	87	42	175
Survivors treated by cryotherapy (N)	18	18	3	39
Patients with acute ROP (%)	49.1	20.5	7.1	22.2†
Survivors treated by cryotherapy among survivors with acute ROP (%)	24.6	5.4	0.5	4.1†

* Beilinson NICU 1977-1982
† Average

TABLE 14–5   Acute ROP and Cicatricial Stage in Relation to Birth Weight in Treated and Untreated Cases*

| | Birth Weight (g) | | | |
Data	<1,000	1,001-1,500	1,501-2,500	Total
Cases of acute ROP	46	87	43	175
Cases of cicatricial Grade I (N)	6	17	5	28
Cases of cicatricial Grade I (%)	13.0	19.5	11.9	16.0†
Cases of cicatricial Grade II (N)	6	4	1	11
Cases of cicatricial Grade II (%)	13.0	4.5	2.3	6.3†
Cases of cicatricial Grade III (N)	0	0	0	0

* Beilinson NICU 1977-1982
† Average

before large masses of fibrovascular tissues have been produced. It is our opinion that the efficacy of cryo-application in preventing further progression of the active process of RLF is well documented and supported by the following data.

DATA BASE

Because with modern techniques employed in the NICU, only very small, very sick babies develop ROP, the incidence of ROP and its sequelae must include information about the survival rate of the very-low-birth-weight groups. Apparently, conflicting statistics regarding incidence of blindness reported at various institutions can often be resolved by comparing the differences in survival rates in the very-low-birth-weight groups (Table 14-6). For example, Campbell et al[5] found much higher rates of cicatricial RLF blindness in the under 1,500-g birth-weight group (survival rate of 69%) than did Kalina and Karr (survival rate of 59%)[6]. However, Beilinson's[7] survival rate of under 1,500-g babies (70.6%) is comparable to that of Campbell et al. (Table 14–1).

TABLE 14–6 Survival Rates by Birth Weight in Three NICUs

	Kalina[6] 1975-1980			Campbell[5] 1976-1977			Beilinson[7] 1977-1982		
	Admitted	Survival		Admitted	Survival		Admitted	Survival	
Birth Weight (g)	(N)	N	%	(N)	N	%	(N)	N	%
<750	73	10	13.7	30	8	26.6	46	9	19.5
751-1,000	226	76	33.6	157	81	51.6	123	64	52.0
1,001-1,250	286	185	64.7	223	163	73.1	188	142	75.5
<1,250	585	271	46.3	410	252	61.4	357	215	60.0
1,251-1,500	353	282	79.9	216	182	84.3	211	186	88.1

METHODS

Methods of Examination

Our current technique follows:

1. We use no sedation or anesthesia even when cryo-application is planned.
2. One hour prior to examination, a nurse instills 1 drop each of tropicamide 1 percent and phenylephrine 2.5 percent. This is repeated twice at 30-minute intervals.
3. We use MIRA (Medical Instruments Research Associates Ltd.) indirect ophthalmoscope (small pupil).
4. When observation of the ora serrata is difficult, Novesin (oxybuprocaine 0.4%) topical anesthetic is applied, and a baby lid speculum is inserted. Fine forceps rotate the eye to the desired location by gently tweezing the limbal conjunctiva.
5. We inspect 360° of the fundus periphery with special emphasis on the following points: location of the avascular zone, state of vessels, presence of ridge, amount of fibrovascular proliferation, plus disease and signs of early cicatrization or involution.

We decide whether to apply cryotherapy after recording the results on a specially developed chart similar to the one presented in the International Classification of ROP[2].

When to Examine the Fundus

In 1974 the American Academy of Pediatrics recommended that the first examination be performed at the time of the infant's discharge from the nursery; this is not acceptable if treatment according to our method is to be considered. Furthermore, Palmer's[8] recommendation that if a single examination is to be made, it should be done between 7 and 9 weeks of age, is directed toward maximum case finding and cannot be accepted by ophthalmologists who plan to treat the infants. We have seen patients from elsewhere although rarely, who have already developed secondary glaucoma from cicatricial RLF at the age of 6 weeks. Therefore, our present recommendations for timing of examinations are as follows:

1. The first examination should be made at 2 to 3 weeks of age.
2. When no signs of active ROP are discovered, examination should be performed every 2 weeks.
3. When a large avascular area is located in Zone I or II, or when active ROP is definitely diagnosed, examination is performed once a week or even more often if rapid progression is suspected.
4. After discharge from the nursery, and if no signs of active ROP are present, we examine the infant once monthly until full vascularization has occurred in the temporal periphery
5. If ROP is present, the child is seen every 1 or 2 weeks.

CRYOTHERAPY

Considerations and Indications for Cryotherapy

The criteria we use are these:

1. When disease progression within Stage 3 is rapid
2. When the amount of fibrovascular proliferation is moderate to severe (according to the International Classification)
3. When there are signs of plus disease accompanying the above two criteria.

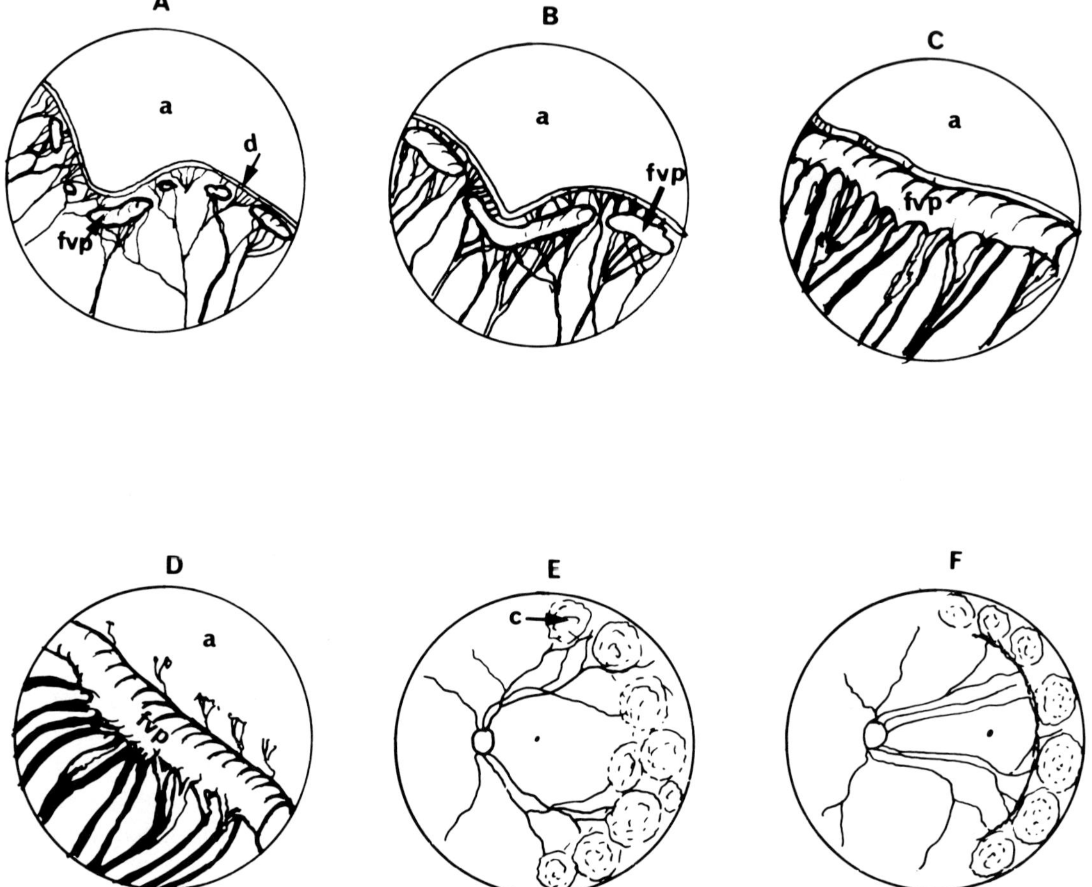

Figure 14–1 Fundus periphery in progressive, active Stage 3 RLF. A. Mild *Stage* 3; *a*, avascular retina; *d*, demarcation line; *fvp*, fibrovascular proliferation. B. Moderate Stage 3. At this stage we perform most of our cryotreatment (see E). C. Severe Stage 3 with confluent fibrovascular proliferation of more than two clock hours, too late for cryotreatment (see F). D. Severe fibrovascular proliferation with early signs of cicatrization and contraction, as seen from the convergence of the engorged retinal vessels approaching the fibrovascular band. Treatment by cryopexy is contraindicated. E. Complete regression of the disease without retinal dragging, when treated as in B; *c*, cryoscars. F. Some contraction of thick fibrovascular band causes retinal dragging if cryotreatment is done in C.

We perform cryoapplication only if more than two clock hours are occupied by a confluent fibrovascular proliferation. Separate fibrovascular proliferations, each of which is less than two clock hours, do not warrant cryotreatment, even if the disease is in Stage 3 progressive and Zone II —i.e., 360° of Stage 3 but separate fibrovascular bands (Fig. 14-1).

Methods of Cryotreatment

1. Treatment is performed in the operating room.
2. Dilation of the pupils is as described for fundus examination.
3. The incubator is brought into the operating theater.
4. If the child cannot be taken out, the child remains in the incubator for surgery.
5. Usually we place the child on a warm mattress that covers the operating table. A trained anesthesiologist and the physician from the NICU stand by and continuously monitor the vital signs.
6. After instillation of local anesthetic eyedrops, a baby lid speculum is inserted.
7. We gently insert a retinal cryoprobe under the lids.
8. We monitor the position of the cryoprobe tip through the indirect ophthalmoscope.
9. Freezing is applied to cover the entire avascular zone that is anterior to a fibrovascular proliferation of more than two clock hours (Fig. 14-2).
10. The ice ball should not reach the fibrovascular proliferation but, rather, cover only the avascular retina.
11. No incision of the conjunctiva is necessary, and freezing is done transconjunctivally. If the disease is more posterior, the conjunctiva near the limbus is incised 2 to 3 mm and the probe inserted through this opening. No sutures are required to close the conjunctival opening.
12. In a very young or small baby, it is sometimes impossible to place the cryoprobe under the lids without elevating the intraocular pressure above the ophthalmic arterial blood pressure. In this case, the eye should be rotated to expose the area to be treated between the lids and cryoinstrument, which is done without simultaneous monitoring.
13. No postoperative treatment is given.

Effects Observed after Cryotherapy

1. Within 12 to 24 hours, the signs of plus disease disappear. The vessels are less engorged, and the pupils are less rigid.
2. Lid edema disappears in 2 to 3 days.
3. In 1 week, the neovascular ridge involutes, and blood vessels are seen to advance between the cryoscars.
4. Two weeks later the cryoscars are well pigmented, and the eye is practically normal except for the scars in the periphery (Fig. 14-2).

Precautions and Prevention of Complications

Accidental freezing of fibrovascular tissue can occur and can result in small vitreous hemorrhages. Excessive pressure on the eye's periphery can also initiate hemorrhage from the engorged fibrovascular proliferation. Care should be taken not to occlude the blood flow through the central retinal artery by excessive pressure on the eye. We have not encountered a severe vitreous hemorrhage from the previously mentioned accidents, but extreme precautions are recommended in handling these extremely delicate and tiny eyes.

RESULTS

Data from the Beilinson Medical Center

Since 1976 we have treated over 100 eyes by cryotherapy: For the purpose of this chapter, however, the results given are only for those infants who came from the Beilinson NICU. Since exact data from 1983 are not available at present, and data from 1976 are also incomplete, we have presented data for 6 years, 1977 to 1982 (Tables 14-1 to 14-5).

No eye has progressed beyond cicatricial Stage 2, i.e., there is no blind or severely handicapped eye among the 942 surviving infants during these years. According

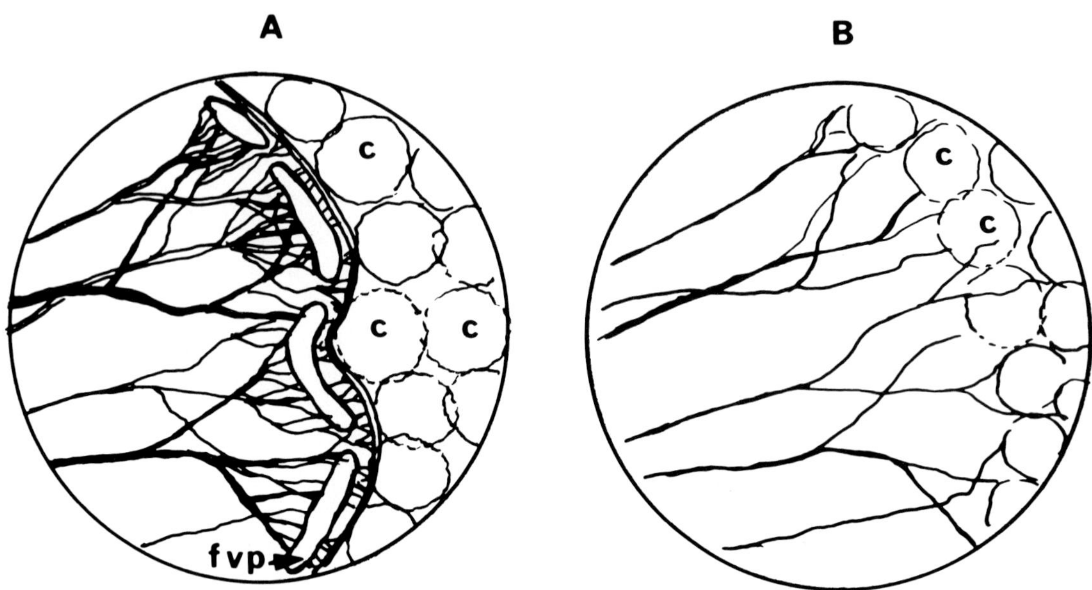

Figure 14–2 Typical stage III active ROP and confluent fibrovascular proliferation (*fvp*) of less than two clock hours. A. Operative plan with multiple cryoapplications (*c*) on avascular retina only. B. Same site two weeks later shows complete resolution of *fvp*, and normal retinal blood vessels extend between the cryoscars.

to various estimates, in such a population with a relatively high survival rate we would have expected 7 to 17 blind or severely visually handicapped children. Although there is no group control, the accurate documentation and the continued good results year after year are sufficient evidence of the efficacy of this treatment.

Data from the Institution for the Blind in Israel

Statistics from the Institution for the Blind in Israel (Table 14-7) indicate that from 1976 to 1981 there were 118 registrations of new blind children, 26 of them blind from RLF, the most common cause of blindness in children in Israel[9]. None of these came from the Beilinson NICU.

Results of 10 Unilaterally Treated Babies

Table 14-8 contains the results of 10 patients who were treated unilaterally. This is not a randomized study; rather, the more severely affected eye of each infant having bilateral symmetrical ROP was chosen for treatment. Although there are only a few eyes in each group, there is an evident difference in the results of the treated versus the control group (Figs. 14-3 and 14-4).

LATE COMPLICATIONS OF ROP AND CRYOTREATMENT

In examining the late complications of the study group, it must be remembered that the follow-up is rather short (median 3 to 4 years). Therefore, complications such as late retinal detachment or glaucoma, although not found so far, might still appear over the years.

TABLE 14-7   Causes of Blindness in Children in Israel 1976-1981

Cause of Blindness	No. of Children
RLF*	26
Brain damage	19
Optic atrophy	15
Congenital cataract	12
Retinitis pigmentosa	8
Congenital glaucoma	5
Unspecified syndromes	5
Viral infections	4
Anophthalmos	4
Lebers amaurosis	3
Microphthalmos	3
Retinoblastoma	2
Iris colomba	2
Albinism	2
Macular degeneration	2
Usher's syndrome	1
Benign familial mucopolysaccharidosis	1
Stevens Johnson	1
Marfan syndrome	1
Corneal dystrophy	1

* None of the children with RLF blindness came from the Beilinson NICU.

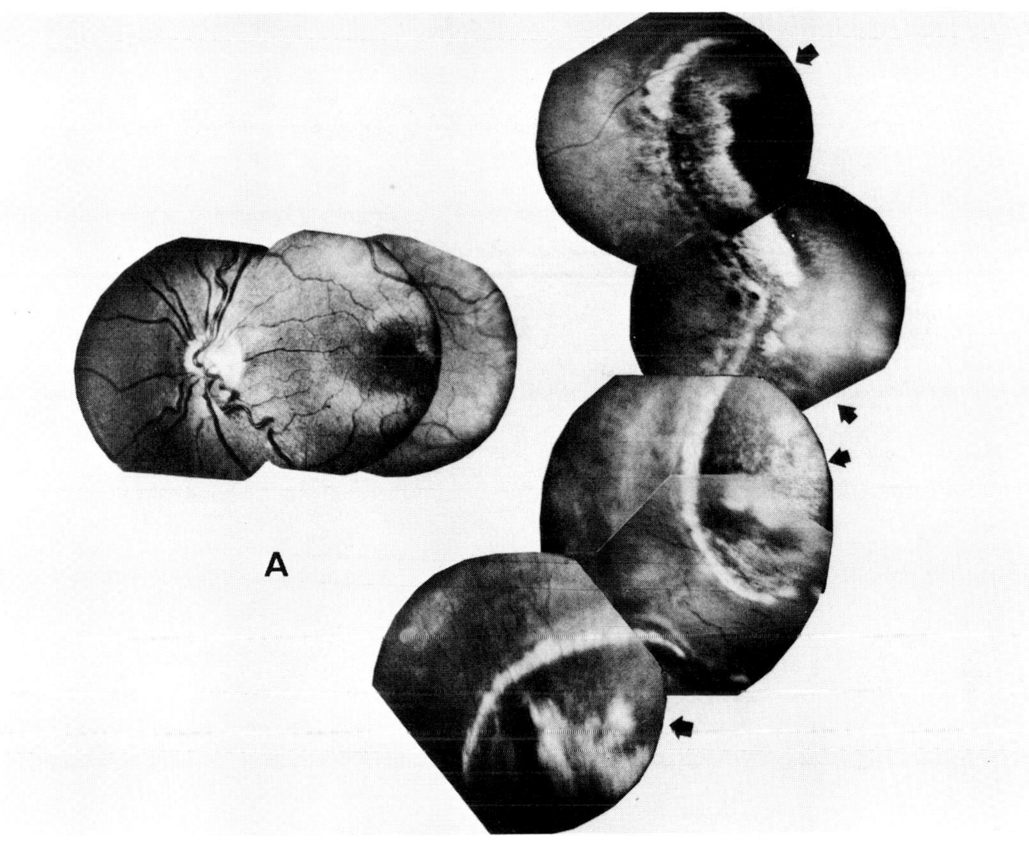

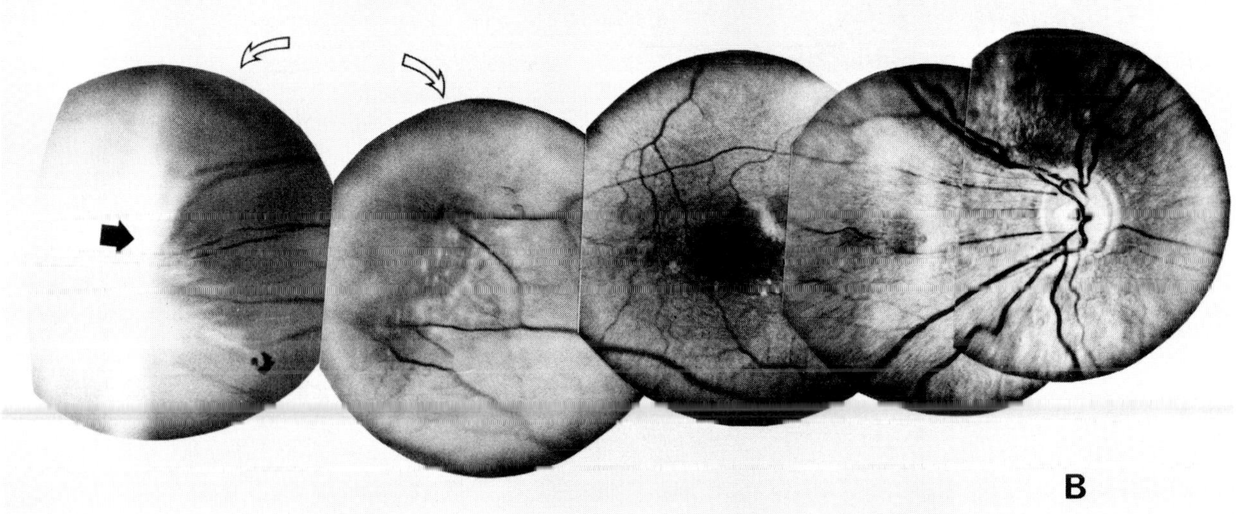

Figure 14–3 Composite of patient 3 in Table 14-8, who had unilateral treatment of symmetrical disease. A. Treated eye has normal architecture and peripheral cryoscars (black arrows). B. Untreated control eye with cicatricial Stage 2*3+ RLF. Retrolental mass (black arrow) caused detachment of peripheral retina (curved white arrows).

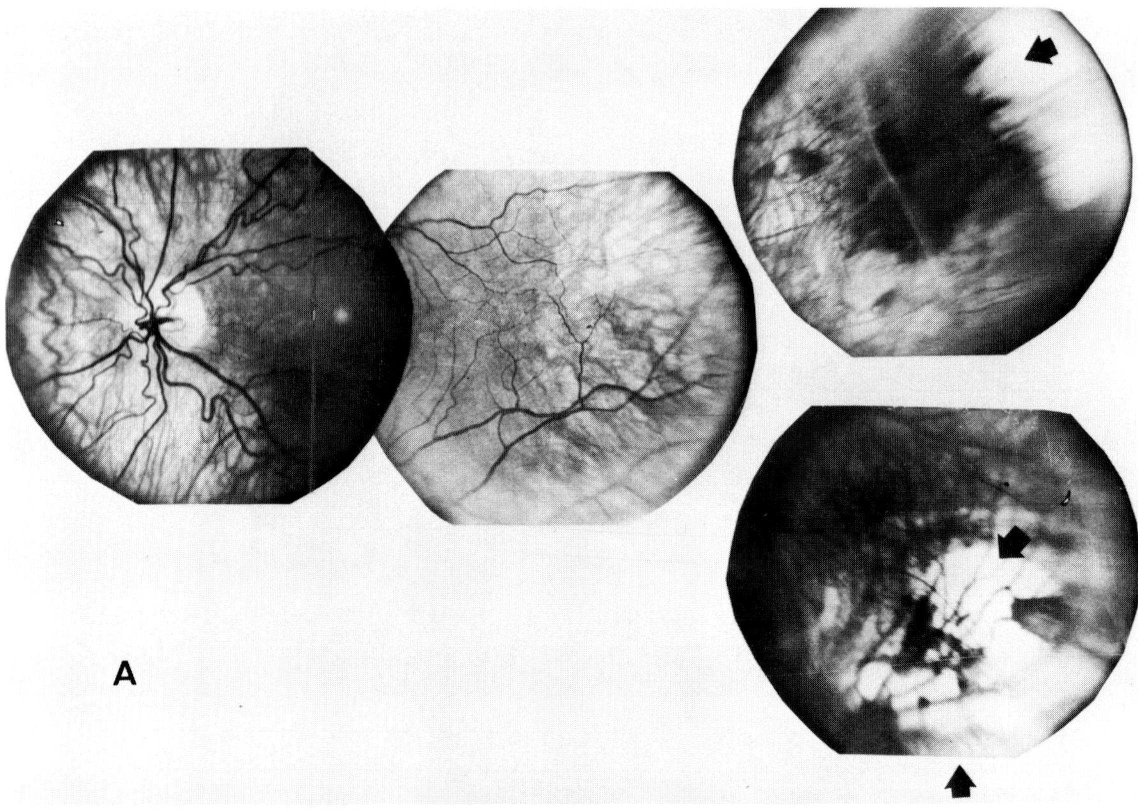

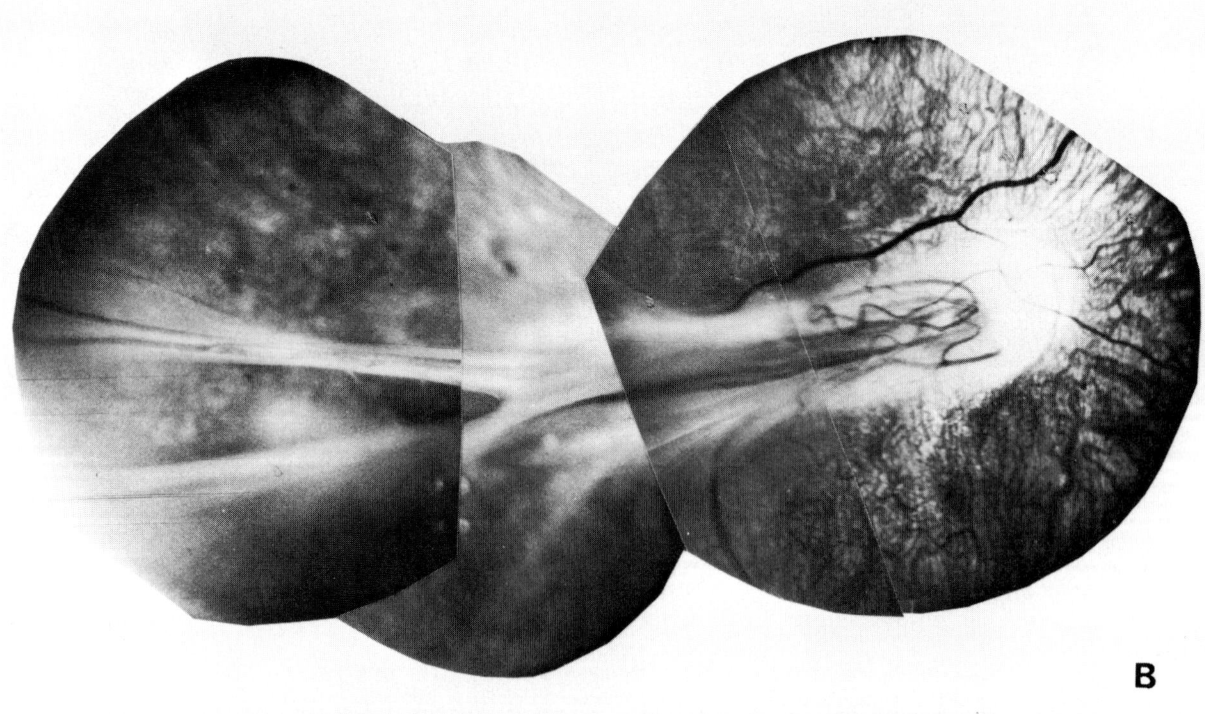

Figure 14–4 Composite of patient 4 in Table 14-8. A. Treated eye with 6.00 D myopia, normal retinal architecture and cryoscars in the periphery (black arrows). B. Untreated control eye has Stage 3 cicatricial RLF (falciform retinal fold); has poor vision.

TABLE 14–8 Results of Unilateral Treatment (of the most severely affected eye) in Symmetrical Stage 3 RLF[*]

Patient	Birth Weight (g)		RLF Stage	Extent of Main-Vessel Involvement	Myopia	Amblyopia
1	1,080	T[**]	1	>120°	+ [§]	
		C[†]	2	100°	+ +	
2	850	T	1	>120°	−	
		C	1	>120°	−	
3	1,270	T	1	120°	+	
		C	2 + 3 +	80°	+	+
4	1,115	T	1	>120°	+	
		C	3	30°	−	+ + +
5	1,600	T	1	>120°	+	
		C	1	> 120°	+	
6	1,020	T	2	110°	+	
		C	1	120°	+	
7	870	T	1	120°		
		C	1	120°		
8	700	T	1	>120°		
		C	2	100°	+	+
9	1,130	T	1	>120°		
		C	1	>120°		
10	1,000	T	1	>120°		
		C	1	>120°		

* Patients were either born elsewhere or were from Beilinson NICU and the parents refused bilateral treatment.
** T – treated eye (more severely affected eye)
† C = control (other untreated eye)
§ + – mild myopia < −3.0 D,   + + = moderate myopia > −3 < −6,   + + + = high myopia > −6,   − = no myopia

Myopia

In 155 premature infants born from 1974 to 1980, we found myopia in 50 percent of the babies who had ROP; only 16 percent of the babies without ROP were myopic. Moreover, we found a positive correlation between the degree of myopia and the severity of the cicatricial stages[10].

Clinico-Pathological Correlation

Only one patient (2 eyes) was available for pathologic examination[11]. This patient had been treated by cryotherapy on the avascular peripheral retina O.D. at Stage 3 in Zone II (six clock hours) and O.S. in Stage 3, Zone II (nine clock hours) + Stage 4 posteriorly, i.e., retinal detachment. In both eyes the ROP involuted rapidly, with eventual cicatricial Stage 1 O.D. and cicatricial Stage 2 without macular displacement O.S. Three months later, at age 6 months, the child died, and we examined the eyes. Figure 14-5 is a macroscopic view of the open left-globe periphery, showing 3 confluent cryocoagulation areas. The posterior border of the cryoscars is limited by an artifactual retinal fold. Further details are published elsewhere[11]. A careful histologic study revealed only a limited area of proliferation of new capillaries,

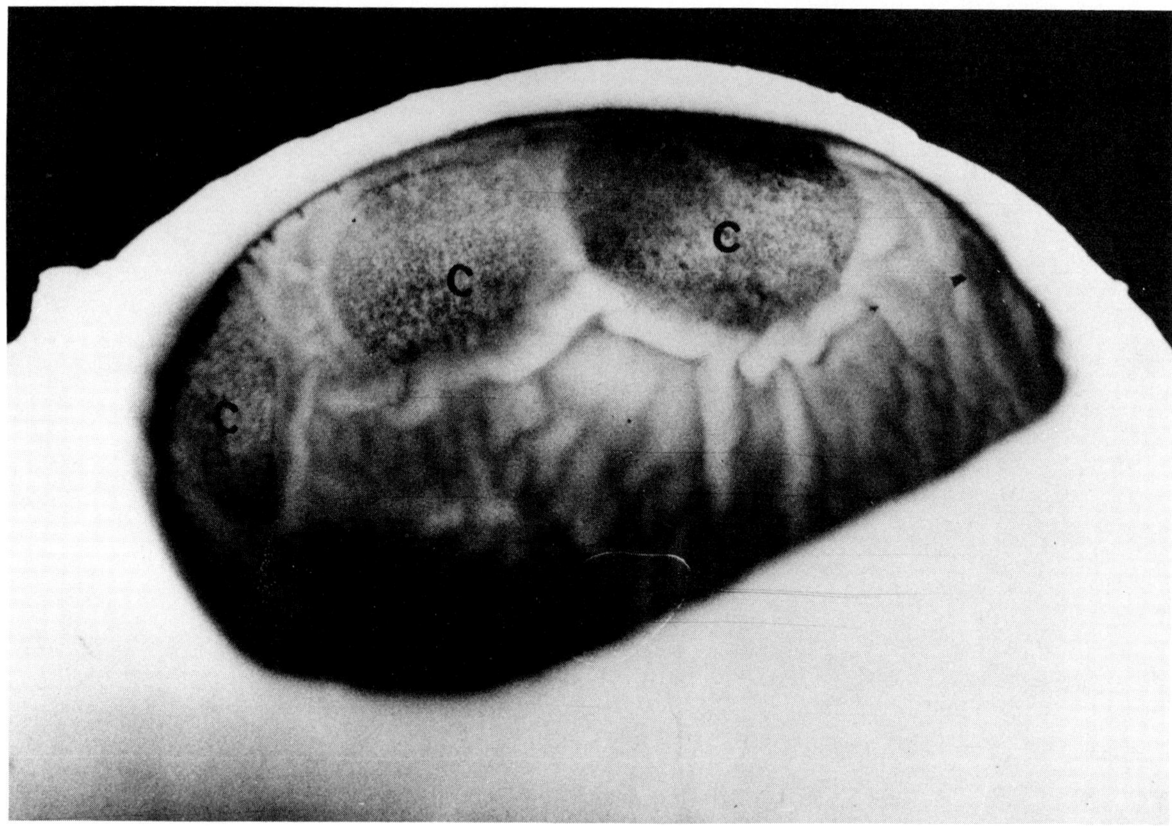

Figure 14–5 Open globe showing 3 confluent cryocoagulated areas (*c*) in retinal periphery. Posterior border of cryoscars is limited by artifactual retinal folds.

whereas most of the retina appeared to be normal (Fig. 14-6).

DISCUSSION

In his introductory remarks to the section on treatment, A. Patz[12] wrote: "Recognizing the high degree of spontaneous resolution, one must exercise extreme care in interpreting any therapeutic modality that has an apparent beneficial effect." Today the indirect small pupil ophthalmoscope facilitates examination of the preterm infant's fundus every week or two and makes it possible to obtain more accurate figures on the incidence of all forms of ROP. Increased survival of extremely-low-birth-weight infants in critical health has created a much larger population at risk of developing severe complications of retrolental fibroplasia.

Better recording of the ocular findings (careful retina drawings in each case, and definitions of zones and clock hours of the affected segments) using a chart similar to that presented in the new International Classification, and serial examinations, together with better understanding of the natural course of the disease, will enable us to reach firm conclusions regarding efficacy of cryotreatment in Stage 3 ROP. Ideally, a randomized double-blind controlled study is the goal of each clinical investigation. In ROP, this is not feasible for many reasons, not least of which is the relatively few patients in a single institution who might be available for testing of any specific therapeutic modality. However, our large data base, with relatively high survival rates of small babies over many years of continuous study, rigid documentation of the findings, and the extremely good results obtained enable us to conclude that our method of treatment is beneficial in preventing severe forms of RLF. Also, our method of treatment has no subsequent complications. In addition, cryotherapy is simple to perform, of short duration, does not need anesthesia, and requires no special postoperative treatment.

Data Base

It is essential in any discussion of the natural history of ROP and the incidence of sequelae, including blind-

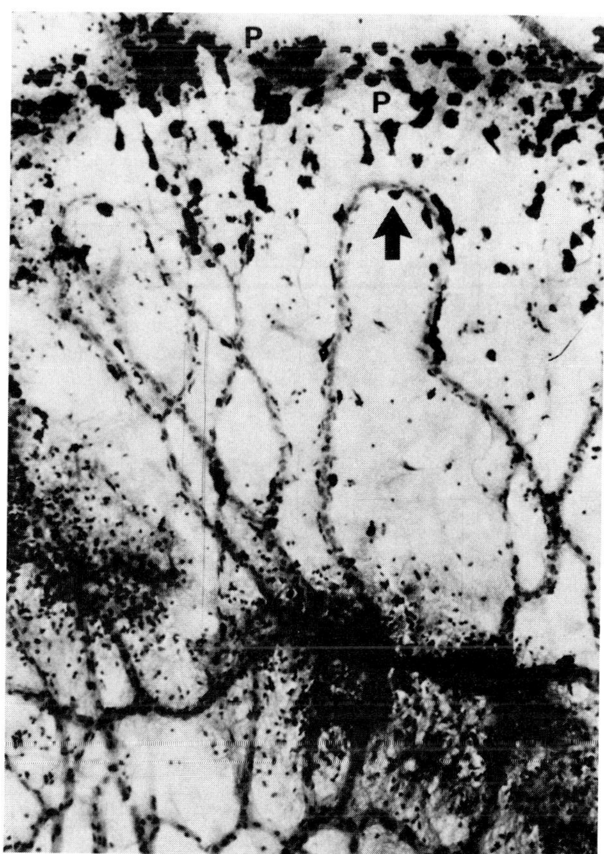

Figure 14–6 Retinal digest preparation showing capillary loops (black arrows) or "shunts" without active proliferation at the retinal periphery. Distally, pigment granules (*p*) are seen at cryotherapy sites.

ness, to study carefully the statistics of the population at risk. Nagata[13] reported on treatment of 17 cases over the past 15 years. Although most of this treatment was by xenon-arc photocoagulation, his method and his indications were similar to ours. His results are also very good in that only one of 17 patients developed blindness. Nagata did not supply data on the percentage of survival for each birth-weight group, but calculation from his overall survival rate of under 2,500 g discloses a comparatively low incidence of survival in the less than 1,500-g birth-weight group. Only 73 of 544 survivors weighed less than 1,500 g at birth, i.e., 13.2 percent as compared to our data, in which 401 infants, or 42.5 percent of a total of 942 survivors, weighed less than 1,500 g.

Kalina and Karr[6] reported a very low incidence of severe cicatricial RLF without any surgical treatment. However, in addition to the 34 infants affected by proliferative RLF that they lost to follow-up, a glance at the survival rate in Table 14-6 immediately discloses that even their best survival figures during recent years still average 10 to 15 percent lower than those of the Beilin-

son NICU or Indiana University Hospital[5]. For example, analysis of recent statistics from Kalina and Karr discloses a survival rate of only 46.3 percent for infants weighing less than 1,250 g, as compared to 60 percent at Beilinson Hospital.

Timing of Examination

Since ROP can develop rather rapidly, we strongly recommend that the first examination be performed at 2 to 3 weeks of age. To first examine the child upon discharge from the nursery would mean a delay in examination of the tiniest and sickest baby, who is in the greatest danger of developing a severe form of the disease while still in the incubator and receiving oxygen treatment. Follow-up examinations should be performed every week or two for most infants, and every week or even 2 to 3 days for rapidly developing ROP.

Cryoapplication on the Avascular Area Only

Foos[14] described an abnormal proliferation of spindle cells in the avascular retina in active ROP, which he designated "vanguard reactions." On the border between the vascularized and avascularized retina, in the area of the demarcation line (D line), he found abnormal proliferation of endothelial cells, which he called "rearguard reactions."

In studying ultrastructure of abnormal spindle cells, Kretzer and associates[4] found an increase in gap junctions of these spindle cells in the avascular retinas of preterm infants receiving continuous oxygen. It is precisely these abnormal spindle cells that are destroyed by our method of almost total ablation of the peripheral avascular retina anterior to the neovascular ridge. The routine observation of rapid regression of the neovascular proliferation after cryoapplication to this area raises the possibility that cryoapplication suppresses production of a vasoformative substance from the avascular retina. Nagata[13] also found that photocoagulation of the D line and avascular area causes disappearance of the vasoproliferative tissue, and commented that direct coagulation of newly-formed vessels, or coagulation of retinal areas posterior to the ridge, is not only unnecessary but rather harmful.

In treating active ROP, all other investigators except for Nagata and us place the application directly over the ridge and the vasoproliferative tissue. Such a direct application can result in minute to mild vitreous hemorrhage from the fibrovascular ridge, which will increase the fibrovascular contraction and cicatrization. We therefore do not recommend this form of therapy.

Analysis of the Results

Our small quasi-comparative study on 10 babies, although very encouraging, is inconclusive because of lack of randomization, and because of the small data base. However, the negative results of similar small quasi-controlled studies, comparing one eye against the other[15-17], should be interpreted along the same lines. On the other hand, the lack of any severe eye damage over 8 years, in a population at high risk of developing ROP, is an indication that our technique of cryotherapy is most effective in preventing the severe complications of RLF. All of the other studies on comparable patients disclose a relatively high percentage of severely visually handicapped or blind children. Comparing Campbell's[5] statistics to ours, we should have seen at least 17 patients with cicatricial Grade III or more, and at least 7 blind babies. Although statistically still feasible, it is quite unlikely that it is purely accidental that we have had no cicatricial Grade III or worse. We, therefore, believe that a double-blind controlled study on the results of cryotherapy is unnecessary, and have refused to participate in such a study.

Comparison of Treatment Methods and Results

We treat only advanced Stage 3 ROP when there are more than two clock hours of confluent fibrovascular proliferation. We do not allow a confluent fibrovascular element to enlarge. It is our impression that when a fibrovascular ridge involves more clock hours, especially if this ridge is thick, its circumferential contraction will cause retinal dragging, some degree of stretching of the temporal vessels, and even some macular heterotropia.

Keith[17] applied cryotherapy directly on the fibrovascular ridge confluent for more than two clock hours, which in 9 eyes resulted in rapid shrinkage and scarring of the ridge, with retinal dragging. In our opinion, he treated the wrong place at too late a stage in the disease, when contraction of fibrovascular elements is unavoidable.

Conversely, we believe that Nagata perhaps undertook treatment earlier than we did. Hindle's and Layton's[18] technique of treating the ridge and the neovascularization behind it is very different from ours; they

conclude that one should treat at Stage 3+. They and Mousel and Hoyt[19] treat directly on the D line and the neovascular ridge. McCormick[15] treated both the avascular zone and the newly formed vessels. He did not believe there was beneficial effect of cryotherapy in the 10 eyes he treated. Kingham[16] treated directly in Stage 4 or late Stage 3, which is very late, in our opinion. Hence his impression that treatment at this stage is ineffective or even harmful seems logical.

CONCLUSIONS

ROP will increase in its prevalence and severity because of the improved techniques for preserving the life of extremely small preterm infants. Early cryotherapy of the avascular retina halts the progression of ROP in every case. Cryotherapy is the only means presently available to prevent blindness or disability in progressive ROP cases.

True, we lack complete information on the natural history of ROP, and the proper time for cryoapplication has not yet been established. This situation should improve in coming years as additional investigators add their data to ours. Nevertheless, we recommend the use of this method in at least one eye, even by those who do not believe in its efficacy. The lack of complications and the data presented in this chapter constitute a good argument for not withholding this mode of therapy from the extremely delicate survivor in the nursery.

Our thanks go to the staff of the Department of Ophthalmology and the Department of Neonatology, Beilinson Medical Center, for their continuous help and cooperation. Mrs. Ruth Fradkin provided editorial assistance.

REFERENCES

1. Patz A. The continuing role of the ophthalmologist in the premature nursery. Arch Opthalmol 1971; 85:129-130.
2. Committee for the classification of retinopathy of prematurity. An international classification of retinopathy of prematurity. Pediatrics 1984; 74:127-133.
3. Ben-Sira I, Nissenkorn I, Grunwald E, Yassur Y. Treatment of acute retrolental fibroplasia by cryopexy. Br J Ophthalmol 1980; 64:758-762.
4. Kretzer FL, Mehta RS, Johnson AT, Hunter DG, Brown ES, Hittner HM. Vitamin E protects against retinopathy of prematurity through action on spindle cells. Nature 1984; 309:793-795.
5. Campbell PB, Bull MJ, Ellis FD, Bryson CQ, Lemons JA, Schreiner RL. Incidence of retinopathy of prematurity in a tertiary newborn intensive care unit. Arch Ophthalmol 1983; 101: 1686-1688.
6. Kalina RE, Karr DJ. Retrolental fibroplasia; experience over two decades in one institution. Ophthalmology 1982; 89:91-95.
7. Reisner S, Amir J, Shohat B, et al. Retinopathy of prematurity: incidence and treatment. Arch Dis Child 1985; 60:698-701.

8. Palmer EA. Optimal timing of examination for acute retrolental fibroplasia. Ophthalmology 1981; 88:662-668.

9. Wysenbeek I, Nissenkorn I, Cohen S, et al. Causes of blindness in children in the years 1976 to 1981 in Israel. Pediatr Ophthalmol Strabis (submitted).

10. Nissenkorn I, Yassur Y, Mashkowski D, Sheref I, Ben-Sira I. Myopia in premature babies with and without retinopathy of prematurity. Br J Ophthalmol 1983; 67:170-173.

11. Nissenkorn I, Kremer I, Ben-Sira I, Cohen S, Garner A. A clinico-pathological case of retinopathy of prematurity (ROP) treated by peripheral cryopexy. Br J Ophthalmol 1984; 68:36-41.

12. Patz A. Treatment of the acute proliferative phase (discussion leader introduction). Retinopathy of Prematurity Conference Syllabus 1981; 2:769-771.

13. Nagata M, Yamagishi N. Treatment of acute proliferative retinopathy of prematurity with xenon-arc photocoagulation. Retinopathy of Prematurity Conference Syllabus 1981; 2:772-783.

14. Foos RT. Acute retrolental fibroplasia. Albrecht von Graefes Arch Klin Exp Ophthalmol 1975; 195:87-100.

15. McCormick AQ. The retinopathy of prematurity in the newborn. Curr Probl in Pediatr 1977; 7:1-28.

16. Kingham JD. Acute retrolental fibroplasia. II. Treatment by cryosurgery. Arch Ophthalmol 1978; 96:2049-2053.

17. Keith CG. Visual outcome and effect of treatment in Stage 3 developing retrolental fibroplasia. Br J Ophthalmol 1982; 66:446-449.

18. Hindle NW, Leyton J. Prevention of cicatricial retrolental fibroplasia by cryotherapy. Can J Ophthalmol 1978; 13:277–282.

19. Mousel DK, Hoyt CS. Cryotherapy for retinopathy of prematurity. Ophthalmology 1980; 87:1121-1127.

Location and Timing of Intervention with Cryotherapy

N. *Warren Hindle*, M.D.

There is no stronger stimulus to understanding a disease than the potential for ameliorating the ill effects of that disease.

The frustration of observing an infant's eyes develop retinopathy of prematurity (ROP) and seeing distortion of the retina and even the whole globe from the resulting retrolental fibroplasia (RLF) provoked many investigators to attempt to alter what is perceived to be the likely outcome. After watching several infants become blind from ROP, in 1975 I attempted to abort serious ROP with cryotherapy. That first attempt failed, and I concluded that for treatment to be possible, the disease process had to be stopped prior to the onset of significant cicatricial disease.

Shortly thereafter, an infant arrived from another area with what I now recognize as severe Stage 3 ROP. I consulted Dr. Gordon Harris in Vancouver, asked him to accept the infant for treatment, and recommended ablation of the avascular retina in both eyes. By the time he saw the patient, both eyes had sectors of serous detachment, or Stage 4 ROP. He applied cryotherapy to the peripheral retina of each eye and placed a band around the eye having the most advanced detachment. The retinas were reattached, and there was no significant peripheral fibrosis; both eyes had a retinal pigment epitheliopathy into the posterior pole. The child's mental retardation interfered with subjective visual assessment, but it was quite evident that there was a field of vision, and that the anatomic state was much better than the Grade III to V RLF that was the expected natural outcome.

The third patient manifested Stage 3 + ROP for 360° in both eyes and was treated by Dr. G.E.M. Kirker, a retina surgeon and colleague, and by me. In our ignorance, we discussed how the eyes should be treated. I favored ablation of the avascular retina; he favored treatment of the extraretinal fibrovascular proliferation (EFP). As a compromise, we measured the location of the EFP from the ora serrata and applied cryotherapy to the avascular retina and to the EFP. The first few applications were accomplished under visualization with indirect ophthalmoscopy, and we timed the appearance of several ice balls. We found that a retina probe was too large and instead used an Amoils cataract pencil. We placed two rows of cryotherapy throughout the entire circumference, mostly without visualization.

When the lid edema had subsided sufficiently to allow examination, there had been a dramatic disappearance of iris hyperemia and posterior pole vascular engorgement; the "plus" disease had disappeared. The EFP could not be distinguished. Later it became apparent that both eyes had cryotherapy scars and no fibrosis, except in the superonasal quadrant of the left eye where peripheral preretinal fibrosis was evident. That infant died several months later of central nervous system complications, and Leyton and I made a clinical pathological correlation.[1] From the documented location of vessels running circumferentially immediately behind the ridge-EFP prior to treatment, and from the relationship of those vessels to the fibrosis and the cryotherapy scars in the postmortem specimen, it was precisely determined that the cryotherapy had been applied anterior to the ridge-EFP structure in the area of residual fibrosis. In all other areas of both eyes, there was no anatomic abnormality other than the cryotherapy scars.

By the time that analysis had been completed, I had treated one or both eyes of three more patients, with encouraging results. On the basis of the analysis, all subsequent patients were treated following the principle of straddling the ridge-EFP with cryotherapy. Some avascular retinas and some vascular retinas were, in fact, treated by the straddle, but usually the treatment spared variable amounts of avascular retina, depending upon the location of the ridge.

The prospect that intervention would be beneficial

necessitated a precise and frequent observation and documentation of ROP. Several excellent publications reassured me that the disease was not unique in our area and that the previous descriptions of ROP were not adequate.[2,3] Upon finally reading several key English translations from the Japanese literature regarding treatment, I was even more encouraged.[4,5] However, being cognizant of the possible hazards of treatment to the whole infant (in addition to the destructive nature of the treatment and the wide-ranging disparity of opinion about it), I attempted to be more critical and selective of cases requiring treatment.

Following the limited protocol of location of treatment, I have reached some tentative conclusions regarding the efficacy of treatment and the quality and quantity of disease that should be treated. Accordingly, the following describes my current methods of examination, documentation, therapy, and criteria for treatment based on results, with necessary digression to give a theoretical or practical rationale for the management of ROP.

TERMINOLOGY

Subdivision of Stage 3 ROP

The terminology used herein is that of the International Classification of Retinopathy of Prematurity.[6] However, in the deliberation that established the classification, problems were encountered in reaching a consensus in certain areas. In particular, there were problems with the subdivision of Stage 3 ROP. In this Stage the ROP reaches a critical mass that will, upon involution or regression, leave sufficient cicatricial disease, so that visual function and the integrity of the retina and eye are partially or completely compromised.

It is fundamental that the subdivision of Stage 3 ROP be based on extraretinal fibrovascular proliferation (EFP) at the ridge, at its posterior aspect and internal to it, and not at any distance behind and separate from the ridge.

Whereas the International Classification of Retinopathy of Prematurity subdivides Stage 3 in a subjective, qualitative fashion into mild, moderate, and severe, it is fundamental to my management that a distinction be made between three identifiable anatomic substages of Stage 3.

The first, Stage 3a, is the earliest manifestation of EFP at the posterior edge of the ridge and not detached from the ridge. Small EFPs accumulate along the posterior aspect of the ridge and remain in contact with it. This

is distinguished from the small EFPs that can be seen posteriorly displaced from the ridge, lying close to the retina, that are not considered sufficient to classify the disease as Stage 3. However, if the small aggregations from the posterior crest of the ridge remain in contact with it, they fungate outside the confines of the retina in the less restrictive vitreous. These small, isolated accretions are the mildest manifestation of Stage 3 disease. The substage might be very short-lived and can easily be missed. It is equally difficult to photograph; a black-and-white photograph does not show these accretions well enough for reproduction here.

The second or middle substage, Stage 3b, is anatomically identifiable as a coalescence of the many small aggregates into a confluent mass attached to the posterior aspect of the ridge. This confluent mass can cover part of a sector, or clock hour, or run from several to many clock hours. The confluent EFP can expand internally and posteriorly to the ridge. It can have irregular projections strung out posteriorly but continuous with the main mass at the posterior aspect of the ridge. Figure 15–1 shows Stage 3b ROP.

When the growth of small structures from the internal aspect of the confluent EFP can be identified, this heralds the onset of Stage 3c ROP, or the late manifestation of the stage. These small structures frequently appear to grow as a sheet or membrane into the vitreous, perpendicularly to the retina or posteriorly. With continued growth, the membrane extends retrolentally. When this intact structure fibroses, the contracting retrolental sheet pulls the retina into that sector produc-

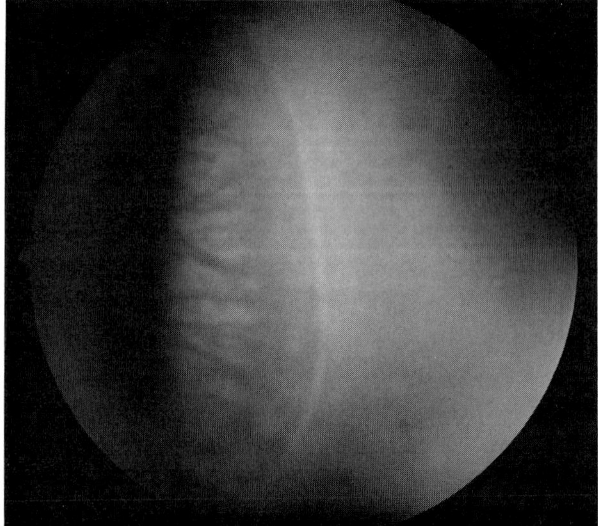

Figure 15–1 Stage 3b ROP. The confluent extraretinal fibrovascular proliferation is collected at the posterior aspect of the ridge.

ing Grade II to IV RLF. If the retrolental sheet is present for 360°, the retina is pulled into a funnel behind the lens to produce Grade V RLF.

This latest substage is the most "severe" manifestation of Stage 3 ROP. It is difficult to see in its earliest phases and can become invisible on examination if indentation collapses the vascular flow. Because of the angle of projection, it is difficult to photograph. James Kingham has contributed the superb photograph in Figure 15–2, showing Stage 3c+ ROP. The absence of color detracts from the excellence of the photograph, but it is evident that the camera focus is internal to the plane of the retina, and the arrow shows the fimbriated projections from the internal surface of the confluent ROP Stage 3b. I discovered these vascular projections when applying cryotherapy to the EFP. With indentation I could not see the vessels, but spikes of freezing were observed to shoot out from the confluent EFP into the vitreous.

The ridge-EFP structure is a vascular sponge that, in proportion to its mass, shunts blood from arteriolar to venous circulation. We first see evidence of the changes in vascular flow in vessels just behind the ridge; the dilated arterioles become indistinguishable from the venules. When the changes in vascular flow affect the vessels in Zone I, producing tortuous arteries and dilated veins, the term "plus" disease is added to the stage. The intravascular incompetence of plus disease in Stage 3 ROP, related directly to the mass of EFP and the vascular shunting, can produce serous detachments or Stage 4 disease prior to the cicatrizing process.

MONITORING AND DOCUMENTATION OF ROP

Methods of Examination

Contrary to most investigators, I do not screen for this disease with indirect ophthalmoscopy. Instead I use the Layden infant gonioscopy lens and a direct ophthalmoscope that can give single diopter steps from +6D to +14D. As in Figure 15–3, the lens splints the lids, can control ocular position with gentle maneuvering, and does not distort the disease. The entire retina can be seen to the ora serrata without indentation. There is a compromise of binocular impression. Using the indirect ophthalmoscope through the infant gonioscopy lens, with and without the condensing lens, gives additional

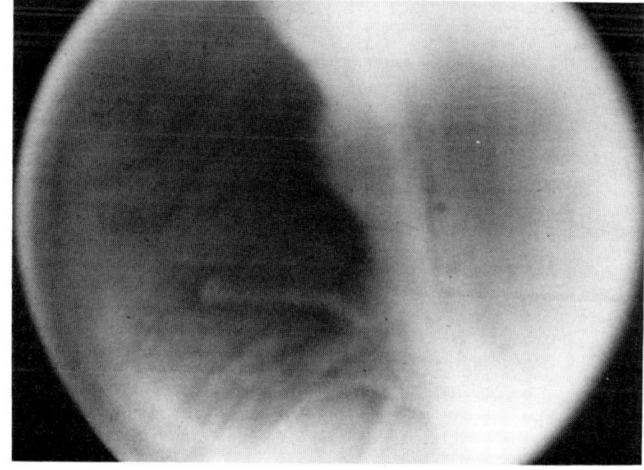

Figure 15–2 Stage 3c+ ROP. Arrow indicates the fibrovascular extensions from the confluent extraretinal fibrovascular proliferation of Stage 3b ROP. Photo courtesy of J. Kingham.

information. I do not indent the eyes in the nursery. Photography is possible with a hand-held camera through the same lens.

The pupils are dilated with 0.2% cyclopentolate and 1.0% phenylephrine, 45 minutes and 30 minutes prior to the examination; topical anesthetic is applied to the cornea. The examination is atraumatic locally or systemically, and can be performed on the smallest infants under almost any circumstances. It can also be effectively used in follow-up of infants up to 4 months of adjusted age, without sedation.

Examination Schedule

I currently follow the examination schedule outlined in Table 15–1. In order to be selective in treatment, to avoid treating eyes unnecessarily, it is fundamental that disease progression be documented and examination be frequent once Stage 3 ROP is observed.

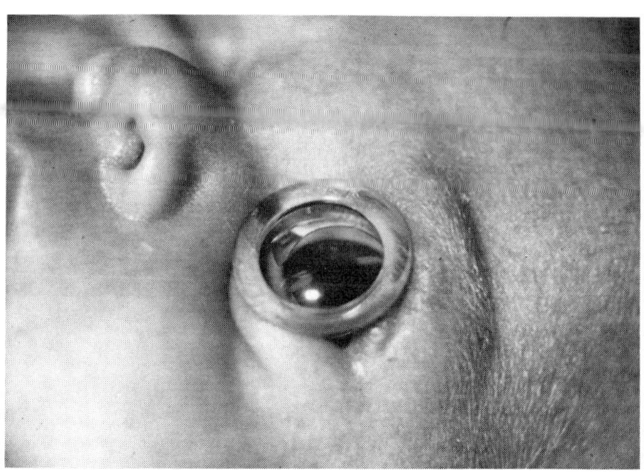

Figure 15–3 Layden infant gonioscopy lens.

TABLE 15-1   Examination Schedule for ROP

Gestational Age at Birth	First Examination Chronological Age	Subsequent Examination
≥ 34 weeks	6–8 weeks	None if no ROP and retina nearly or fully vascularized
< 34 weeks	4–5 weeks	Every 2 weeks if no ROP; every 1 week if ROP
Any age with Stage 3 ROP		Every 2–7 days, depending on severity and rate of progression
Any age with resolving ROP		Every 2–4 weeks to complete resolution
Any age with iris hyperemia	Immediate	Dictated by findings

Documentation of Findings

Since December 1981, I have documented the disease not only by its qualitative appearance or stage, but also by the location of the ROP and associated findings in the eye, employing a coding system.[7] The system allows quantification of the ROP. At each examination it enables a comparison to previous observations, and facilitates documentation of disease progression in terms of stages or quantity. The process also allows one to verify observations when significant differences of location or staging of disease are identified from one examination to the next. The International Classification of Retinopathy of Prematurity describes a simplified version of this documentation system (see Chapter 3); I adjusted my previously reported system to the staging of the International Classification.

SELECTION OF EYES FOR TREATMENT

The problem of selecting eyes for treatment is the primary obstacle in this disease. If we could be certain which eyes were destined to develop visually disabling RLF, there would be little controversy about subjecting these eyes to treatment that is less destructive. That the majority of ROP regresses with little to no visible trace of its prior existence is not in question. *Under no circumstances should Stage 1 or 2 ROP require treatment.* Also, I have not seen significant cicatricial disease result from eyes that have Stage 3a or 3a+ disease as the maximum stage. Accordingly, Stage 3a is not an indication for treatment.

I have presented and submitted for publication a retrospective analysis of 30 eyes treated in 17 patients, following the protocol of treatment of the ridge-EFP. In some of the eyes, the avascular retina was also partially treated. The treated eyes were in three groups, according to severity of ROP at the time of treatment: early Stage 4 to 4+, Stage 3c+, and Stage 3b+ ROP. Early Stage 4 refers to only those eyes with shallow detachment just posterior to the ridge-EFP, and still peripherally located.

Better visual function in terms of acuity and field and RLF less than Grade II was found in the group with Stage 3b+ disease than in the groups treated with Stage 3c+ or Stage 4 to 4+ ROP. In both instances there was a high degree of statistical significance.

Comparing the results of Stage 3c+ and Stage 4 to 4+ groups showed that this method of therapy did not yield significantly better results statistically. However, the results from the Stage 4 to 4+ ROP group were significantly better than in a group of eyes with Stage 4 ROP that had had no treatment as reported by McCormick.[3] Finally, the number of eyes treated was approximately 7.6 percent of all eyes that had any stage of ROP, well within the range of eyes in that population that would be expected to have visual disability due to RLF.

Given that the goal of intervention is the preservation of visual function and the reduction of visually disabling RLF, the following conclusions could be made:

1. Any eye with any Stage 4 ROP should be treated.
2. Any eye with any Stage 3c+ ROP should be treated.

However, a definitive statement with respect to treatment of Stage 3b+ ROP is not possible at this time. *The simple presence of any Stage 3b+ ROP is not an indication for treatment.* Several factors must be considered. Selection for treatment of eyes with Stage 3b+ ROP is based upon:

1. Progressive accumulation of confluent EFP.
2. The presence of plus disease.
3. The location of the ridge-EFP. The more posterior the disease and accordingly the greater the area of avascular retina, the more serious the disease.
4. The uninterrupted circumferential extent of the confluent EFP.

While absolute indications for treatment of progressive Stage 3b+ ROP are not possible, some events encourage withholding treatment. It seems that one or two clock hours, perhaps even three clock hours of confluent EFP will lift away from the ridge and resolve with little or no evidence of cicatrization. This seems to occur with the following signs:

1. Progressive lifting of the confluent EFP, first observed at the end of the continuous segment.
2. Fading of the pink congested color of the EFP, and subsidence of vascular dilatation behind the EFP, and of the plus in Zone I.
3. Separation of the confluent EFP from the ridge, such that it sits as a sinusoid or cloud in the vitreous posterior, and internal to the ridge. As a result, the ridge is evident anterior to the EFP. Feeder vessels from the posterior retina can elevate to the sinusoid and should not be interpreted as a retinal detachment or Stage 4 ROP. The sinusoid fades away, leaving a wispy gray skeleton that eventually disappears. The feeder vessels simultaneously disappear.

Completion of vascularization in other sectors of the eye is also a favorable sign. As the area of avascular retina decreases, the stimulus for proliferation also seems to decrease. (The theoretical basis for this phenomenon is supported by Kretzer's observation on angiogenic factors in the avascular retinas.)[8]

However, if the EFP remains at the site of the ridge, frequently obscuring it, and turns white with the disappearance of the vascular congestion, while retaining a solid appearance, then cicatrization and distortion of the adjacent posterior retina is likely to occur. In that case, the EFP should have been ablated prior to that appearance. Additionally if any part of the confluent EFP shows progression to Stage 3c+ or Stage 4 ROP, I interpret that as an absolute indication for treatment and that I should have treated before those developments. Accordingly, I ablate all of the Stage 3c+ or 4 ROP and any Stage 3 ROP in continuity with it.

An exception to the above indications for selection is the occurrence of the rare disease labeled "rush" ROP.[5] I have only experienced one case of this type of ROP. After a delay in diagnosis, treatment efforts with photocoagulation and cryotherapy were futile, probably because of improper timing and lack of aggressive treatment.

OPERATIVE MANAGEMENT

Anesthesia

I would personally find treatment impossible unless the infant was under a general anesthetic. Perhaps because we treat more posteriorly than those who treat the avascular retina only, we find that control using a general anesthetic is necessary. Additionally, in the one case in which we used local anesthesia, the infant's response and Valsalva with crying might have been sufficient to cause excessive hemorrhage from the treated EFP. Accordingly, I advise treatment by this method only if the child is paralyzed, intubated, and narcotized or anesthetized.

Instrumentation

Because we treat posteriorly, I recommend that the cataract probe be used. I insulate it by pulling a piece of 19-gauge intracath silicone over the shaft, leaving 1.5 to 2 mm of tip exposed. The probe should have a mild curve to avoid shaft indentation of the globe and incorrect placement of the cryotherapy.

Technique

Under visualization with indirect ophthalmoscopy, the probe is passed over the avascular retina until the ridge-EFP structure is indented. I apply cold until the internal extent of the EFP is frozen. The conjunctiva has not had to be opened on any cases to date; accordingly, nonsterile operating conditions are sufficient.

All Stage 3 ROP, contiguous with the Stage 3 b+ or worse ROP, is treated. We try to place one spot adjacent to the next, i.e., avoiding gaps. With defrosting, a small hemorrhage might occur at the internal extent of the EFP. Separate areas of Stage 3a ROP are not treated, nor is any lesser stage of ROP.

At the end of the procedure, atropine 1 percent ophthalmic ointment and chloromycetin hydrocortisone ophthalmic ointment are applied to the operated eye. The infant is returned to the intensive care nursery for postanesthetic recovery.

POSTOPERATIVE FINDINGS AND MANAGEMENT

The atropine 1 percent ointment is continued once daily, and the chloromycetin hydrocortisone ointment twice daily for 5 days postoperatively.

I re-examine the eyes as soon as the subsidence of lid edema allows. A successfully treated eye shows a disappearance of the plus disease and fading or absence of iris hyperemia, if that was present preoperatively. Within 3 days, a retinal pigment epithelial reaction to the cryotherapy is evident. The EFP that was treated is usually indistinguishable, overlying the cryo spot. The small hemorrhages that might have occurred at the cessation of freezing usually remain localized and disappear over 2 to 4 weeks. A small serous detachment posterior to the cryotherapy is sometimes seen, particularly following treatment of Stage 4 or Stage 3c+ disease. Small areas of 3b+ (less than one clock hour) that were inadvertently missed between cryo spots are watched for progression. Areas of Stage 3a ROP or less that were not treated because they were not contiguous with the Stage 3b+ or worse disease are watched closely for progression. If sufficient Stage 3b+ is reached, or if any quantity of Stage 3c+ is observed, I treat those areas.

The eyes are examined closely at intervals dictated by the state of disease and the response to cryotherapy. Once the retina is fully vascularized and any residual ROP is clearly resolving, unexpected or sudden changes in the state of the eye do not occur.

COMPLICATIONS

Intraoperative

Conjunctival tears are sometimes produced; they have required no treatment. Hemorrhage from the treated EFP usually is small and remains localized. On two occasions, bradycardia was encountered during the procedures. In the first instance, the condition was resolved with cessation of treatment and stabilization of the patient by the anesthesiologist; in the second, the anesthesiologist requested that the procedures be abandoned because of recurrent bradycardia. I treated this infant 5 days later without a recurrence of the problem.

Postoperative

Once when the retina probe was used on anteriorly located ROP, bilateral hyphemas occurred. That was the only case treated with the retina probe. The hyphemas cleared spontaneously, with some peripheral iris atrophy in areas, but there was no other evidence of anterior segment damage. I presumed that the ice ball had inadvertently encroached on the peripheral iris. This instance occurred after considerable experience with the cataract probe, and we have returned to using only the

cataract probe. Two infants had to be maintained on a respirator for up to 12 hours postoperatively, but no systemic problems have persisted as a result of the anesthetic or the procedure.

LONG-TERM RESULTS

Successfully treated eyes showed peripheral cryotherapy scars and no gross evidence of preretinal fibrosis. Retinal drag was absent or minimal, such that macular heterotopia still allowed corrected acuity of better than 20/60. In those eyes that had peripheral fibrosis and retinal drag, the degree of drag at the disc was less than the degree of drag described in the Reese classification of Grade II RLF.

Table 15–2 summarizes the results of treatment from each group. All of the eyes with a field of vision only had macular pigment epitheliopathy. Possibly this condition is aggravated by the treatment. Its infrequency in the Stage 3b+ treated eyes, and the fact that vascular incompetence and serous effusion are more extensive in the Stage 3c+ or 4+ eyes, even to the posterior pole, somewhat reassure us that the treatment might not have contributed to this compromise of central acuity.

Optic atrophy was found in four eyes of two patients, and suspected in two eyes of one patient. Two patients were from the Stage 3c+ ROP group, and one from the Stage 4 ROP group. Compression of the eyes during treatment could contribute to optic atrophy. The paired distribution, and optic atrophy from cerebral hypoxia and other causes in these high-risk infants, make it less likely that the treatment caused the optic atrophy, but the treatment could have been a contributing factor. Accordingly, compression of the eyes at treatment should not be sustained.

CONCLUDING REMARKS

This has been one investigator's method of ROP management. The methods and opinions from other authors cited in this text indicate that there are several treatment options. I look forward to collaborative, controlled studies using the common language and the location and qualification of disease inherent in the International Classification of Retinopathy of Prematurity. Such studies will more accurately identify that critical mass of ROP that is intolerable, give us more

TABLE 15-2 Results of Cryotherapy in 30 Eyes with ROP

Stage of ROP	No. of Eyes	RLF Grade II	Functional Acuity and Field	Functional Field Only	Blind
3b+	13	13	12	1	0
3c+	7	3	2	5	0
4 to 4+	10	1	2	7	1

accurate indications for intervention, and identify the least destructive methods of intervention that will effectively abort the progression of those eyes to visual disability, ocular morbidity, and blindness.

REFERENCES

1. Hindle NW, Leyton J. Prevention of cicatricial retrolental fibroplasia by cryotherapy. Can J Ophthalmol 1978; 13:277–282.
2. Kingham JD. Acute retrolental fibroplasia. Arch Ophthalmol 1977; 95:39–47.
3. McCormick AQ. Retinopathy of prematurity. Curr Probl Pediatr 1977; 7(11):1–28.
4. Nagata M. Treatment of acute proliferative retrolental fibroplasia with xenon-arc photocoagulation: its indication and limitations. Jpn J Ophthalmol 1977; 21:436–459.
5. Uemura Y. Current status of retrolental fibroplasia: report of joint committee for the study of retrolental fibroplasia in Japan. Jpn J Ophthalmol 1977; 21:366–378.
6. The Committee for The Classification of Retinopathy of Prematurity. An international classification of retinopathy of prematurity. Arch Ophthalmol 1984; 102:1130–1134.
7. Hindle NW. The Calgary code. A numerical and alphabetical nosography of retrolental fibroplasia. Can J Ophthalmol 1982; 17:110–112.
8. Kretzer FL, Mehta RS, Johnson AT, Hunter DG, Brown ES, Hittner HM. Vitamin E protects against retinopathy of prematurity through action on spindle cells. Nature 1984; 309:793–795.

Treatment of Acute Retinopathy of Prematurity by Cryotherapy and Photocoagulation

16

Makoto Tamai, M.D.

The incidence of acute retinopathy of prematurity (ROP) has been dramatically reduced because of strict control in the concentration of oxygen used and advanced technology in nursing premature neonates.

Consequently, fewer infants require surgical treatment to prevent progression of retinopathy of prematurity (ROP) to retinal detachment and severe RLF. But it is also true that in neonates who have idiopathic respiratory distress syndrome (IRDS), pediatricians must frequently administer oxygen at high concentration. That means ROP in IRDS neonates is sometimes inevitable, and new cases continue to appear.

Nagata[1] used photocoagulation for acute ROP and Yamashita et al[2-3] used cryotherapy in Japan, where their experiences and results have been published. Unfortunately, the effectiveness of these surgical treatments, particularly cryotherapy, has been controversial, and the results conflicting[1-14].

Here I present our experience with ROP in premature neonates, and the results of treatment of active stages by cryotherapy and/or photocoagulation at Tohoku University Hospital and Sendai Red Cross Hospital. Our belief is that cryotherapy or photocoagulation is effective in decreasing the incidence of severe cicatricial grades of RLF.

CLASSIFICATION USED IN OUR CLINIC

Some results reported in Japan have not been understood or accepted in other countries, because we have not described our classification of acute and cicatricial RLF. To better understand the present results, it would be worthwhile to desribe briefly these classifications. From the early 1960s to the early 1970s, most Japanese ophthalmologists classified their patients according to Owen's system[15]. But they felt keenly the need to revise it and to establish a new classification system,

and the Joint Committee for the Study of ROP in Japan, sponsored by the Ministry of Health and Welfare, was formed in 1974. The committee announced a new classification system in 1977[16]. Even though it was revised by the same committee in 1981, we have been using the system reported in 1977; the present report is also based on it. As a result, the data previously reported from our clinic are compatible with this report.

Active Stages of Retinopathy of Prematurity

Stage 1. There is tortuosity and dilation of retinal vessels at the peripheral retina. They run parallel and branch into small vessels. No abnormality is found in the posterior retina.

Stage 2. A white ridge is formed by the terminal area of branching temporal vessels. It is an intraretinal proliferation. Nagata[17] in 1970 called this structure the demarcation line (D line). It was called the mesenchymal band by O'Grady and associates[4], the mesenchymal ridge by Hindle and Leyton[10], and the shelf, or vasoformative ridge, by Keith[18]. In this report we call it the D line after Nagata: it is formed at the margin of vascularized and unvascularized retina.

Stage 3. New vessels project into the vitreous, and exudates from these vessels reach into the vitreous along the D line. This structure progressively extends through one or two quadrants. Few vessels with proliferative mesenchymal cells extend widely. If the retinopathy becomes more active, the D line, with vessels and mesenchymal cells, greatly proliferates and approaches the posterior lens surface. Dilated, tortuous vessels with proliferative mass extend from the disc to the top of the D line through the vitreous cavity. In the revised classification, this stage was divided into three substages.

Stage 4. There is partial or total retinal detachment and retrolental fibrous mass formation. In the revised classification, this stage is also divided into Stages 4 and 5, depending upon the amount of retinal detachment.

Cicatricial Grades of Retrolental Fibroplasia

Grade I.   There is atrophy of the peripheral retina, and white scar tissue. The atrophic area consists of pigmentation, retinal atrophy, and abrupt disappearance of the retinal vessels. Sometimes retinoschisis is found, and myopia is common.

Grade II.   A dragged disc is observed in most cases. The macula is temporally displaced. If the macula is intact, vision is usually normal. Myopia (sometimes high) is common, as is astigmatism. In the revised classification, this grade is divided into three subgrades by the degree of dragged disc.

Grade III.   The dragged disc, with partial tentlike extension of the fibrous tissue into the temporal periphery, forms a retinal fold. The retinal vessels are incorporated into the fold. A peripheral ring-shaped retinal detachment can be present.

Grade IV.   Partial or total RLF formation is present. This grade is also subdivided into Grades IV (partial RLF) and V (total RLF) in the revised classification.

MATERIALS AND METHODS

From 1976 to 1983, 372 premature babies were born at the Obstetric Ward of the Tohoku University Hospital, and acute ROP was found in 108. Their active ROP stages and birth weights of gestational ages are shown in Tables 16-1 and 16-2. At Sendai Red Cross Hospital, 92 premature babies were born between April 1982 and

TABLE 16-1   ROP Stages Compared with Birth Weights (1976-1983) at Tohoku University Hospital

	Birth Weight (g)			
Active Stage	< 1,000	1,000-1,500	> 1,500	Total
0	1	18	245	264
1	0	12	61	73
2	4	11	5	20
3	1	13 (cryo and/or phc:9)*	1	15
4	0	0	0	0
Total	6	54	312	372

* Cryotherapy and/or argon laser photocoagulation

TABLE 16-2   ROP Stages Compared with Gestational Ages (1976-1983) at Tohoku University Hospital

	Gestational Age (wk)				
Active Stage	23-27	28-30	31-35	36-40	Total
0	2	12	97	153	264
1	1	10	39	23	73
2	4	8	7	1	20
3	2 (cryo:1)	12 (cryo* and/or phc:8)	1	0	15
4	0	0	0	0	0
Total	9	42	144	177	372

* Cryotherapy and/or argon laser photocoagulation

September 1983 at the Neonatal Intensive Care Unit (NICU). Their active ROP stages and birth weights or gestational ages are shown in Tables 16-3 and 16-4.

Delivery of Cryotherapy

Cryotherapy is easy to deliver if we customarily observe the fundus through the binocular indirect ophthalmoscope; we routinely use local anesthesia with 1 percent procaine hydrochloride, or topical anesthesia with lidocaine. General anesthesia is used only in exceptional cases, such as for babies having severe asphyxia. We use the cryopencil for retinal detachment surgery (Keeler-Amoils Co., England), through the conjunctiva under direct control through the binocular indirect ophthalmoscope. Freezing must be directed at the D line and extend on both sides of it. Repeating a freeze-thaw cycle in one spot must be avoided. When the media were hazy, and it was difficult to confirm the location of the

TABLE 16-3   ROP Stages Compared with Birth Weights (April 1982 - September 1983) at Sendai Red Cross Hospital

	Birth Weight (g)			
Active Stage	< 1,000	1,000 - 1,500	> 1,500	Total
0	2	19	46	67
1	5	4	3	12
2	3	5	0	8
3	2 (cryo:2)*	2 (cryo:1)	0	4
4	1 (cryo:1)	0	0	1
Total	13	30	49	92

* Cryotherapy

TABLE 16-4   ROP Stages Compared with Gestational Ages (April 1982 - September 1983) at Sendai Red Cross Hospital

Active Stage	Gestational Age (wk)				Total
	23-27	28-30	31-35	36-40	
0	0	14	42	11	67
1	5	2	5	0	12
2	3	4	1	0	8
3	4 (cryo:3)*	0	0	0	4
4	1 (cryo:1)	0	0	0	1
Total	13	20	48	11	92

* Cryotherapy

cryopencil tip, and treatment was urgent, we extrapolated its location from the visible area. In such cases, we never coagulated more than two spots in one quadrant. When there was a wide avascular area anterior to the D line, one more row of cryotherapy was required from the periphery to the line. If the retinopathy progressed in spite of cryotherapy, we repeated cryotherapy but carefully selected one location. The second session could be done by photocoagulation if the media became clear and the peripheral retina could be examined in detail.

Delivery of the Photocoagulation

We use Mizuno's binocular argon laser photocoagulator[19] (Nidek Co., Tokyo). Using general anesthesia, we delivered one or two rows of photocoagulation posterior to the D line, one spot diameter apart, then one or two rows anterior to the D line. Coagulation was done in 600 to 1,000 μm spots, using 400 to 700 mW of power for 0.1 to 0.2 seconds. Great care was taken not to treat too much posterior retina. In active Stage 3, or a more advanced stage, the D line and the macula are very close to each other, and photocoagulation spots can unexpectedly reach too far posteriorly, resulting in macular damage. If the media were still too hazy to apply photocoagulation, we would prefer to treat with cryotherapy.

RESULTS

The incidence of active ROP by birth weight and gestational age is listed in Table 16-5. Fifteen cases in the Tohoku University Hospital and four in the Red Cross Hospital were diagnosed as active Stage 3. One case in Red Cross Hospital was treated in Stage 3, but developed to the active Stage 4. We maintain that neonates having active Stage 3 retinopathy and a D line progressing through more than two quadrants must be surgically treated. If the Stage 3 retinopathy was not progressive or gradually slowed, as observed by daily funduscopy, we did not treat surgically and only observed. Under these guidelines, we treated nine neonates in Tohoku University Hospital and four in Sendai Red Cross Hospital.

Unfortunately, two treated active Stage 3 patients in the University Hospital, and one untreated Stage 3 patient in the Red Cross Hospital, could not be followed up. Accordingly, 11 treated and six untreated patients were analyzed in this report. All other patients, at both hospitals, with acute ROP in active Stages 1 and 2 had a normal fundus or Grade I cicatricial retinopathy.

We describe in full our treatment of the following two patients, listed as cases 9 and 10 in Table 16-6.

Patient 9

A female was born on February 10, 1983 at 23-weeks gestation, weighing 674 g. She developed IRDS and required mechanical ventilation for 5 days and was kept in the oxygen-enriched environment for 361 days. She developed hydrocephalus and underwent several shunt procedures. At 62 days, her fundus showed marked vascular dilation and a prominent D line around almost

TABLE 16-5   Incidence of Retinopathy of Prematurity (ROP)

Facility	Birth Weight (g)			Gestational Age (wk)			
	<1,000	1,000-1,500	>1,500	23-27	28-30	31-35	36-40
Tohoku University Hospital	83.3%	66.7%	21.5%	77.8%	71.4%	32.6%	13.6%
Sendai Red Cross Hospital	84.6%	36.7%	6.1%	100.0%	30.0%	12.5%	0%

TABLE 16–6 Stage 3 Patients Treated Surgically

Case	Sex	Gestational Age (wk)	Birth Weight (g)	Days in Oxygen	Max. PaO₂ (%)	Eye	Active Stage	Treatment	Age when Treated (wk)	Duration of Follow-up yr (mo)	Cicatricial Grade
1	M	29	1,090	40	-	OD	3	cryo	8	5 (2)	II
						OS	3	cryo + phc	8		II
2	M	28	1,080	28	103.0	OD	3	cryo	7	2 (5)	I
						OS	3	phc + cryo	7		I
3	F	29	1,440	39	98.0	OD	3	cryo	7	3 (3)	II
						OS	3	cryo	7		II
4	M	29	1,180	24	-	OD	3	cryo	10	3	II
						OS	3	cryo	10		II
5	M	29	1,060	24	-	OD	3	cryo	10	3	II
						OS	3	cryo	10		I
6	M	29	1,000	35	-	OD	3	cryo	10	3	II
						OS	3	cryo	10		II
7	F	29	1,160	13	-	OD	3	phc	9	2 (5)	I
						OS	3	-	-		I
8	M	24	826	68	57.4	OD	3	cryo	9.5	1 (1)	I
						OS	3	cryo	14		II
9	F	23	674	361	100.2	OD	3	phc + cryo	12	1 (2)	II
						OS	3	-	-		I
10	F	25	860	70	55.6	OD	3	cryo	10	(9)	I
						OS	3	-	-		I
11	F	24	724	123	136	OD	3	cryo	9	1 (8)	IV
						OS	3	cryo	10		IV

360°, with arteriovenous shunts posterior to the line. On May 4, hemorrhages appeared on the line, and there was early traction on the posterior retina. By May 16 the condition was still advancing; photocoagulation was done using Mizuno's binocular indirect argon laser photocoagulator, under general anesthesia, in 50 spots delivered for 0.2 seconds at 500 to 700 mW, diameter 900 μm. But the peripheral vitreous was still hazy, and the coagulation was not satisfactory. Cryotherapy was then delivered on May 17 under local anesthesia, in 12 spots for 10 seconds each. The fundus examination revealed an uncoagulated area in the periphery of the line, and still active ROP; the same procedure was repeated in 10 spots on May 25. During these processes, the left eye showed acute ROP in active Stage 3, but neovascularization around the line was less active, and no treatments were done.

On April 28, 1984, the fundus photographs were taken, as shown in Figures 16-1A (OD), and 16-1B (OS).

The right eye showed Grade II cicatricial retinopathy. A mild dragged disc was observed; the macula was displaced temporally; but the structure seemed to be normal. Cryotherapy scars were found at the midperiphery (Fig. 16-1A). There was fibrous tissue on the retina's surface and in the adjacent vitreous in the temporal periphery. The cryotherapy in this case was incorrectly placed, as shown, too posteriorly.

The left eye had Grade I cicatricial retinopathy. There was no dragged disc, but a minimum temporal displacement of the macula was found. Irregular, abnormal retinal vessels were prominent, as shown in Figure 16-1B. We must follow the patient's progress to determine if she can have normal visual function in the future. Vitreoretinal adhesions formed a fibrous membrane covering 360° in the midperiphery. More peripheral to this membrane, there were no retinal vessels within the wide avascular area. Skiascopy revealed myopic astigmatism H: −3.5 D, V: −2.0 D, OD, and H: −3.5 D, V: −4.5D, OS. She is

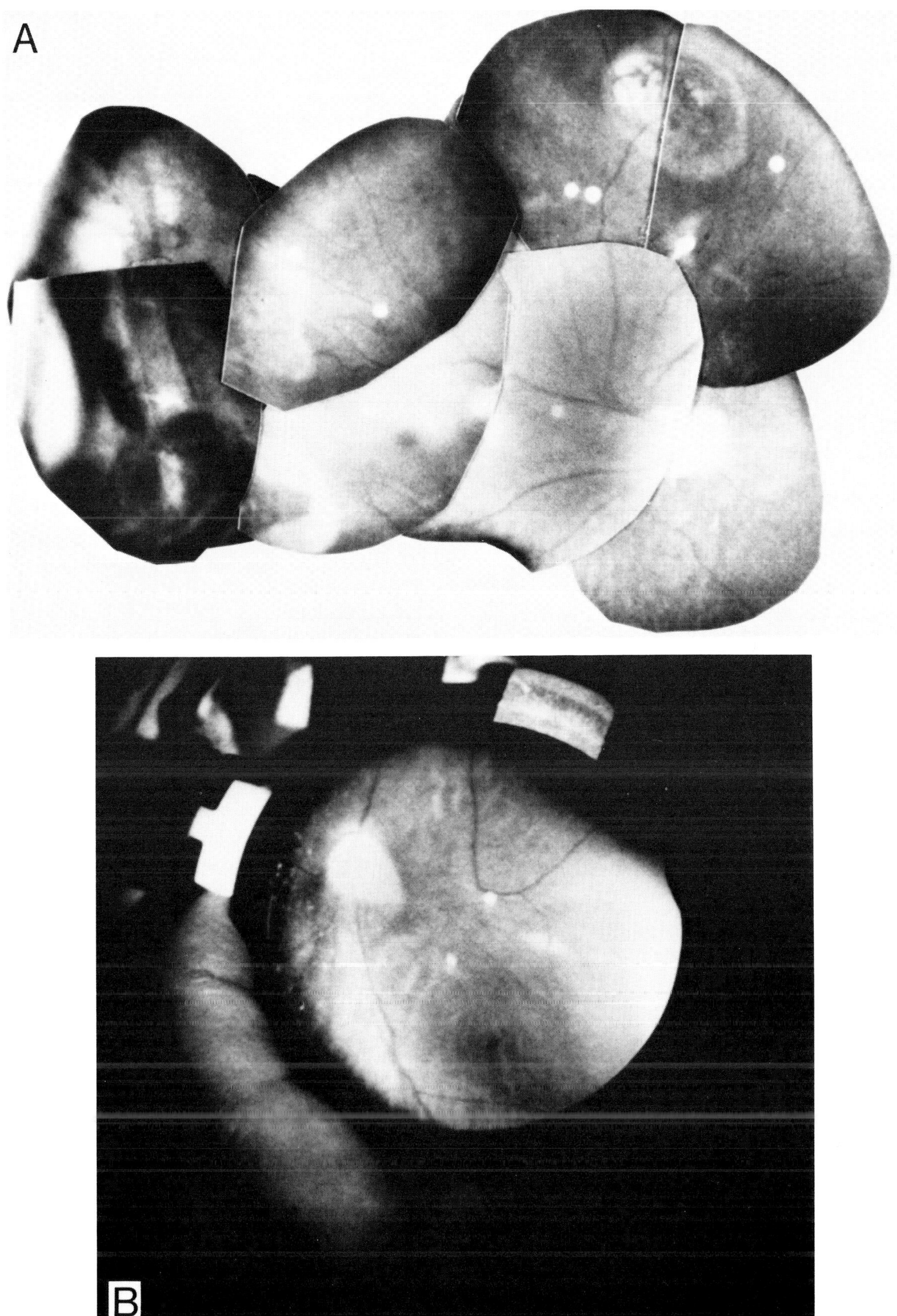

Figure 16-1 *A.* Fundus of the right eye of patient 9. Chorioretinal scars by cryotherapy in the temporal and upper nasal peripheral retina, mild dragged disc and temporal dislocation of the macula. *B.* Fundus of the left eye (same patient). Cryotherapy was not performed; there was no dragged disc, but abnormal vessels and slight dislocation of the macula can be observed.

still hospitalized in the pediatric department of the Sendai Red Cross Hospital, having difficulty eating and receiving nourishment through a nasal catheter.

Patient 10

A female was born in September 1983 at 25-weeks gestation, weighing 860 g. She developed IRDS and required an oxygen-enriched environment for 70 days. On November 18, she had active Stage 3 in both eyes. On November 25, it was still progressing, and she received cryotherapy of 11 spots on the D line in the temporal periphery of the right eye. Although a similar D line was found in the left eye, this eye was not treated. The fundus pictures (Figs. 16-2A and B) were taken April 16, 1984. A dragged disc in the treated eye was very slight, and a peripheral white vitreous membrane was mild. Chorioretinal atrophy was pronounced in the coagulated area, but in other areas it was mild. This eye had Grade I cicatricial retinopathy.

In the left eye, a dragged disc was also very slight, but the macula was dislocated slightly temporally. The structure was normal. Abnormal vessels were more pronounced in the peripheral retina of the untreated eye, and a thick vitreous membrane was found in the temporal midperiphery. A pronounced pigmented avascular area had abrupt disappearance of retinal vessels and retinal atrophy. Refraction showed myopic astigmatism in both eyes (H: −6.5 D, V: −8.0 D, OD, and H: −12 D, V: −5.0 D, OS). We are unable to determine her subjective visual function at present.

The incidence of acute ROP in both hospitals is compared in Table 16-5. Higher rates of acute ROP in low-birth-weight premature neonates coincided with increasing prematurity, but the incidence of ROP in Tohoku University Hospital was higher than that in the Sendai Red Cross Hospital. When premature neonates were born at 23- to 27-weeks gestation and weighed less than 1,000 g, most in both groups suffered acute ROP. Fortunately, there were relatively few severe cases in active Stages 3 or 4 in either hospital.

Clinical data and results of surgical treatments are contained in Table 16-6. All patients had active progressive Stage 3 when they received cryotherapy and/or photocoagulation. Eight patients were treated bilaterally, the remaining three unilaterally. Patient 11 was treated in active Stage 3, but her retinopathy progressed to active Stage 4, and a retrolental fibrous mass finally formed. Treatment results are summarized in Table 16-9. Nine of 22 eyes had Grade I cicatricial retinopathy and normal

maculae. Eleven eyes had Grade II and mild-to-moderate dragged discs without retinal folds. Both eyes in patient 11 were Grade IV.

Six patients with ROP in active Stage 3 (10 eyes) and Stage 2 (2 eyes) were observed and received no surgical treatment. Their clinical data are shown in Table 16-7. They all had cicatricial Grade I retinopathy and showed no changes in the posterior retinas.

DISCUSSION

In Japan, the incidence of acute ROP in the 1960s and early 1970s was believed to be higher than that in the later 1970s to 1980s. But this was not true. The incidence of acute ROP at Tohoku University in 1970 to 1971, which Yamashita reported[20] in 1972, was almost the same as currently reported (Table 16-8). Recent trends toward increasing incidence of ROP were also reported from other institutions in Japan[21] and in the United States[22]. In both the Tohoku University Hospital and Sendai Red Cross Hospital the criteria for surgical treatment of active ROP stages have not changed. During these 10 years we have become more cautious about treatment and have tried to wait as long as possible, even if the acute ROP was in active Stage 3. As a result, we did n ot treat six of 20 cases in active Stages 3 and 4. Three were unilateral, and the remaining 11 were treated bilaterally with cryotherapy and/or photocoagulation. In the last series from our clinic, Sasaki et al[7] reported that only four cases were unilaterally treated, and all other cases were bilaterally treated. Their results were almost the same (Table 16-9). All patients in active Stage 3 without surgical treatment had Grade I cicatricial RLF in the present series.

These results suggest that, even if the D line were formed at the temporal periphery, new vessels projected into the vitreous cavity, and exudates and hemorrhages were to appear, the acute ROP in active Stage 3 would still be self-limiting in a certain number of cases, and their fundi would show Grade I cicatricial RLF without surgical intervention. In other words, the standards for the application of surgical treatments to active Stage 3 ROP in 1970 to 1973 were too easy. This was reflected in the large number of patients who were surgically treated with cryotherapy and had Grade I cicatricial RLF in the 1970 to 1973 series, compared to the small number currently. The incidence of spontaneous regression of ROP was already reported at other Japanese clinics[8]. Kinsey and Hemphill[23] reported that 45 percent of neonates reaching active Stage 3 regressed to normal.

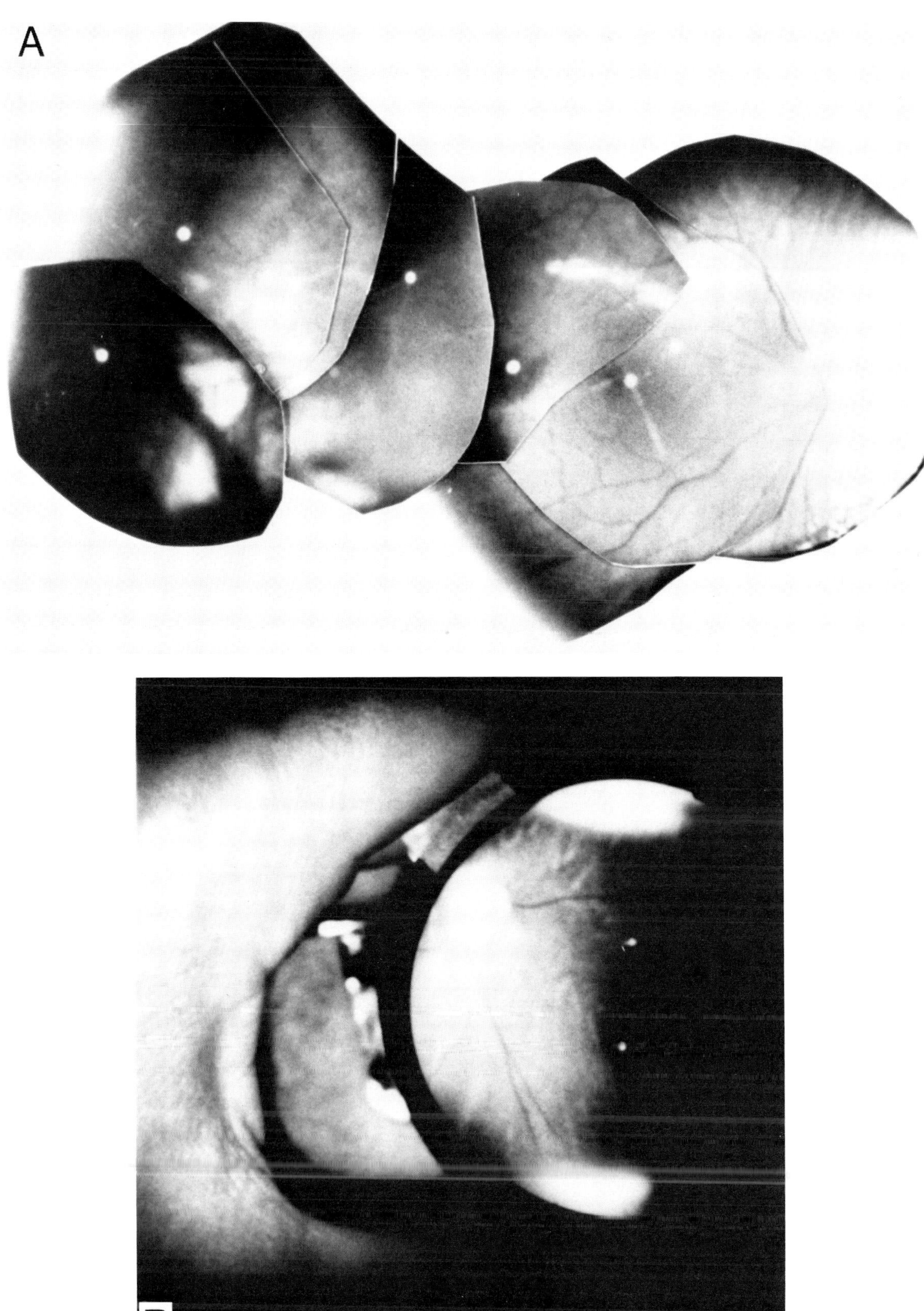

Figure 16-2 *A.* Fundus of the right eye of patient 10. This eye was treated with cryotherapy. There was no dragged disc or dislocation of the macula. *B.* Fundus of the left eye (same patient). No surgical treatment was delivered. There is a very slight dragged disc and temporal dislocation of the macula.

TABLE 16–7   Active Stage 2 and 3 Receiving No Surgical Treatment

Case	Sex	Gestational Age (wk)	Birth Weight (g)	Days in Oxygen	Eye	Active Stage	Duration of Follow-up (mo)	Cicatricial Grade
1	M	24	1,300	6	OD	3	10	I
					OS	3		I
2	F	28	940	69	OD	2	7.5	I
					OS	3		I
3	F	26	1,200	28	OD	2	7	I
					OS	3		I
4	M	31	1,420	5	OD	3	8	I
					OS	3		I
5	M	29	1,450	34	OD	3	4	I
					OS	3		I
6	F	30	1,704	7	OD	3	3	I
					OS	3		I

Then how do we decide which patients will be surgically treated? The fundus examination must be careful and accurate. But the present results suggest that we cannot make this decision based only on funduscopy. First, systemic conditions are important. Up to now, the PaO_2, the degree of prematurity, and the duration of the final active stage of ROP were known to affect the incidence and severity of RLF[24,25]. But these factors cannot explain in every case why the retinopathies became severe. For example, why did patient 9 (Table 16-6) not develop severe cicatricial retinopathy? If we compare her with patient 11, the prematurity was much greater, the birth weight lower, and oxygen administration was longer than for patient 11. If we can accumulate experience with such cases, we can establish definite criteria to decide which patient can be observed without surgery and which one urgently requires surgical treatment.

Second, we have to accumulate the long-term follow-up data concerning the complications of cryotherapy or photocoagulation in eyes having cicatricial retinopathy. If the incidence of retinal detachment[26], myopia[27] and

TABLE 16-8   Incidence of Premature Retinopathy at Tohoku University Hospital

	1970 - 71*		1976 - 83	
Total	42/133	(31.6%)	108/372	(29.0%)
Active Stage 1	29/133	(21.8%)	73/372	(19.6%)
2	10/133	(7.5%)	20/372	(5.4%)
3	3/133	(2.3%)	15/372	(4.0%)

* Data from Yamashita (1972)

TABLE 16-9   Treatment Results

	Tohoku University Hospital (1970-1973)*						Tohoku University (1976-1983) and Sendai Red Cross Hospital (April 1982 - September 1983)					
Active Stage	No. of Cases						No. of Cases					
3	15						16					
4	1						1					
Treatment with Cryo and/or Phc.		Cicatricial Grade (Eyes)						Cicatricial Grade (Eyes)				
		0	I	II	III	IV		0	I	II	III	IV
Bilateral	12	0	16	6	1	1	8	0	5	9	0	2
Unilateral Treated	4	0	3	1	0	0	3	0	2	1	0	0
Untreated		0	3	1	0	0		0	3	0	0	0
Observation	0	-	-	-	-	-	6	0	12	0	0	0
Total	16	0	22	8	1	1	17	0	22	10	0	2

* Sasaki et al. Jpn J Ophthalmol 1976; 20:384-395.

other factors were lower in treated eyes, or the same in both treated and untreated groups, early surgical treatment to prevent the occurrence of Grade IV cicatricial retinopathy would have to be accepted. If the incidence of complications were higher in the operated group, we would have to carefully observe then decide the indications for treatment. Faris and Brockhurst[28] reported that two-thirds of patients having rhegmatogenous retinal detachment in the cicatricial stages of RLF were between 6 and 15 years of age. The patients treated with cryotherapy between 1970 and 1973 in our Tohoku University Hospital have fortunately shown no rhegmatogenous retinal detachment up to now. But they must be closely followed up.

If the retina is detached and a retrolental mass is formed, both cryotherapy and photocoagulation are absolutely contraindicated. Recently scleral buckling[29,30] or closed-[31] and open-sky vitrectomy (Hirose, personal communication 1982) for both active and cicatricial stages of RLF have succeeded in some cases. Although we tried open-sky vitrectomy for patient 11, the result was not satisfactory.

At present, it is clear that the high incidence of cicatricial retinopathy in Grades III or IV occurs if acute ROP advances to the late phase of active Stage 3[32]. But it is also true that if ROP is limited to the early phase of active Stage 3, most have Grade I cicatricial retinopathy, and physiological function is normal. We suppose the cryotherapy and photocoagulation would be beneficial to prevent progression of ROP to retinal detachment and RLF formation. But we don't agree to applying these statements to acute ROP in active Stage 2, even if the results are apparently good[13].

Appreciation is extended to Professor K. Mizuno for his suggestions and critical reading of the manuscript. The author is also grateful to Drs I. Takahashi and M. Honda for their help in this work.

REFERENCES

1. Nagata M, Kobayashi Y, Fukuda H, Suekane K. Photocoagulation for the treatment of retinopathy of prematurity. Jpn J Clin Ophthalmol 1968; 22:419-427.
2. Yamashita Y. Studies on retinopathy of prematurity (III). Cryocautery for retinopathy of prematurity. Jpn J Clin Ophthalmol 1972; 26:385-393.
3. Sasaki K, Yamashita Y, Hata T, Mizuno K. Cryocautery for retinopathy of prematurity. Acta Fifth Afro-Asian Congress of Ophthalmology 1972:403-407.
4. O'Grady GE, Flynn JT, Herrera JA. The clinical course of retrolental fibroplasia in premature infants. South Med J 1972; 65:655-658.
5. Nagata M, Tsuruoka Y. Treatment of acute retrolental fibroplasia with xenon-arc photocoagulation. Jpn J Clin Ophthalmol 1972; 16:131-143.
6. Oshima K, Nishimura N, Kano M, Mukuno T, Kumano S, Takagi I, Nakama T. Photocoagulation treatment on rapidly progressive cases of retinopathy of prematurity. Jpn J Clin Ophthalmol 1974; 28:217-223.
7. Sasaki K, Yamashita Y, Maekawa T, Adachi T. Treatment of retinopathy of prematurity in active stage by cryocautery. Jpn J Clin Ophthalmol 1976; 20:384-395.
8. Majima A, Takahashi M, Hibino Y, Kamao N, Takai M. Clinical observations of photocoagulation on retinopathy of prematurity. Jpn J Clin Ophthalmol 1976; 30:93-97.
9. Harris GS, McCormick AQ. The prophylactic treatment of retrolental fibroplasia. Mod Probl Ophthalmol 1977; 18:364-367.
10. Hindle NW, Leyton J. Prevention of cicatricial retrolental fibroplasia by cryotherapy. Can J Ophthalmol 1978; 13:277-282.
11. Kingham JD. Acute retrolental fibroplasia. II. Treatment by cryosurgery. Arch Ophthalmol 1978; 96:2049-2053.
12. Kalina RE. Treatment of retrolental fibroplasia. Surv Ophthalmol 1980; 24:229-236.
13. Ben-Sira I, Nissenkorn I, Grunwald E, Yassur Y. Treatment of acute retrolental fibroplasia by cryopexy. Br J Ophthalmol 1980; 64:758-762.
14. Stark DJ, Manning LM, Lenton L. The incidence and the results of active treatment of acute retrolental fibroplasia. Aust J Ophthalmol 1982; 10:135-140.
15. Owens WC. Retrolental fibroplasia: clinical course. Am J Ophthalmol 1955; 40:159-162.
16. Uemura Y. Current status of retrolental fibroplasia. Jpn J Clin Ophthalmol 1977; 21:366-378.
17. Nagata M. Retinopathy of prematurity. Jpn J Clin Ophthalmol 1970; 24:1327-1333.
18. Keith CG. Retrolental fibroplasia, a new classification of the developing and cicatricial changes. Aust J Ophthalmol 1979; 7:189-194.
19. Mizuno K, Takaku Y. Dual delivery system for argon laser photocoagulation. Improved techniques of the binocular indirect argon-laser photocoagulator. Arch Ophthalmol 1983; 101:648-652.
20. Yamashita Y. Studies on retinopathy of prematurity. Jpn Rev Clin Ophthalmol 1972; 66:727-734.
21. Tanaka S, Majima A, Kato T, Kamao N. Statistical analysis of relationships between active changes and cicatricial residua of retinopathy of prematurity, based on the newly amended classification in Japan. Jpn J Clin Ophthalmol 1983; 37:1137-1142.
22. Akeson N, Hatlen P. Retrolental fibroplasia is increasing in California. Pediatrics 1982; 69:388.
23. Kinsey VE, Hemphill FM. Etiology of retrolental fibroplasia. Am J Ophthalmol 1955; 40:166-174.
24. Yamamoto M, Tabuchi A. Management of the retinopathy of prematurity. Jpn J Clin Ophthalmol 1976; 20:372-383.
25. Majima A. Problems on retinopathy of prematurity. Acta Soc Ophthalmol Jpn 1976; 80:1372-1419.
26. Minoda K, Ozeki S, Shimizu H. Rhegmatogenous retinal detachment in retinopathy of prematurity. Folia Ophthalmol Jpn 1976; 27:162-169.
27. Schaffer DB, Quinn GE, Johnson L. Sequelae of arrested mild retinopathy of prematurity. Arch Ophthalmol 1984; 102:373-376.
28. Faris BM, Brockhurst RJ. Retrolental fibroplasia in the cicatricial stage. The complication of rhegmatogenous retinal detachment. Arch Ophthalmol 1969; 82:60-65.
29. Tasman W. Retinal detachment in retrolental fibroplasia. Albrecht V. Graef's Arch Klin exp Ophthalmol 1975; 195:129-139.
30. McPherson A, Hittner HM. Scleral buckling in two and one-half to 11-month-old premature infants with retinal detachment associated with acute retrolental fibroplasia. Ophthalmology 1978; 86:819-835.
31. Merritt JC, Lawson EE, Sprague DH, Eifrig DE. Lensectomy-vitrectomy for stage V cicatricial retrolental fibroplasia. Ophthalmic Surg 1982; 13:300-306.
32. Nagata M. Treatment of acute proliferative retinopathy of prematurity with xenon-arc photocoagulation. Acta Soc Ophthalmol Jpn 1976; 80:1453-1475.

Treatment of Acute Retinopathy of Prematurity with Cryotherapy

Alice R. McPherson, M.D.
Helen M. Hittner, M.D.
Frank L. Kretzer, Ph.D.

HISTORICAL DATA BASE

Seventeen reports document the utilization of cryotherapy to induce regression of severe ROP,[1-17] as applied either to the avascular retina, or the ridge with intravitreal neovascularization, or the proliferating posterior vessels. The timing and extent of the cryotherapy, when stated, is highly variable. Historically, the data base involves the following reports: O'Grady, et al[1] (n = 1 eye, n = 1 failure); Payne and Patz[2] (n = 3 eyes, n = 3 successes); Yamashita[3] (n = 16 eyes, n = 16 successes); Sasaki, et al[4] (n = 28 eyes, long-term outcome not stated); Harris and McCormick[5] (n = 10 eyes, long-term outcome not stated); Hindle and Leyton,[6] and Hindle[7] (n = 21 eyes; n = 16 successes); Kingham[8] (n = 14 eyes, n = 1 success); Mousel and Hoyt,[9] and Mousel[10] (n = 6 eyes; n = 1 success); Koerner[11] (n = 21 eyes; no long-term difference); Ben-Sira, et al[12] and Nissenkorn, et al[13] (n = 20 eyes; n = 17 successes); Keith[14] (n = 9 eyes; no long-term difference); Stark, et al[15] (n = 16 eyes, n = 13 successes); Topilow, et al[16] (n = 12 eyes; n = 10 successes); Tasman[17] (n = 17 eyes; n = 12 successes).

ULTRASTRUCTURAL INTERPRETATION OF CRYOTHERAPY

Theoretically, cryotherapy halts the development of severe ROP either by obliteration of peripheral, ischemic retina caused by vaso-obliteration and endothelial necrosis,[18] or by ablation of peripheral, hyperoxic, gap junction-linked spindle cells that are secreting angiogenic factors prior to myofibroblast invasion into the vitreous from the ridge,[19] or by ablation of peripheral gap-junction-linked spindle cells and destruction of the ridge when significant myofibroblast invasion into the vitreous has occurred.[20] Morphologically, the ridge and peripheral retina are transretinal to immature photoreceptors and, thus, are in a hyperoxygenated environment postnatally. Further, there is no ultrastructural evidence of vaso-obliteration or endothelial necrosis.[19] Therefore, placement and timing of transretinal cryotherapy to obliterate spindle cells, including or excluding the ridge, is of critical importance in interpreting the successes and failures reported in the literature.

Cryotherapy must be applied to full retinal thickness to ablate spindle cells at the retina-vitreous interface (Fig. 17–1). Destruction of the choroid, retinal pigment epithelium and outer neural retina, with ablation of some spindle cells, may be sufficient to decrease the production of angiogenic factors to a critical level, or such destruction may create a retina-choroid bond in regressing disease with traction (Fig. 17–2). However, destruction of the choroid, retinal pigment epithelium and outer neural retina, with ablation of some spindle cells, is not sufficient to reduce the number of spindle cells to a critical level (Fig. 17–3B) in order to prevent retinal detachment (Fig. 17–3A) caused by severe traction of myofibroblasts in advancing disease.

As predicted by the spindle cell pathogenesis of ROP, placement of cryotherapy can be incorrect in the following three ways: (1) If only the proliferating vessels are destroyed, the peripheral, gap junction-linked spindle cells continue to secrete angiogenic factors. (2) If only the far peripheral retina is obliterated, but the region adjacent to the shunt is spared, the highest density of spindle cells continues to secrete angiogenic factors. (3) If only the peripheral retina containing spindle cells is obliterated, but the shunt is spared after a significant invasion of myofibroblasts has occurred, a self-perpetuating traction ensues.

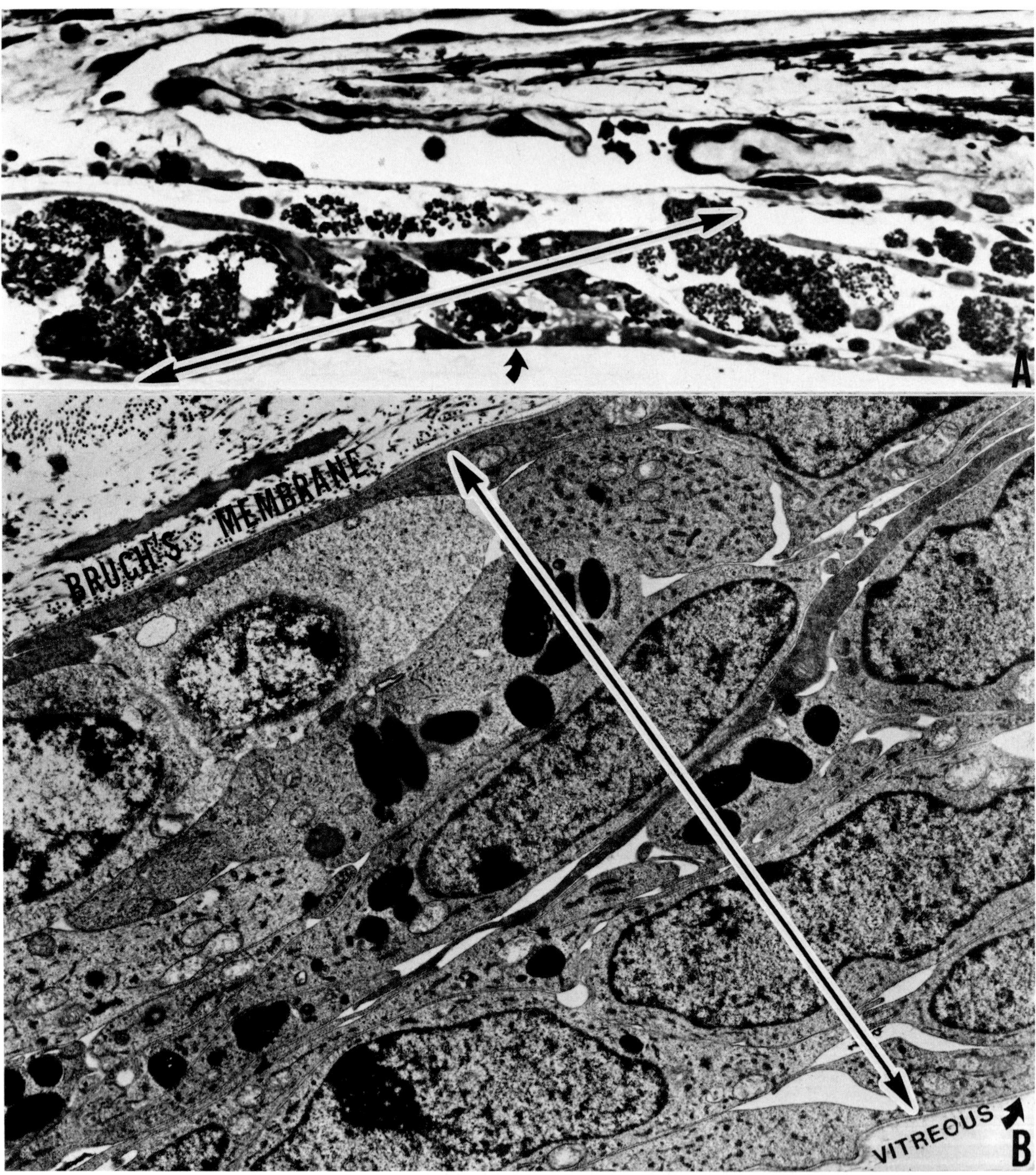

Figure 17–1 Light micrograph A and transmission electron micrograph B of left eye of patient 21 (Table 17–1), who weighed 940 grams at birth, demonstrating full thickness cryoapplications. The retina is totally obliterated into amorphous cells interspersed with pigment. (⟷) delineates the obliterated retina between Bruch's membrane and the retina-vitreous interface (⬆). This infant received insufficient vitamin E supplementation. Cryoapplications were applied at 8-weeks post partum, at Stage 3b ROP, to the gap junction-linked spindle cells, which were still secreting angiogenic factors in the avascular, peripheral, vanguard retina. Clinically, this resulted in retinal quiescence at the time of death, at 11- weeks post partum. Thus, all the spindle cells were obliterated, and there was no source of angiogenic factors. A=740×. B=10,600×.

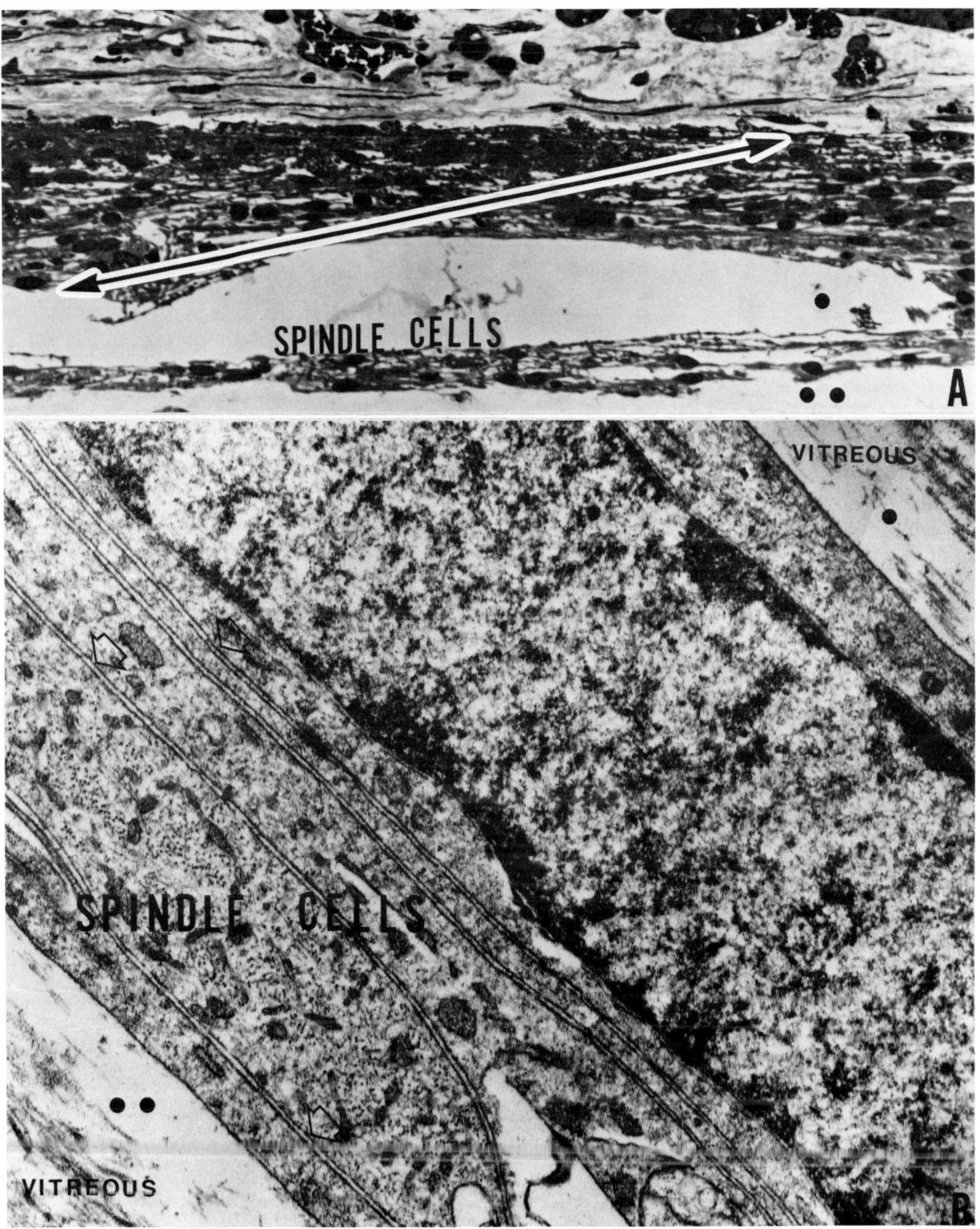

Figure 17–2   Light micrograph A and transmission electron micrograph B of right eye of patient 21 (Table 17–1), demonstrating cryoapplications that are not full thickness. The retina is not completely obliterated. (◄——►) delineates the obliterated retina between Bruch's membrane and the vitreous. A sheet of spindle cells resides within the vitreous. The two surfaces of the sheet are marked by (●) and (● ●). The residual spindle cells within the sheet demonstrate no gap junctions (▽), indicating down modulation of previously activated spindle cells. Cryoapplications were applied at 8-weeks post partum, at Stage 3a ROP, to the gap junction-linked spindle cells that were still secreting angiogenic factors in the avascular, peripheral, vanguard retina. Clinically, this resulted in retinal quiescence at the time of death, at 11-weeks post partum. This occurred despite incomplete destruction of spindle cells, achieved by decreasing to a critical level the production of angiogenic factors. A=440×. B=38,000×.

TABLE 17–1 Cryotherapy Performed at 12 Weeks or Less Postnatal Age

Patient Number	Case Number	Birth Weight (g)	Stage ROP[†]	Postnatal Age at Surgery (wks)	Number of Treatments	Number of Marks	Success/ Failure	Visual Acuity	Follow-up (mos)	Figures
1	1	500	3	9	1	39	S	CF	69	
	2		3		2	39	S	CF	69	
2	3	610	3	11	3	38	F	HM	11	
	4[o/oo]		3	10	1	63	F	HM	11	
3	5[*]	610	3	10	5	48	F	HM	14	17–13,14
	6[o]		3		5	44	F	NLP	14	17–15,16
4	7	630	3	12	1	34	S	UN	8[‡]	
	8		3		3	36	S	UN	8[‡]	
5	9	650	3	12	1	47	S	UN	44	
	10		3		1	65	S	UN	44	
6	11	680	3	10	1	40	F	UN	1[‡]	
	12[o]		3		1	40	F	UN	1[‡]	
7	13[*]	680	3	11	4	53	F	UN	3[‡‡]	17–5,7,9
	14[*]		3		4	42	F	UN	3[‡‡]	17–6,10,12
8	15	740	3	12	1	41	S	HM	22	
9	16[*]	750	3	8	2	26	F	20/400	39	
	17		3		4	40	S	20/30	39	
10	18	750	3	8	1	17	F	NLP	38	
	19[o]		3		3	28	F	LP	38	
11	20[oo]	750	4	12	2	45	F	UN	13	
	21[o]		4		2	66	F	UN	13	
12	22	775	3	11	2	55	S	HM	13	
	23		3		2	30	S	HM	13	
13	24	790	3	10	1	34	S	UN	14	
	25		3		3	36	S	UN	14	
14	26[**]	800	3	6	2	47	F	LP	19	
	27[*]		3		2	65	F	LP	19	
15	28	810	3	9	2	21	S	20/30	67	
	29[*]		3		1	20	F	20/30	67	
16	30	870	3	12	2	60	F	HM	21	
	31[*]		3		3	57	F	HM	21	
17	32	880	3	11	2	22	S	LP	15	
	33		3		2	24	S	LP	15	
18	34	890	3	10	3	45	S	20/400	60	
	35		3		3	44	S	20/100	60	

19	36*	890	3	9	1	19	F	CF	58	
	37		3		2	5	S	CF	58	
20	38	930	3	8	4	15	S	20/80	65	
	39		3		5	20	S	HM	65	
21	40	910	3	8	1	50	S	UN	1‡‡	17–2
	41		3		1	50	S	UN	1‡‡	17–1
22	42**	950	3	11	4	65	F	CF	30	
	43 o/oo		3		3	60	F	LP	30	
23	44	1,000	3	10	1	40	S	UN	1‡	
	45		3		1	40	S	UN	1‡	
24	46°	1,000	3	8	3	48	F	UN	2‡‡	
	47°		3		3	54	F	UN	2‡‡	
25	48	1,040	3	8	2	19	S	LP	41	
	49		3		2	24	S	LP	41	
26	50	1,060	3	11	2	45	S	20/200	54	
	51		3		2	37	S	20/25	54	
27	52*	1,090	3	9	2	36	F	UN	7	
	53 o/oo		4		1	40	F	UN	7	
28	54	1,110	3	10	3	33	S	CF	62	
	55		3		3	22	S	20/80	62	
29	56°	1,110	4	9	1	19	F	UN	43	
30	57	1,180	4	12	3	19	S	HM	90	
	58		4		3	23	S	HM	90	
31	59*	1,195	3	11	3	30	F	LP	60	
	60°		3		3	21	F	LP	60	
32	61	1,230	3	11	6	UN	S	UN	54	
	62		3		6	UN	S	UN	54	
33	63	1,250	4	8	1	6	F	LP	100	
	64		3		1	20	F	LP	100	
34	65	1,310	3	8	3	25	S	20/70	69	
	66		3		3	40	S	20/50	69	
35	67	1,540	3	7	2	11	S	NLP	119	
	68		3		2	12	S	NLP	119	

* Underwent scleral buckle: success (See Table 1, Chapter 18)
° Underwent scleral buckle: failure (See Table 1, Chapter 18)
** Underwent open-sky vitrectomy: success (See Table 1, Chapter 19)
oo Underwent open-sky vitrectomy: failure (see Table 1, Chapter 19)

† Retrospectively classified
‡ Lost to follow-up
‡‡ Deceased

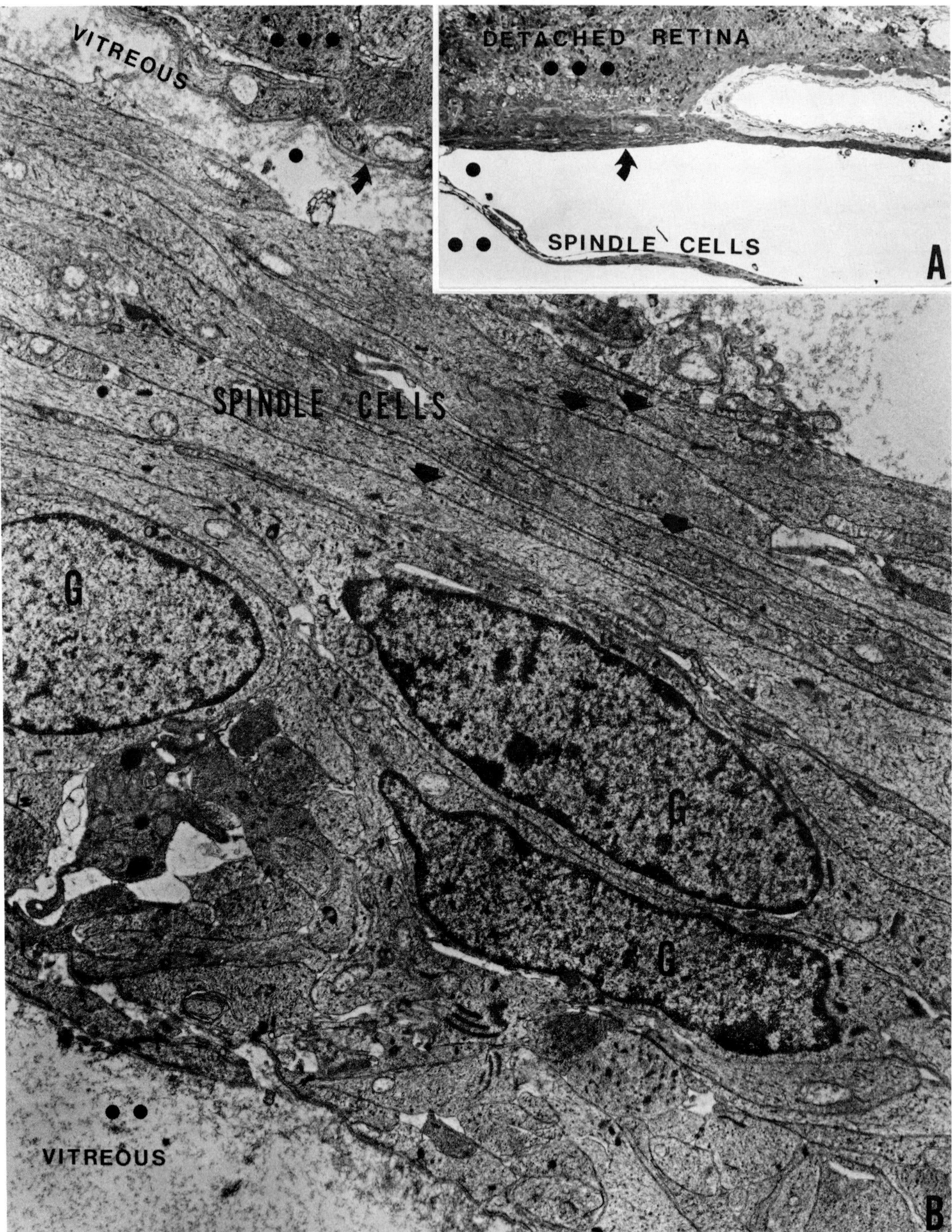

Figure 17–3 Light micrograph A and transmission electron micrograph B of right eye of patient 17 (Table 17–2), who weighed 1,350 grams at birth, demonstrating cryoapplications that are not full thickness. The retina is incompletely obliterated and detached (● ● ●). (⬆) indicates the retina-vitreous interface. A sheet of spindle cells and ganglion nuclei resides within the vitreous. The two surfaces of the sheet are marked by (●) and (● ●). The residual spindle cells within the sheet demonstrate extensive gap junction linkage (⬇), indicating persistent secretion of angiogenic factors. This infant received interrupted vitamin E supplementation. Cryoapplications were applied at 14, 16 and 16.5 weeks post partum, at Stages 3c and 4 ROP, to the gap junction-linked spindle cells that were still secreting angiogenic factors in the avascular, peripheral, vanguard retina. Clinically, this did not result in retinal quiescence at the time of death, at 24-weeks post partum. Thus, gap-junction linkage persists with the production of angiogenic factors, long after the natural time course of spindle cell maturation would have occurred. This delay probably relates to the location of free spindle cells within the vitreous. A = 250×. B = 10,000×.

TABLE 17-2 Cryotherapy Performed at 13- to 15-Weeks Postnatal Age

Patient Number	Case Number	Birth Weight (g)	Stage ROP[†]	Postnatal Age at Surgery (wks)	Number of Treatments	Number of Marks	Success/ Failure	Visual Acuity	Follow-up (mos)	Figures
1	1[*]	490	3	14	4	26	F	UN	3[‡‡]	
	2		3		4	16	S	UN	3[‡‡]	
2	3[*]	520	4	15	1	102	F	UN	6	
3	4[o/oo]	600	4	13	2	133	F	UN	22	
4	5[*]	660	3	15	2	78	F	UN	3[‡‡]	
	6		4		1	52	S	UN	3[‡‡]	
5	7	740	4	13	2	52	F	UN	1[‡‡]	
	8		4		2	53	F	UN	1[‡‡]	
6	9[o]	760	3	15	1	42	F	UN	86	
	10[*]		3		1	44	F	UN	86	
7	11	765	3	13	3	UN	S	UN	6[‡]	
	12		3		2	UN	S	UN	6[‡]	
8	13[o/**]	800	3	14	3	76	F	UN	20	
9	14	835	3	14	3	19	S	HM	60	
	15		3		3	26	S	HM	60	
10	16[*]	880	3	15	2	17	F	UN	10[‡‡]	
	17[*]		3		2	14	F	UN	10[‡‡]	
11	18	910	3	15	3	19	S	CF	42	
	19		3		3	17	S	CF	42	
12	20[*]	920	3	14	3	43	F	20/60	63	
	21[*]		3		3	40	F	20/60	63	
13	22	940	4	15	2	30	S	CF	61	
14	23	970	3	13	1	39	S	CF	70	
	24		3		1	34	S	CF	70	
15	25[*]	1,015	3	14	1	62	F	20/200	69	
16	26[*]	1,310	4	13	2	34	F	CF	97	
	27		4		1	22	F	NLP	97	
17	28	1,350	3	14	3	60	F	UN	2[‡‡]	17-3
	29[o]		3		1	60	F	UN	2[‡‡]	
18	30	1,360	3	14	2	15	S	20/400	125	
	31		3		2	17	S	20/400	125	
19	32	1,360	3	15	2	29	S	20/30	90	
	33		3		2	28	S	20/30	90	
20	34	1,560	3	15	1	24	S	UN	86	
	35		3		1	32	S	UN	86	

[*] Underwent scleral buckle: success (See Table 1, Chapter 18)
[o] Underwent scleral buckle: failure (See Table 1, Chapter 18)
[**] Underwent open-sky vitrectomy: success (See Table 1, Chapter 19)
[oo] Underwent open-sky vitrectomy: failure (See Table 1, Chapter 19)
[†] Retrospectively classified
[‡] Lost to follow-up
[‡‡] Deceased

Spindle cell maturation (Chapter 4) is delayed by approximately 2 weeks with adequate prophylactic vitamin E supplementation from the first hours of life (between 10 and 12 weeks). The natural time course of spindle cell maturation is unaffected by initial hypoxia or hypothermia or incomplete vitamin E supplementation (between 8 and 10 weeks). Therefore, timing of appropriately placed cryotherapy to destroy spindle cells can explain the successes and failures reported in the literature. Cryotherapy applied only to the peripheral retina, when significant myofibroblast invasion has not occurred (Stage 2 or 3a ROP), can potentially induce regression of moderate ROP (between 8 and 10 weeks in vitamin E unsupplemented infants and between 10 and 12 weeks in vitamin E supplemented infants). This result correlates with destruction of spindle cells prior to their down modulation and with significant myofibroblast invasion into the vitreous. Cryotherapy applied to both the peripheral retina and shunt, when significant myofibroblast invasion has occurred (Stages 3b and 3c ROP), can potentially induce regression of severe ROP (after 8 weeks in vitamin E unsupplemented infants and after 10 weeks in vitamin E supplemented infants). Cryotherapy applied after 16 weeks will predictably fail in severe cases of active ROP, because spindle cell maturation and severe myofibroblast invasion have occurred. Cryotherapy applied after 16 weeks will predictably succeed in mild to moderate cases of active ROP, if a retinal-scleral scar can counterbalance the minimal traction created by scarce myofibroblasts in the vitreous.

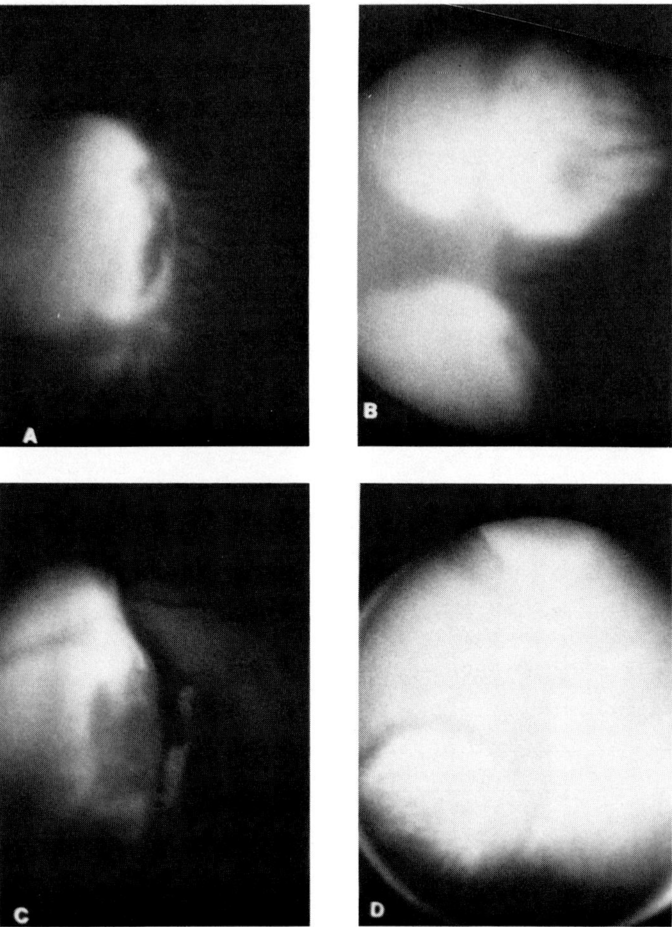

Figure 17–4 Photographs demonstrate the appearance of cryotherapy to the avascular retina and shunt. A Cryo mark applied to the avascular retina and shunt, with minimal hemorrhage. B Cryo marks applied to the avascular retina and shunt, without hemorrhage. C Cryo mark applied to the avascular retina and shunt, with slight hemorrhage of no clinical significance. D Example of multiple cryo marks, with pigment that develops after the first week. (Color plate 1)

SURGICAL TECHNIQUE

Prophylactic cryotherapy should be applied to the peripheral, avascular retina in Zones I and II for Stage 3a ROP and to the peripheral, avascular retina and the ridge for Stages 3b and 3c ROP.

The neonatologist or pediatrician places a peripheral intravenous line prior to the infant's being brought by portable incubator to a prewarmed operating theater for administration of a general anesthetic.

It is imperative that careful fundus drawings be made bilaterally, with particular attention paid to the location of the macula when dragging has occurred, before one begins treatment to document all aspects of the fundus. The cataract probe should have a silicone sleeve to pre-vent unnecessary freezing of adjacent tissues. The cornea should be kept moist with Tissue-sol or BSS (balanced salt solution) and care taken to prevent corneal abrasions. Excessive pressure on the globe raises the intraocular pressure, possibly occluding the central retinal artery. Excessive globe pressure also results in corneal edema and poor visibility.

When cryotherapy is done without any conjunctival incision, the retinal probe can be used when the fornices are deep, while the curve-tipped cataract probe is used to treat farther posteriorly. Sometimes the retinal probe is used if larger cryo marks are to be placed, and if so, fewer marks are needed. The smaller, less bulky cataract probe enables more precise placement of the iceball, particularly posteriorly. Probe selection, as well as the number and location of marks required, are governed by individual circumstances.

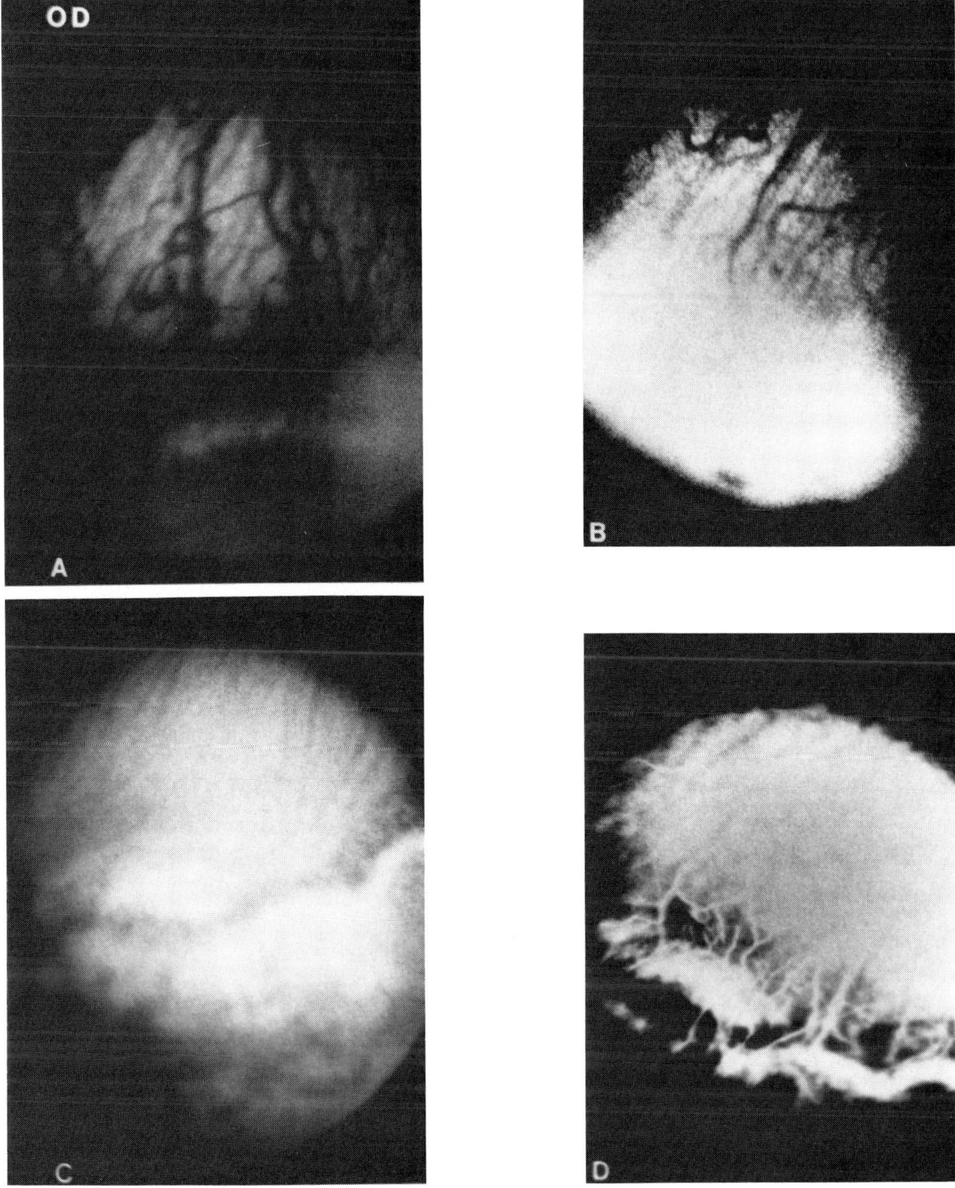

Figure 17-5 Right eye of patient 7 (Table 17 1), demonstrating preoperative and postoperative cryotherapy with corresponding fluorescein angiograms. The preoperative fundus photograph A, taken at 11-weeks post partum, and the corresponding fluorescein angiogram B demonstrate Stage 3b ROP and fluorescein leaking into the vitreous. The postoperative fundus photograph C, taken at 13-weeks post partum, and the corresponding fluorescein angiogram D demonstrate straightening of the vessels and obliteration of the shunt, with absence of fluorescein leakage. (Color plate 2)

In many of these cases, the shunt is far posterior in Zones I and II, and it is impossible to reach the posterior shunt because of the limits of the conjunctival fornices. If the physician decides to treat the shunt, a conjunctival incision is required. There are two possible conjunctival incision methods. One is to make a small incision in one to four of the quadrants. The other is a 360-degree peritomy. When making such incisions, make the first in the quadrant with the more severe disease. If necessary, make additional incisions in other quadrants. There are limitations to the use of quadrant incisions, because often the conjunctiva is torn. Although it can be closed with conjunctival sutures, sometimes the incisions produce unnecessary scars. For better cosmetic closure, it is often preferable to make the incision in a peritomy-like fashion.

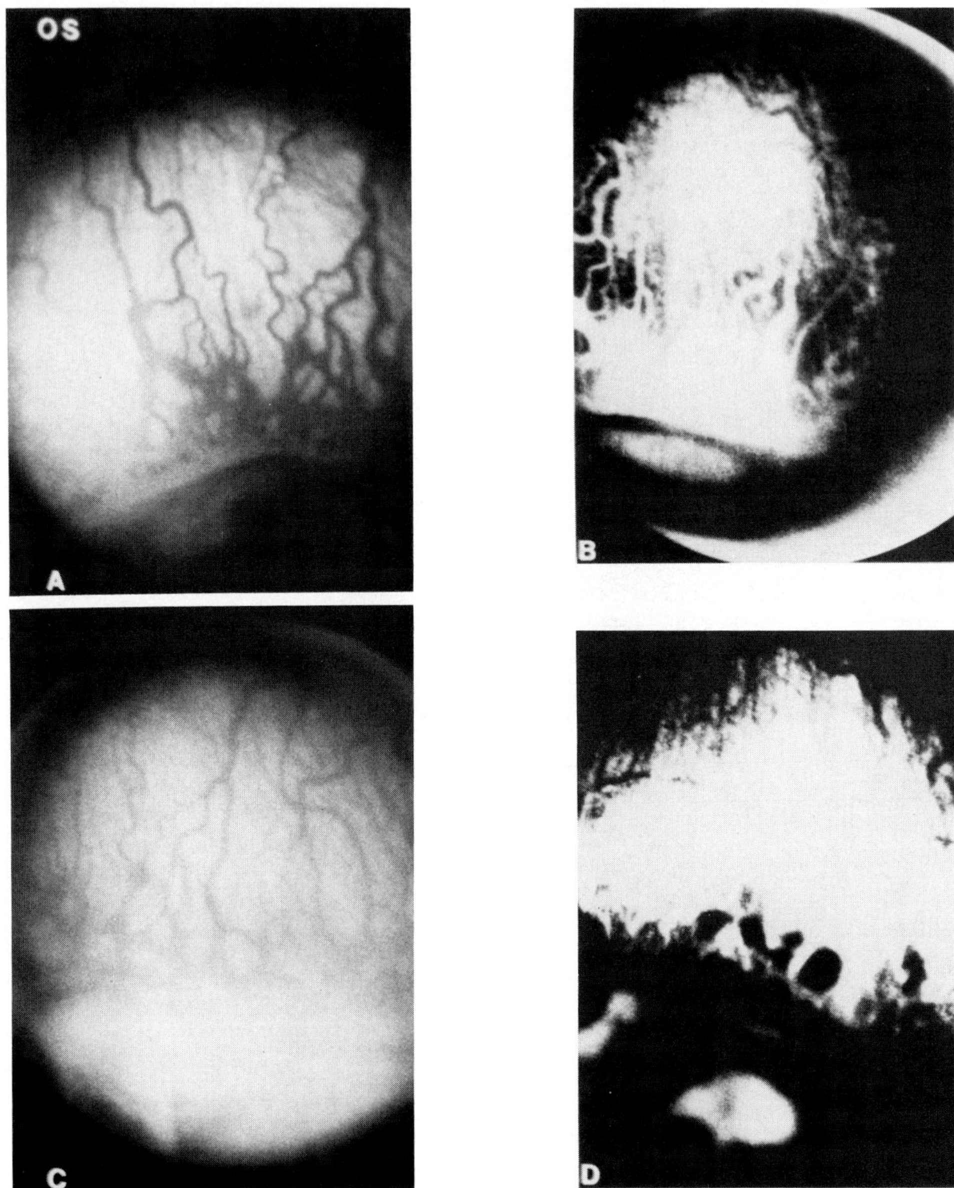

Figure 17–6 Left eye of patient 7 (Table 17–1), demonstrating preoperative and postoperative cryotherapy, with corresponding fluorescein angiograms. The preoperative fundus photograph A, taken at 11-weeks post partum, and the corresponding fluorescein angiogram B demonstrate Stage 3b ROP and fluorescein leaking into the vitreous. The postoperative fundus photograph C, taken at 13-weeks post partum, and the corresponding fluorescein angiogram D demonstrate straightening of the vessels, with persistence of the nonfunctioning shunt but absence of fluorescein leakage. (Color plate 3)

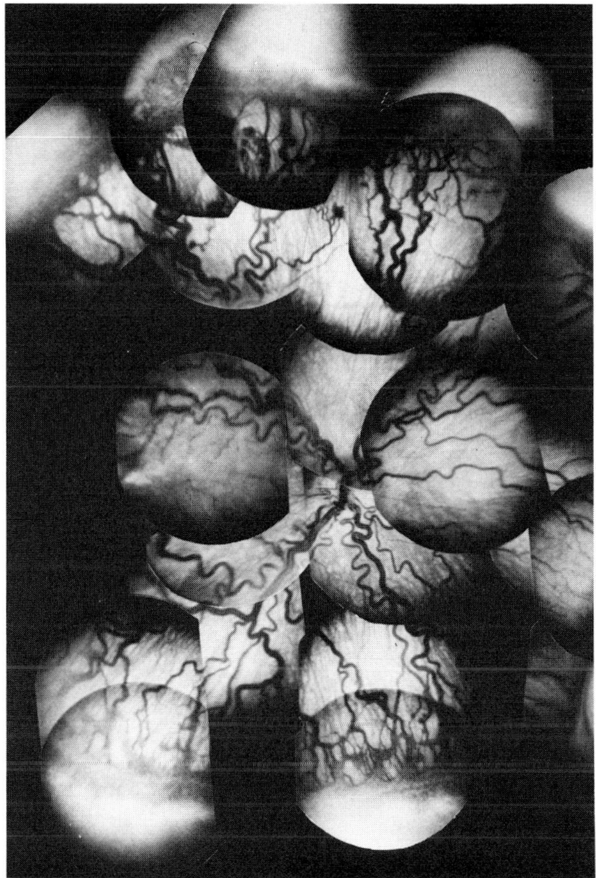

Figure 17–7 Right eye of patient 7 (Table 17–1), who weighed 680 grams at birth and received continuous vitamin E supplementation. However, the distribution of interstitial retinol binding protein (IRBP) at this gestational age is insufficient to establish a favorable oxidant-antioxidant balance in the peripheral retina in order to protect spindle cells. Before treatment, this patient demonstrated Zone I, Stage 3b ROP, with dilated and tortuous posterior polar vessels. This eye was treated with 53 cryo marks at 11-weeks post partum. (Color plate 4A)

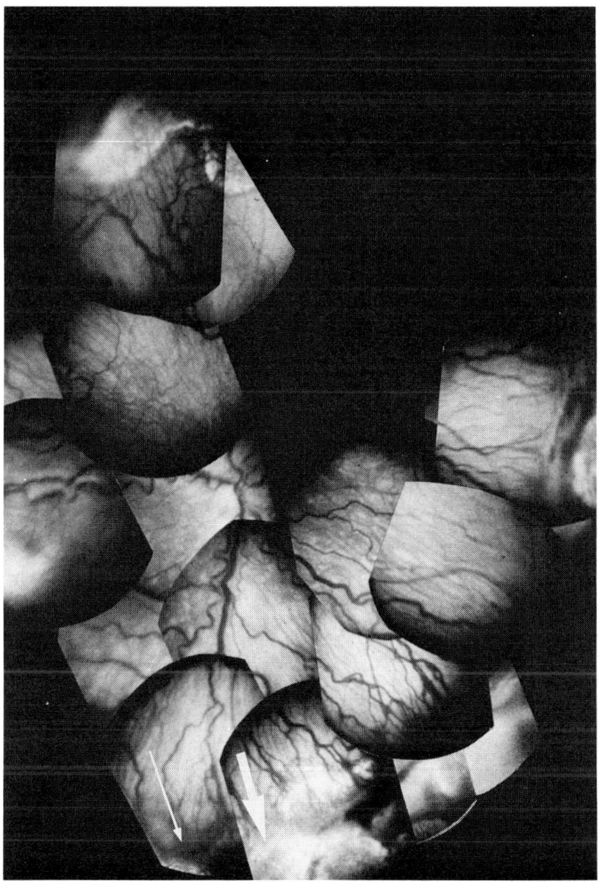

Figure 17–8 Right eye of patient 7 (Table 17–1), shown at 12-weeks post partum, 1 week following initial cryotherapy, when 58 additional cryo marks were added. A significant area of the peripheral retina was not ablated. Therefore, angiogenic factors continued to be secreted, and tortuosity of the posterior polar vessels persisted. Some of these cryo marks obliterated the shunt ( ). However, some areas of the shunt were untreated ( ), and myofibroblasts continued to invade the vitreous. (Color plate 4B)

When cryotherapy is to be performed, use a quick-freezing, quick-defrosting machine, preferably the MIRA cryo unit. When the iceball is formed, the central part freezes and expands circumferentially. As it expands, the center of the iceball rises into the vitreous (Fig. 17–4, Color plate 1). Once you observe this, wait a few seconds and then defrost immediately. Perform complete treatment with approximately 50 to 60 cataract probe marks or approximately 30 retinal probe marks during the first session (Figs. 17–5 and 17–6, Color plates 2 and 3).

Since the spindle cell pathogenesis of ROP is now understood, the placement, timing, and number of cryotherapy sessions has evolved. It is recommended to place contiguous rows of transretinal cryo marks, beginning just anterior to the shunt for 360 degrees. By placing the first row just anterior to the shunt and subsequent rows adjacent anteriorly to the original marks, ablation of that area with the highest density of gap junction-linked spindle cells occurs. The spindle cells do not reach the temporal ora serrata in utero until the child is

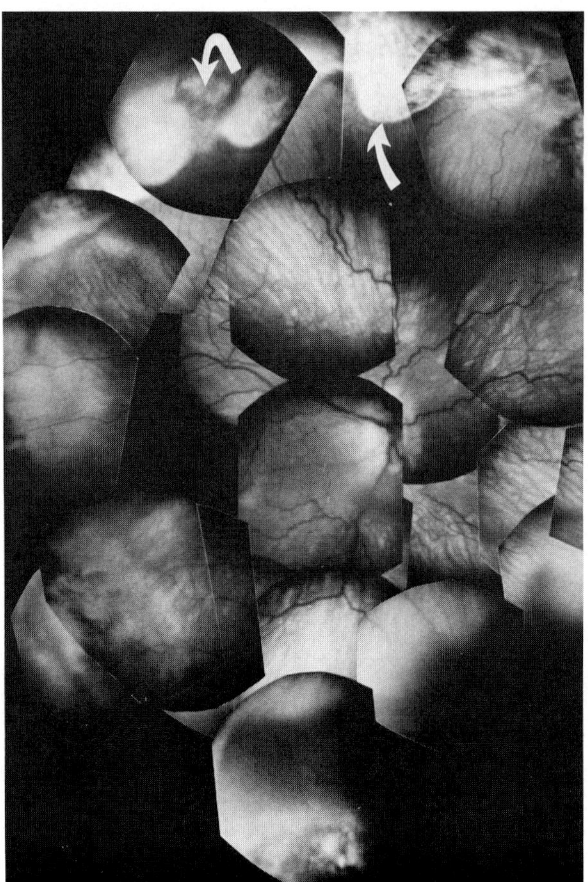

Figure 17–9   Right eye of patient 7 (Table 17–1), shown at 13-weeks post partum, at 1 and 2 weeks following cryotherapy. Additional cryo marks were added. A limited flat retinal detachment was present posterior to the cryo marks in the temporal retina, encroaching upon the displaced macula. Some of the cryo marks were transretinal ( ). Others were not full thickness ( ). This eye successfully underwent scleral buckling (Chapter 18, Table 1, Patient 13, Case 18; Color plate 4C).

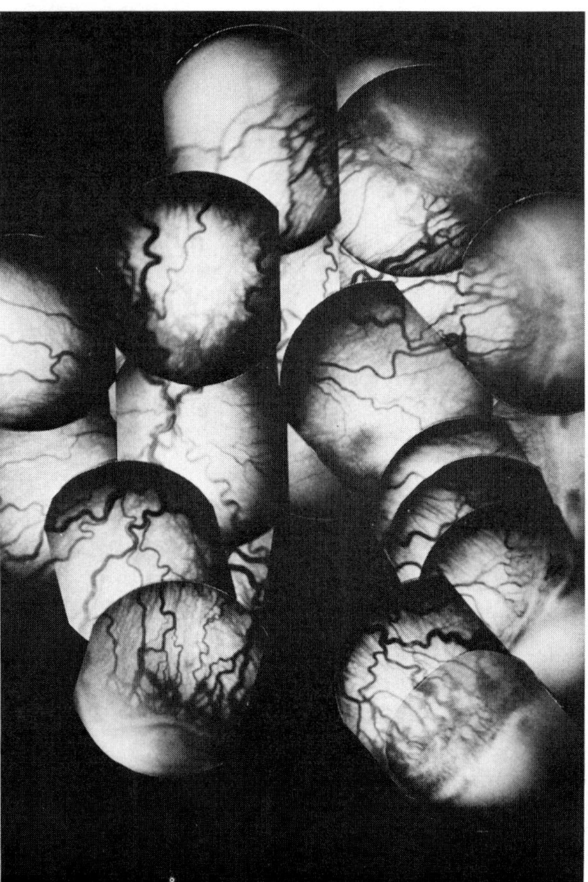

Figure 17–10   Left eye of patient 7 (Table 17–1), who weighed 680 grams at birth and received continuous vitamin E supplementation. However, the distribution of interstitial retinol binding protein (IRBP) at this gestational age is insufficient to establish a favorable oxidant-antioxidant balance in the peripheral retina in order to protect spindle cells. Before treatment, this patient demonstrated Zone I, Stage 3b ROP, with dilated and tortuous posterior polar vessels. This infant was treated with 42 cryo marks at 11-weeks post partum. (Color plate 5A)

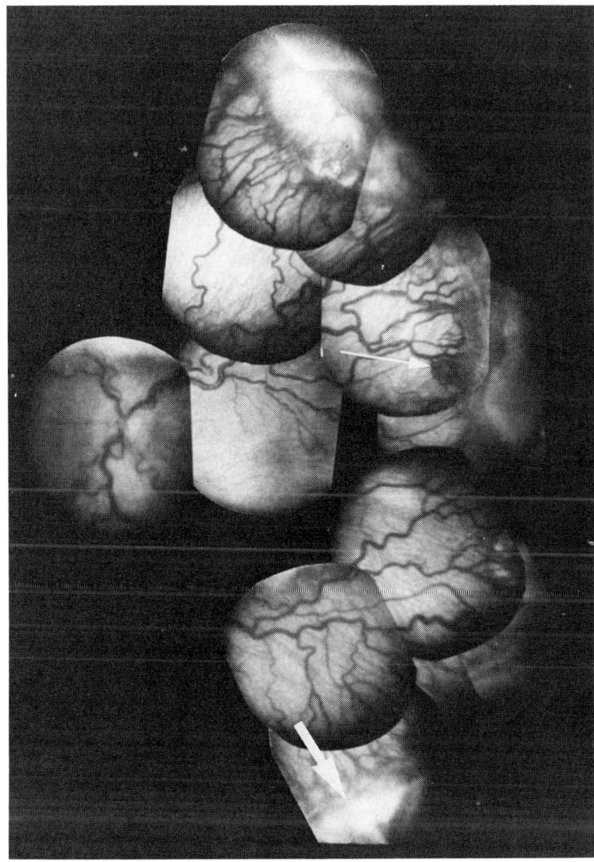

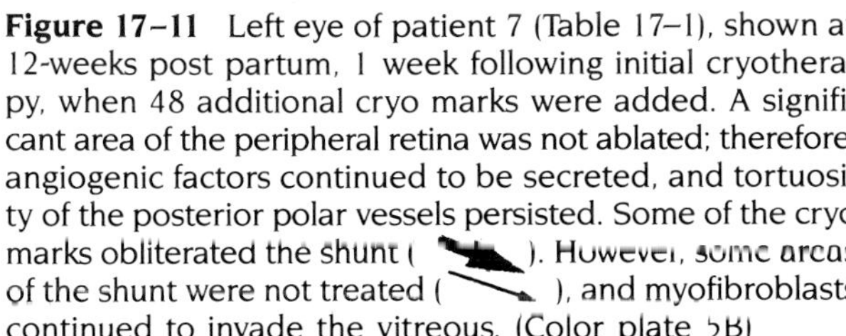

Figure 17–11 Left eye of patient 7 (Table 17–1), shown at 12-weeks post partum, 1 week following initial cryotherapy, when 48 additional cryo marks were added. A significant area of the peripheral retina was not ablated; therefore, angiogenic factors continued to be secreted, and tortuosity of the posterior polar vessels persisted. Some of the cryo marks obliterated the shunt ( ). However, some areas of the shunt were not treated ( ), and myofibroblasts continued to invade the vitreous. (Color plate 5B)

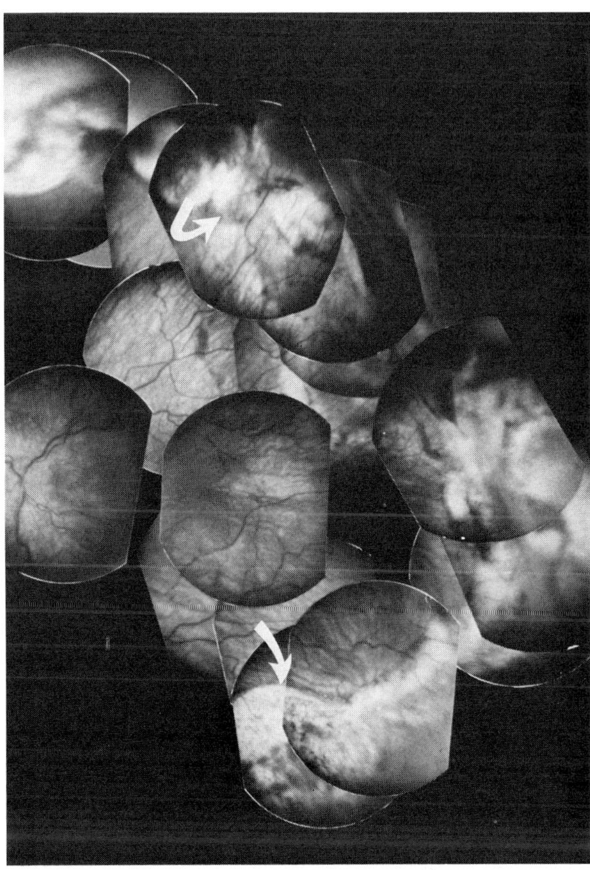

Figure 17–12 Left eye of patient 7 (Table 17–1), shown at 13-weeks post partum, at 1 and 2 weeks following cryotherapy. Additional cryo marks were added. Some of the cryo marks were transretinal ( ). Others were not full retinal thickness ( ). This eye successfully underwent scleral buckling (Chapter 18, Table 1, Patient 13, Case 19; Color plate 5C).

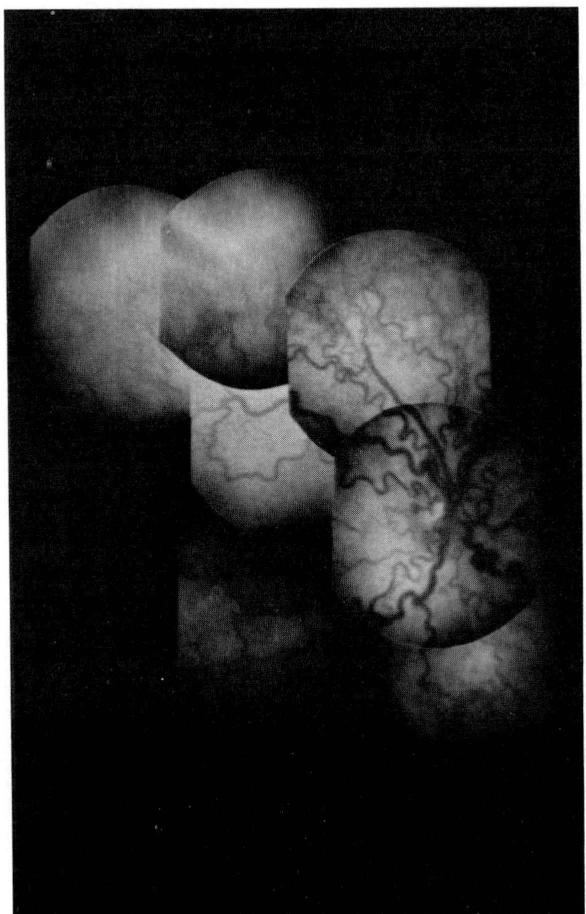

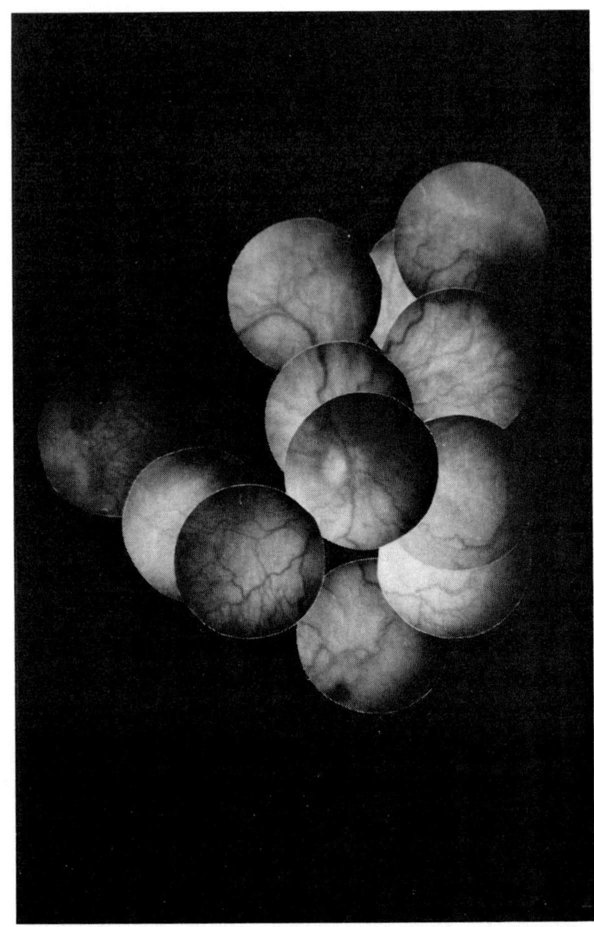

Figure 17–13 Right eye of patient 3 (Table 17–1), who weighed 610 grams at birth and received vitamin E supplementation. Before treatment, this patient demonstrated Zone I, Stage 3c ROP, with dilated and tortuous posterior polar vessels. This eye was treated with 48 cryo marks at 10-weeks post partum. (Color plate 6A)

Figure 17–14 Right eye of patient 3 (Table 17–1), shown at 11-weeks post partum, 1 week following initial cryotherapy, when 49 additional cryo marks were added. The tortuosity of the posterior polar vessels decreased, because a significant amount of the peripheral retina, with gap junction-linked spindle cells that were secreting angiogenic factors, was ablated. However, the shunt was not treated, myofibroblasts continued to invade the vitreous, and retinal detachment ensued. This eye successfully underwent scleral buckling (Chapter 18, Table 1, Patient 7, Case 9; Color plate 6B).

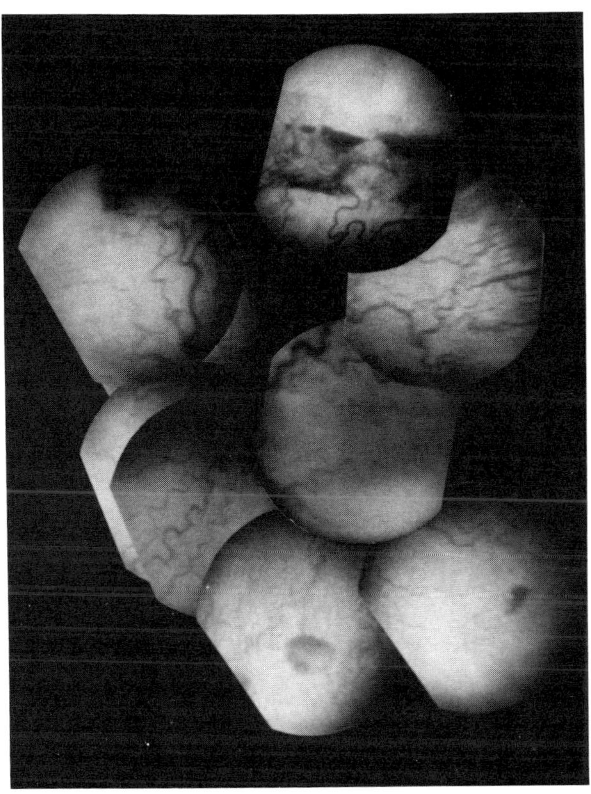

Figure 17–15 Left eye of patient 3 (Table 17–1), who weighed 610 grams at birth and received continuous vitamin E supplementation. Before treatment, this patient demonstrated Zone I, Stage 3c ROP, with dilated and tortuous posterior polar vessels. This infant was treated with 44 cryo marks at 10-weeks post partum. (Color plate 7A)

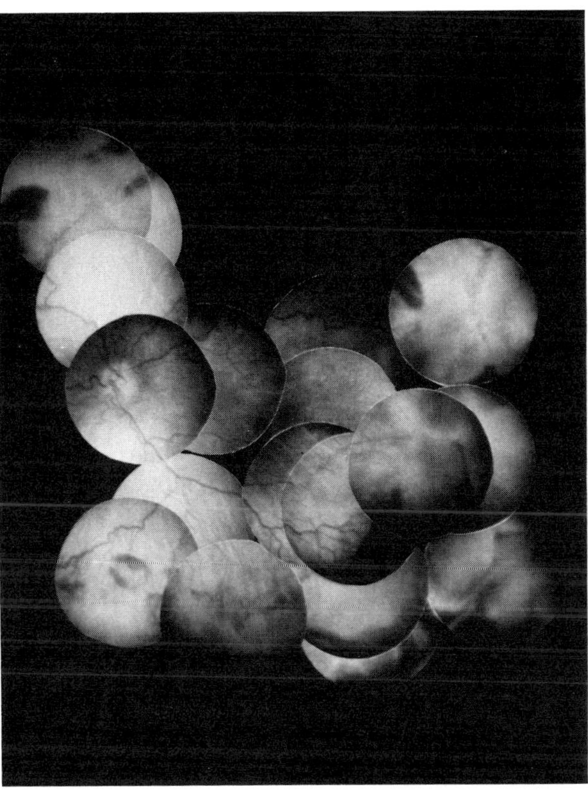

Figure 17–16 Left eye of patient 3 (Table 17–1), shown at 11-weeks post partum, 1 week following initial cryotherapy, when 25 additional cryo marks were added. The tortuosity of the posterior polar vessels decreased, because a significant amount of the peripheral retina, with gap-junction-linked spindle cells that were secreting angiogenic factors, was ablated. However, the shunt was not treated, myofibroblasts continued to invade the vitreous, and retinal detachment ensued. Scleral buckling on this eye was not successful. (Chapter 18, Table 1, Patient 7, Case 10; Color plate 7B)

TABLE 17–3   Cryotherapy Performed at 16 Weeks or More Postnatal Age

Patient Number	Case Number	Birth Weight (g)	Stage ROP[†]	Postnatal Age at Surgery (wks)	Number of Treatments	Number of Marks	Success/ Failure	Visual Acuity	Follow-up (mos)	Figures
1	1	460	4	20	1	14	S	UN	29	
	2		4		1	16	S	UN	29	
2	3	500	4	29	1	18	F	CF	15	
3	4	650	3	17	3	42	S	HM	24	
4	5	700	3	18	1	41	S	HM	20	
	6		4		1	65	F	LP	20	
5	7*	740	3	18	1	47	S	UN	18	
6	8	750	3	18	1	26	S	CF	7	
7	9	775	3	17	7	27	S	CF	18	
8	10	820	4	17	3	12	S	20/80	114	
	11		3		3	30	S	20/80	114	
9	12	860	3	16	2	83	F	UN	3[‡‡]	
	13		3		2	78	F	UN	3[‡‡]	
10	14	880	4	17	1	15	S	UN	5[‡]	
	15		3		1	25	S	UN	5[‡]	
11	16	880	3	20	2	41	S	20/200	70	
	17*		3		2	11	F	HM	70	
12	18	920	3	20	2	25	S	20/200	70	
13	19	940	3	16	1	23	S	20/80	64	
14	20	960	3	17	4	33	S	HM	47	
15	21	1,015	3	18	1	31	S	20/60	69	
16	22	1,030	3	18	1	24	S	20/60	119	
	23		3		2	23	S	20/50	119	
17	24	1,150	3	33	3	12	S	HM	97	
	25		3		3	14	F	NLP	97	
18	26	1,210	3	32	1	18	S	UN	3[‡]	
	27		3		1	13	S	UN	3[‡]	
19	28	1,210	3	16	2	49	S	HM	12	
	29		3		2	57	S	HM	12	
20	30	1,260	3	20	4	29	S	HM	6[‡‡]	
21	31	1,340	3	20	3	UN	S	20/200	43	
	32		3		3	UN	S	HM	43	
22	33	1,350	4	20	3	32	S	HM	45	
23	34	1,420	3	16	1	20	S	20/50	102	
	35		3		1	14	S	20/30	102	

* Underwent scleral buckle: success (See Table 1. Chapter 18)
† Retrospectively classified
‡ Lost to follow-up
‡‡ Deceased

29-weeks gestational age; therefore, in the smallest infants, when spindle cell migration has been halted by premature birth, cryotherapy placed adjacent to the ora serrata will ablate only neuroblastic retina that is not inducing ROP. Lastly, treat the shunt at the time of the first session, when Stage 3b or 3c is present. This should be the last circumferential row, since significant hemorrhaging may occur afterward, preventing direct visualization for further cryotherapy. Not uncommonly, small hemorrhages develop at the time of cryotherapy or in the immediate postoperative period. These do not negate the effect of the therapy.

Previously, cryotherapy was not consistently transretinal (Fig. 17–3), began at the ora serrata, or did not encroach upon or include the shunt (Figs. 17–7 to 17–16, Color plates 4 to 7).

Wait approximately 3 to 5 days, then examine the infant to determine if adequate treatment has been achieved. Successful treatment should provide noticeable blood vessel changes within a few days. By 3 to 5 days, the resolution of residual neovascularization should be quite obvious.

RESULTS

The cryotherapy data base comprises 138 eyes of 78 infants ranging from 460- to 1,560-grams birth-weight. Thirty-one eyes were lost to follow-up, 19 eyes because of patient death. The average follow-up was 43 months. Retrospectively, the fundus photographs were analyzed according to the International Classification.[21] All eyes

TABLE 17–4 Summary of Cryotherapy Data

	Postnatal Age (wks) of Initial Cryotherapy			
	---	---	---	---
	$\leq$12	13–15	$\geq$16	Total
Mean Birth Weight (g)	959	938	952	951
Success	38/68 (56)	17/35 (49)	28/35 (80)	84/138 (61)
Success Following Scleral Buckle	10/21 (48)	10/14 (71)	2/2 (100)	22/37 (59)
Success Following Open-sky Vitrectomy	2/5 (40)	1/3 (33)	0/0 (00)	3/8 (38)
Mean Follow-up (mo)	38	48	46	43
Lost to Follow-up or Deceased	12	12	8	32
Visual Acuity:				
CF	6	6	3	15
20/40–20/400	8	5	10	23
20/20–20/30	4	2	1	7

( ) = Percent

treated were at Stage 3 or 4 ROP in Zones I and II. Success is defined as quiescence at the ridge, decrease in vascular tortuosity of the posterior pole, and no progression to retinal detachment.

The data base is stratified into three groups, according to postnatal age at the time of initial cryotherapy (12 weeks or less, Table 17–1; between 13 and 15 weeks, Table 17–2; and 16 weeks or more, Table 17–3). The overall success rate was 61 percent. Specifically, 56 percent of treatments at 12 weeks or less were successful (Table 17–1); 49 percent of treatments between 13 and 15 weeks (Table 17–2); and 80 percent of treatments at 16 weeks or more (Table 17–3). These three categories are summarized in Table 17–4. The cryotherapy data base is clustered in this manner because, ideally, cryotherapy should be applied in infants aged 12 weeks or less to obliterate gap junction-linked spindle cells and minimize myofibroblast invasion (Stages 3a and 3b ROP). In infants between 13 and 15 weeks postnatal age, Stages 3b and 3c ROP had already developed, and cryotherapy was less effective, because myofibroblast invasion was already significant and spindle cells were not secreting angiogenic factors. In infants of 16 weeks postnatal age or more, it was too late to treat severe, active ROP (Stages 3c or 4) by cryotherapy alone. Successful cases reflected primarily the induction of a chorioretinal adhesion to counterbalance myofibroblast traction that had not produced complete retinal detachment.

Thirty-seven eyes underwent a scleral buckling procedure, of which 22 were successful (Chapter 18). Eight eyes had open-sky vitrectomies, of which three were successful (Chapter 19). Considering the combined procedures, there were 109 successes, a 79-percent success rate.

Visual acuities ranging from 20/20 to counting fingers have been recorded in 45 eyes (Table 17–4). As the children mature, additional assessment of visual acuities will be possible.

Retrospectively, failures are attributed to inadequate spindle cell destruction, because infants were referred too late; multiple sessions that delayed adequate therapy; conservative therapy insufficient to destroy the majority of spindle cells, including or excluding the shunt; or cryo marks not contiguous or not applied to full retinal thickness.

POSTOPERATIVE CARE

Immediate postoperative problems primarily affect the cornea. Haziness can result from abrasion or increased intraocular pressure. Postoperative synechiae can form, and so dilating drops must be given daily (Mydriacyl 1% three times a day for 3 weeks and Neo-Synephrine 2.5% three times a day for 1 week). Topical Econopred 1% is given three times a day for 3 weeks to quiet the eye, and lightweight ice compresses decrease local lid swelling. Garamycin ophthalmic solution is given topically four times a day for 3 weeks after surgery.

If neovascularization persists or progresses, repeat cryotherapy. If the disease progresses with peripheral detachment, scleral buckling is indicated as soon as possible. Delay can result in a reduced final visual acuity, because the retinal neurons quickly die as a result of insufficient nutrition being transported from the choriocapillaris.

COMPLICATIONS

In 138 eyes, occasional minor hemorrhages occurred along the ridge of extraretinal fibrovascular proliferation, which always cleared uneventfully within 1 to 2 months. One case of corneal edema resulted, and one case of corneal erosion resulted in a minimal, corneal scar.

REFERENCES

1. O'Grady GE, Flynn JT, Herrera JA. The clinical course of retrolental fibroplasia in premature infants. South Med J 1972; 5:655–658.
2. Payne JW, Patz A. Treatment of acute proliferative retrolental fibroplasia. Trans Pan Acad Ophthalmol Otolaryngol 1972; 76:1234–1240.
3. Yamashita Y. Studies on retinopathy of prematurity. III. Cryocautery for retinopathy of prematurity. Jpn J Clin Ophthalmol 1972; 26:385–393.
4. Sasaki K, Yamashita Y, Maekawa T. Adachi T. Treatment of retinopathy of prematurity in active stage by cryocautery. Jpn J Ophthalmol 1976; 20:384–395.
5. Harris GS, McCormick AQ. The prophylactic treatment of retrolental fibroplasia. Mod Probl Ophthalmol 1977; 18:364–367.
6. Hindle NW, Leyton J. Prevention of cicatricial retrolental fibroplasia by cryotherapy. Can J Ophthalmol 1978; 13:277–282.
7. Hindle NW. Cryotherapy for retinopathy of prematurity to prevent retrolental fibroplasia. Can J Ophthalmol 1982; 17:207–212.
8. Kingham JD. Acute retrolental fibroplasia. II. Treatment by cryosurgery. Arch Ophthalmol 1978; 96:2049–2053.
9. Mousel DK, Hoyt CS. Cryotherapy for retinopathy of prematurity. Ophthalmology 1980; 87:1121–1127.
10. Mousel DK. Cryotherapy for retinopathy of prematurity: a personal retrospective. Ophthalmology 1985; 92:375–378.
11. Koerner FH. Retinopathy of prematurity: natural course and management. Metab Pediatr Syst Ophthalmol 1978; 2:325–329.
12. Ben-Sira I, Nissenkorn I, Grunwald E, Yassur Y. Treatment of acute retrolental fibroplasia by cryopexy. Br J Ophthalmol 1980; 64:758–762.
13. Nissenkorn I, Kremer I, Ben-Sira I, Cohen S. Garner A. A clinicopathological case of retinopathy of prematurity (ROP) treated by peripheral cryopexy. Br J Ophthalmol 1984; 68:36–41.
14. Keith CE. Visual outcome and effect of treatment in Stage 3 developing RLF. Br J Ophthalmol 1982; 66:446–449.
15. Stark DJ, Manning LM, Lentun L. The incidence and the results of active treatment of acute retrolental fibroplasia. Aust J Ophthalmol 1982; 10:135–140.
16. Topilow HW, Ackerman AL, Wang FM. The treatment of advanced retinopathy of prematurity by cryotherapy and scleral buckling surgery. Ophthalmology 1985; 92:379–387.
17. Tasman W. Management of retinopathy of prematurity. Ophthalmology 1985; 92:995–999.
18. Patz A. Retinal neovascularization: early contributions of Professor Michaelson and recent observations. Br J Ophthalmol 1984; 68:42–46.
19. Kretzer FL, Mehta RS, Johnson AT, Hunter DG, Brown ES, Hittner HM. Vitamin E protects against retinopathy of prematurity through action on spindle cells. Nature 1984; 309:793–795.
20. Kretzer FL, McPherson AR, Rudolph AJ, Hittner HM. Pathogenic mechanism of retinopathy of prematurity: a controversial explanation for the efficacy of oral and intramuscular vitamin E supplementation and cryotherapy. Bull NY Acad Med 1985; 61:883–900.
21. Committee for the classification of retinopathy of prematurity: An international classification of retinopathy of prematurity. Pediatrics 1984; 74:127–133.

Treatment of Acute Retinopathy of Prematurity by Scleral Buckling

18

Alice R. McPherson, M.D.

Helen M. Hittner, M.D.

Frank L. Kretzer, Ph.D.

CLINICAL PRESENTATION OF RETINAL DETACHMENT

For older children who have cicatricial retrolental fibroplasia (RLF) with rhegmatogenous detachments, scleral buckling is an accepted procedure.[1-6] Scleral buckling in infants who have active retinopathy of prematurity (ROP), with tractional and serous detachments, is controversial, because some cases will reattach spontaneously. For active ROP, many authors have reported anatomic reattachment in 50 to 100 percent of cases employing scleral buckling procedures (in infants less than 1-year postnatal age): Koerner[7] (n = 2 eyes, n = 1 success); Yassur, et al[8] (n = 2 eyes, n = 2 successes); McPherson and Hittner[9] (n = 10 eyes, n = 6 successes); Grunwald, et al[10] (n = 3 eyes, n = 3 successes); Bert, et al[11] (n = 7 eyes, n = 7 successes); Baruch, et al[12] (n = 1 eye, n = 1 success); McPherson, et al[13] (n = 32 eyes, n = 24 successes); Topilow, et al[14] (n = 7 eyes, n = 5 successes); Tasman[15] (n = 6 eyes, n = 5 successes).

Retinal detachments for active ROP are primarily of two types, or mechanisms: tractional (Figs. 18–1 to 18–6, Color plates 8 and 9, myofibroblast contraction); and serous (Figs. 18–7 to 18–11, Color plates 10 and 11, subretinal fluid accumulation). These two types can also occur in combination. Rarely, rhegmatogenous detachments occur and are usually produced iatrogenically (Figs. 18–12 and 18–13, Color plate 12).

In tractional detachments, myofibroblasts exert centripetal force at the shunt.[16,17] With extensive myofibroblast contraction, elevation of the retina occurs, producing a peripheral detachment. Peripheral detachments can become complete within a day. With progression, a funnel detachment is created through a pursestring effect, which is gestational-age related. The pursestring is posterior in the most immature infants (Zone I), and an-

terior in the more mature infants (Zone III). As the pursestring contracts, vitreous closure can occur by a circumferential ridge (Figs. 18–14 and 18–15) or by punctate, transvitreal strands (Figs. 18–16 and 18–17, Color plate 13). Within a week, complete detachments can become funnels, at which point scleral buckling techniques alone are no longer effective.

In serous detachments, leakage of plasma from choroidal or neovascularizing retinal vessels causes the accumulation of subretinal fluid, with development of yellowish precipitates. Recent serous detachments have small, white flakes (Fig. 18–8, Color plate 10B), while longstanding serous detachments show large, yellow aggregates (Figs. 18–10, Color plate 11A). Cryo applications to the shunt or posterior vessels can cause partial

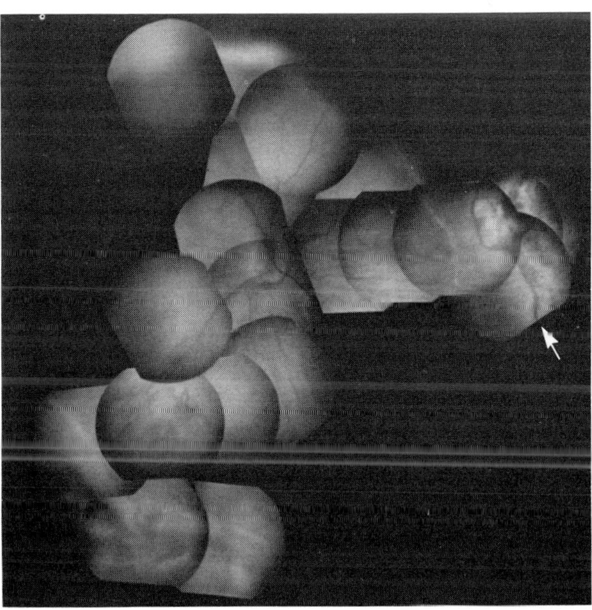

Figure 18–1 Left eye of patient 11, who weighed 660 grams at birth. The eye was treated by cryotherapy at 15- and 16-weeks postnatal age. Prophylactic cryotherapy, (arrow) which did not approach the shunt, was unsuccessful in controlling progression of the disease. These fundus photographs were taken at 16-weeks postnatal age (Color plate 8A).

"

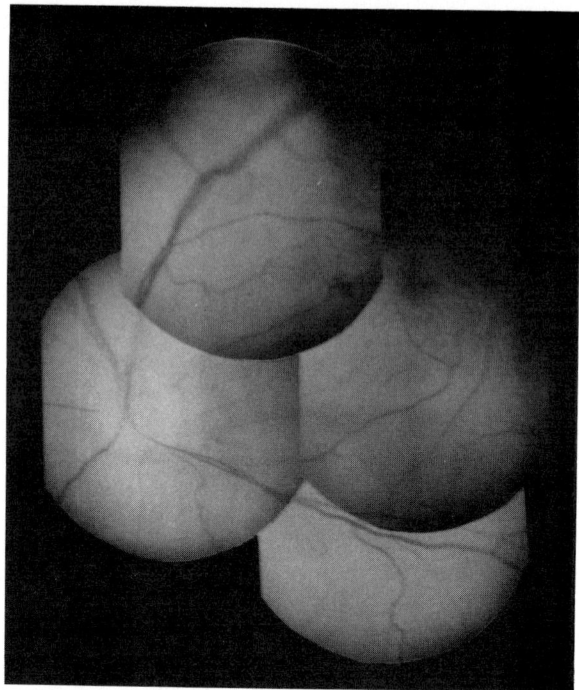

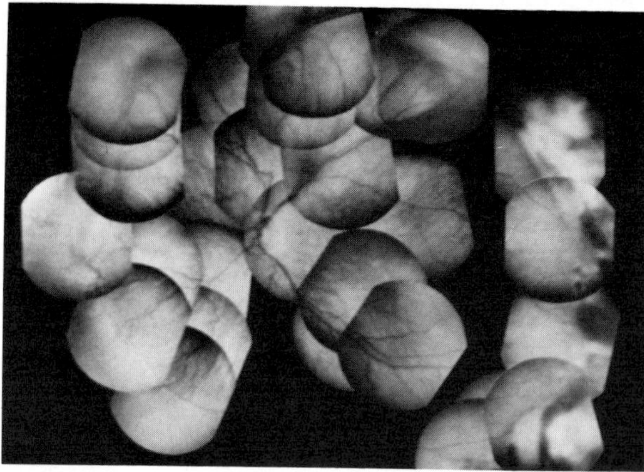

Figure 18–3 Patient 11 shown at 18-weeks postnatal age, left eye demonstrating an anatomic reattachment of the retina (Color plate 8C).

Figure 18–2 Patient 11 shown at 17-weeks postnatal age, left eye demonstrating a tractional retinal detachment. A scleral buckling procedure was performed (Color plate 8B).

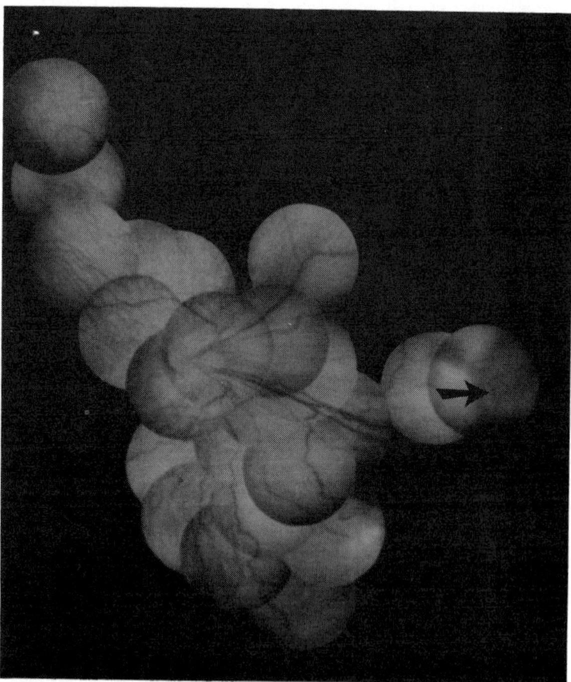

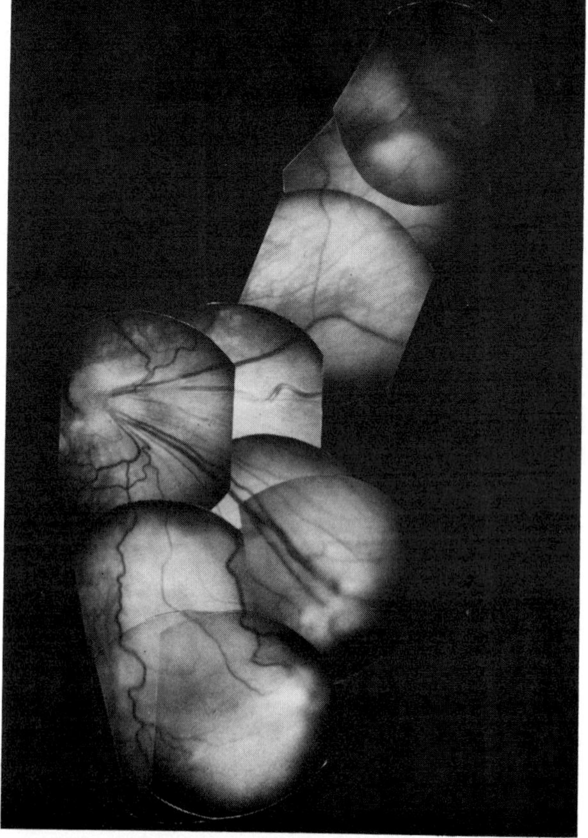

Figure 18–4 Left eye of patient 20, who weighed 740 grams at birth. The eye was treated by cryotherapy at 18-weeks postnatal age. Prophylactic cryotherapy (arrow) was unsuccessful in halting progression of the disease, and a peripheral, tractional retinal detachment (*) developed. These fundus photographs were taken at 19 weeks postnatal age; a scleral-buckling procedure was performed (Color plate 9A).

Figure 18–5 Patient 20 shown at 20-weeks postnatal age, left eye demonstrating reattachment of the retina with significant dragging of the macula (Color plate 9B).

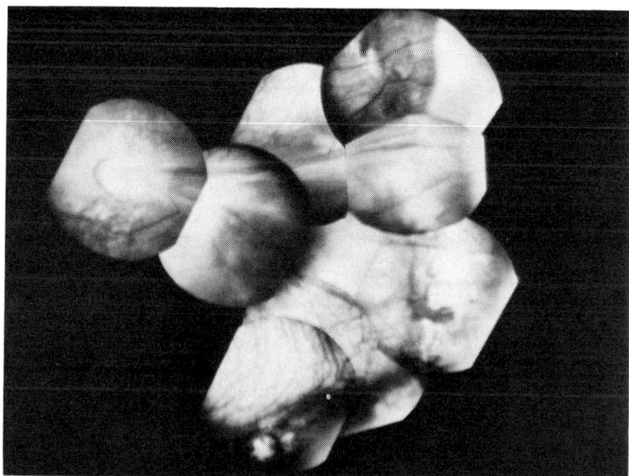

Figure 18–6 Left eye of patient 20, shown at 5-months post scleral buckling, with an anatomically reattached retina with significant dragging of the macula. Additional cryoapplications had been placed during revisions, and the buckle is visible (Color plate 9C).

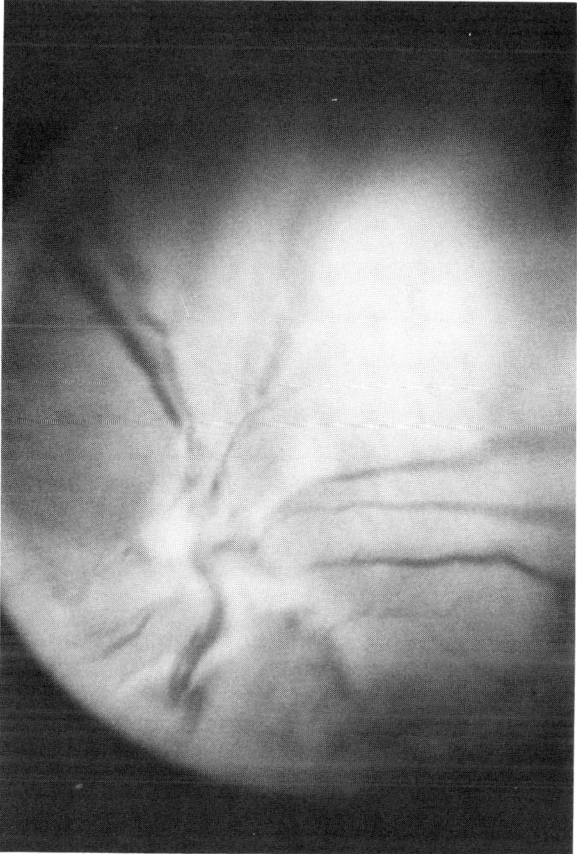

Figure 18–7 Left eye of patient 30, who weighed 840 grams at birth, with a serous, total retinal detachment. Infant is shown at 16-weeks postnatal age. (Color plate 10A).

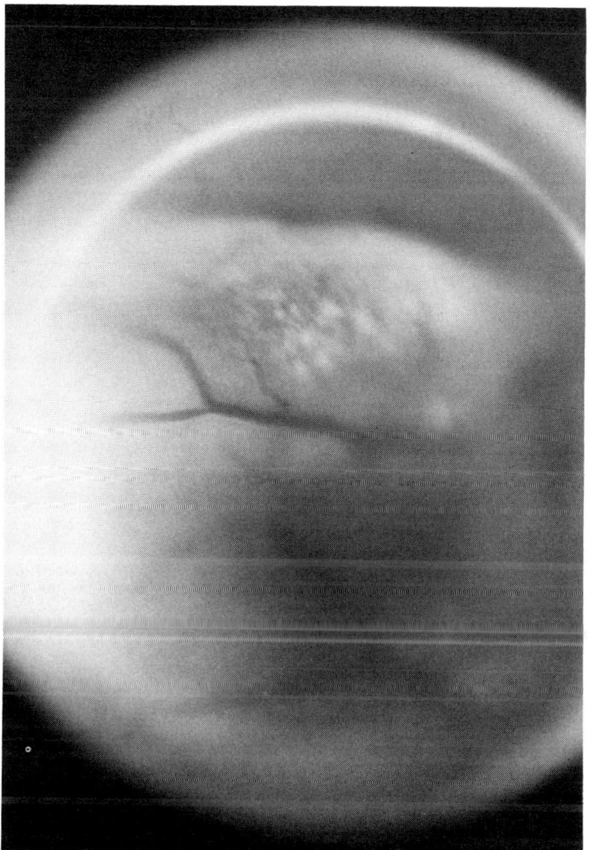

Figure 18–8 Left eye of patient 30 with a serous, total retinal detachment. The infant is shown at 16-weeks postnatal age. The small, white flakes in the subretinal fluid are characteristic of the recent onset of this serous retinal detachment (Color plate 10B).

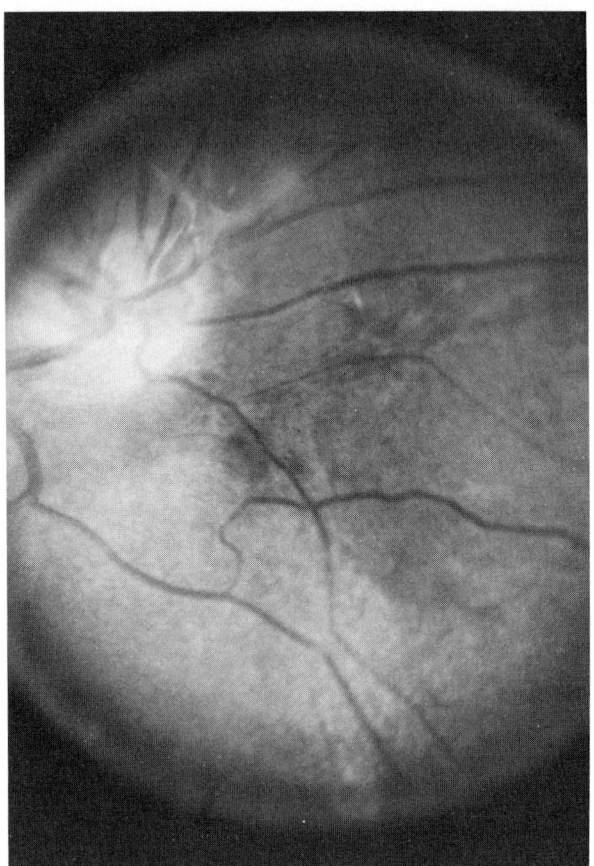

Figure 18-9 Left eye of patient 30, shown at 9-months post scleral buckling, with an anatomically reattached retina with pigment mottling (Color plate 10C).

Figure 18-10 Right eye of patient 19, who weighed 740 grams at birth, the infant shown at 19-weeks postnatal age with a serous, total retinal detachment. The large, yellow aggregates in the subretinal fluid indicate that this serous, retinal detachment was long-standing (Color plate 11A).

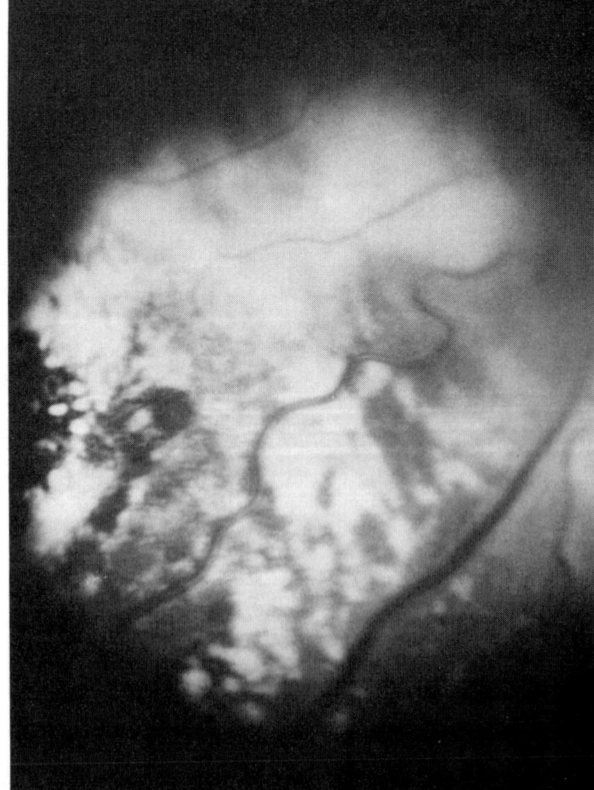

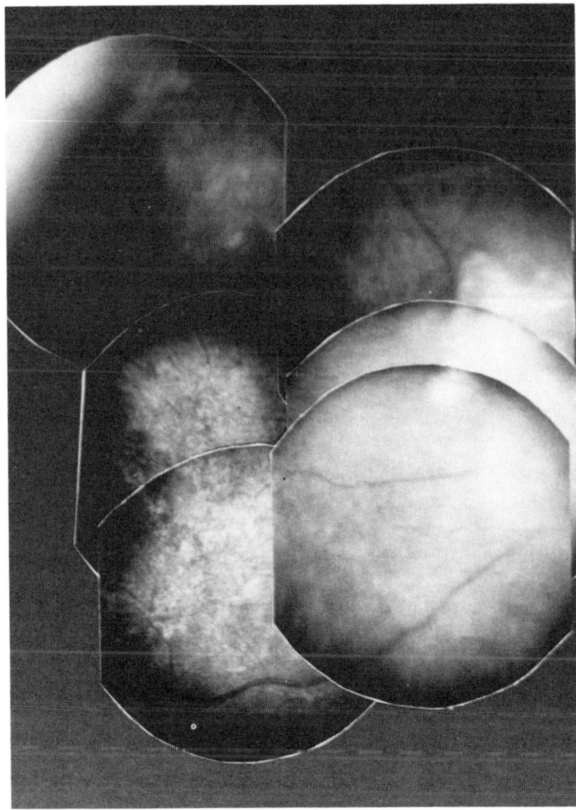

Figure 18–11   Right eye of patient 19, shown at 12-months post scleral buckling, with an anatomically reattached retina with pigment mottling (Color plate 11B).

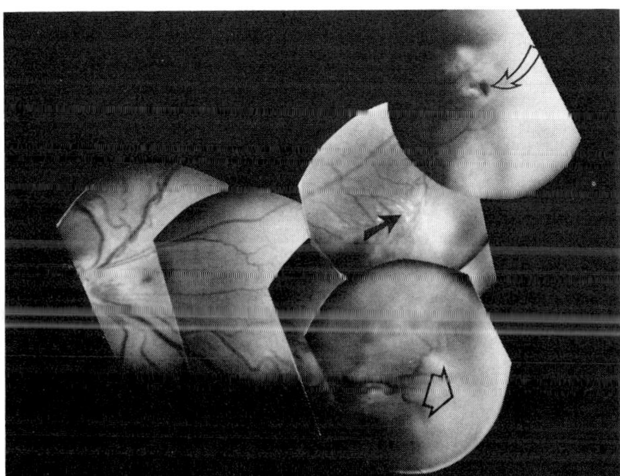

Figure 18–12   Left eye of patient 69, who weighed 1,320 grams at birth and who received no previous cryotherapy. The patient developed a combined tractional (   ) and serous (   ) retinal detachment. During the scleral buckling procedure at 20-weeks postnatal age, an iatrogenic tear was produced (   ) (Color plate 12A).

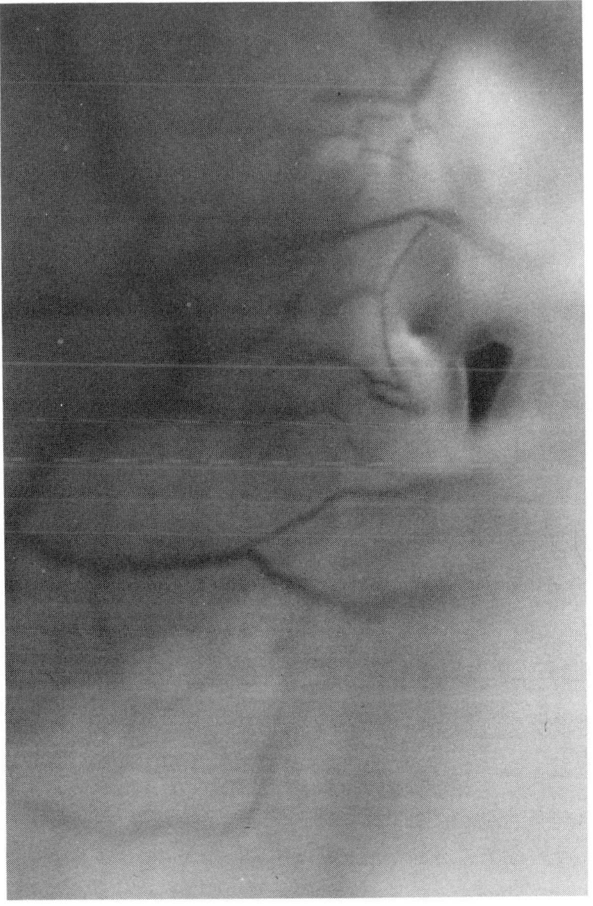

Figure 18–13   Left eye of patient 69 at 20 weeks postnatal age. The eye demonstrates a high magnification of the iatrogenic tear, only rarely produced during the scleral buckling procedure (Color plate 12B).

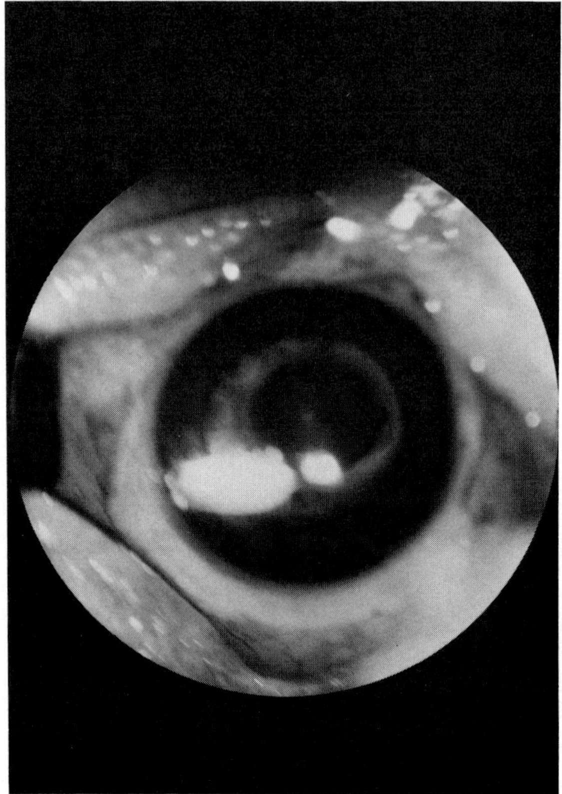

Figure 18–14 Photograph, through the dilated pupil, of the purse-string closure. The closure resulted from myofibroblast contraction at the shunt, creating a tractional detachment with a circumferential ridge.

damage, without obliteration but with induced plasma leakage, from the choroidal and neovascularizing retinal vessels.

In active ROP, when the macula is threatened by extensive peripheral detachment, or when the detachment involves the posterior pole, scleral buckling is performed

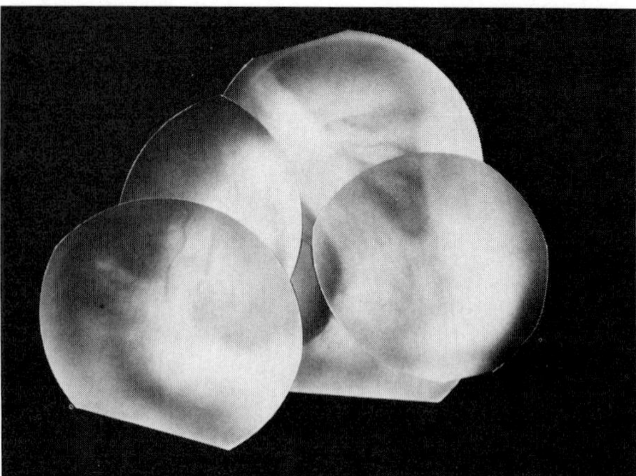

Figure 18–16 Photograph demonstrating transvitreal strands contracting at the shunt, creating a funnel (Color plate 13A).

immediately, because settling over a long time will only result in anatomic attachment of a dysplastic retina.

SURGICAL TECHNIQUE

Scleral buckling should be utilized when retinal detachment develops. This can occur in infants who are supplemented prophylactically with vitamin E, but whose systems are not able to adequately utilize the supplemented vitamin E to suppress spindle cell activation (infants 27-weeks gestational age or less), in infants who have suffered initial hypothermia and/or hypoxia, or in infants who have received improperly timed or placed cryotherapy.[18]

Preoperative dilating drops include Mydriacyl (tropicamide) 1 percent and Neo-Synephrine (phenylephrine hydrochloride) 2.5 percent eyedrops every 15 minutes, repeated four times prior to surgery.

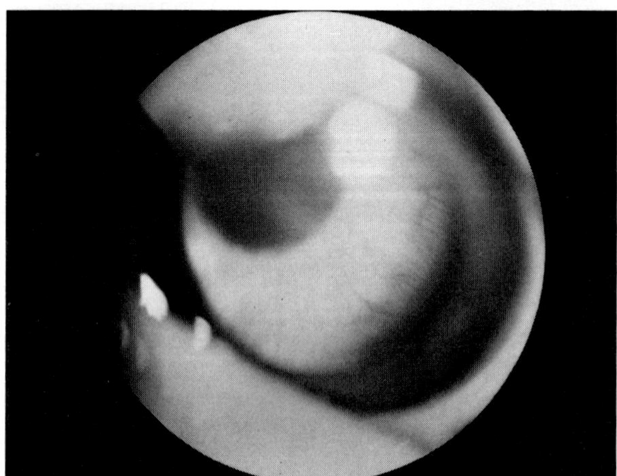

Figure 18–15 Photograph, through the dilated pupil, showing progression of the pursestring closure. This resulted from myofibroblast contraction at the shunt, creating a funnel.

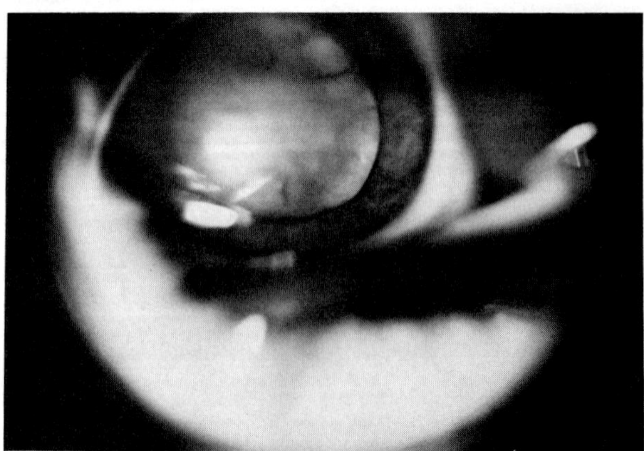

Figure 18–17 Photograph, through the dilated pupil, showing contraction of vitreous strands, creating a closed funnel (Color plate 13B).

The neonatologist or pediatrician places a peripheral, intravenous line prior to the infant being brought by portable incubator to a prewarmed operating theater for administration of a general anesthetic.

Betadine and soap are used for preoperative preparation of the surgical field, and then Chloroptic solution (chloramphenicol 0.5%) is utilized to irrigate the eye. The drapes are then placed on the infant. As surgery begins, Decadron (dexamethasone) 1 mg per kilogram, as a steroid, and Ancef (cefazolin sodium) 25 mg per kilogram, as an antibiotic, are administered intravenously.

Materials used for adult scleral buckling are too cumbersome. The basic surgical tray includes at least two pediatric needle holders, a fine Bishop forceps, a small mosquito hemostat (Fig. 18–18), a Ballen orbital retractor, a small Halsted malleable retractor, pediatric muscle hooks (Fig. 18–19), pediatric tenotomy scissors (Stevens), either a Sauer, Cook, or Alfonso pediatric speculum, and a 20- and 30-diopter indirect aspheric lens.

Tissue-Sol keeps the cornea moist to maintain corneal clarity. When the surgeon is not using the indirect ophthalmoscope, a Gelfoam sterile sponge, soaked in balanced salt solution (BSS) or Tissue-Sol, keeps the cornea moist.

A 360-degree conjunctival perilimbal peritomy is performed. A relaxing incision is made in the conjunctiva at either the 5 and 11 o'clock or at the 1 and 7 o'clock meridians. The edges are tagged with 5–0 silk or Mersilene suture to assist in locating the conjunctival edges at the end of the procedure (Fig. 18–20). Blunt dissection is done with scissors in each quadrant.

The horizontal and vertical muscles are isolated with a pediatric muscle hook or tenotomy hook (Fig. 18–21). A cannulated muscle hook passes a 2–0 silk suture un-

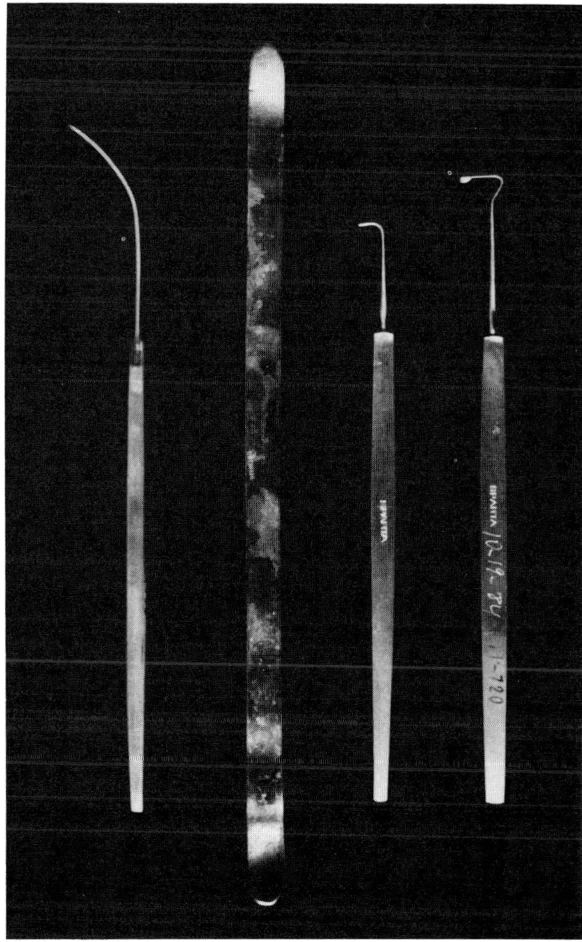

Figure 18–19   Instruments used for infant scleral buckling: small retractors and pediatric muscle hooks.

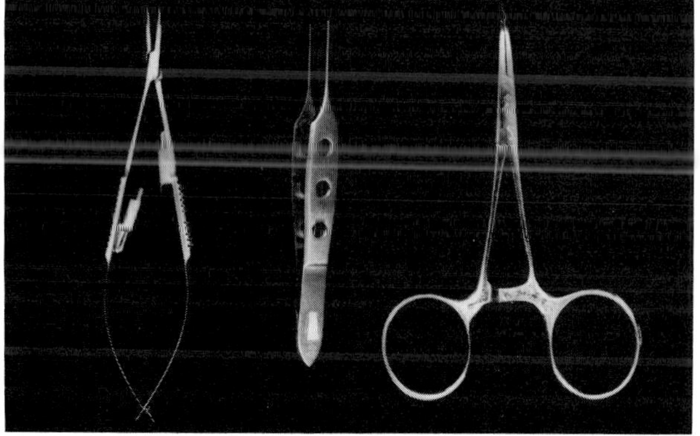

Figure 18–18   Instruments used for infant scleral buckling: pediatric needle holder, fine Bishop (toothed) forceps, and small mosquito clamp.

der the muscle as a traction suture. Excessive traction on the muscle can cause bradycardia or avulse the muscle from the globe.

Under direct visualization, cryotherapy is applied confluently to the shunt and the adjacent peripheral avascular retina in order to destroy any remaining activated spindle cells in the nerve fiber layer, as well as myofibroblasts in the vitreous that may create traction. Multiple, full-thickness cryo applications covering the 360-degree detachment will not damage the globe. To reduce the chance of iatrogenic, choroidal cracks or retinal tears, the iceball should thaw totally before the probe is removed. If there is marked, temporal dragging of the macula, avoid cryo applications or buckling in that area. Occasionally, mild vitreous haze develops from inflammation caused by cryotherapy.

Because such an infant has a thin, fragile sclera, episcleral silicone is used for the buckle. In a smaller infant, the number 40 solid silicone band is used; in a larger infant, the wider number 240 band is preferable.

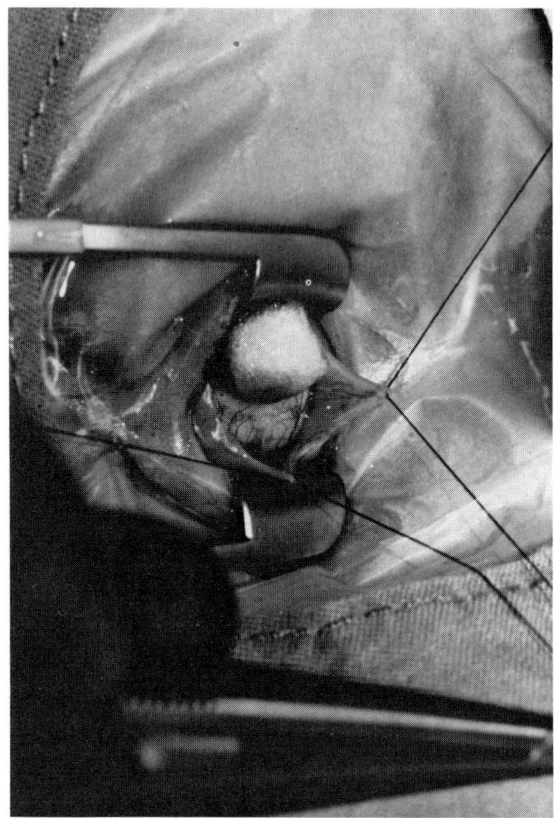

Figure 18–20 A 360-degree perilimbal, conjunctival peritomy is done. Relaxing incisions are made at 5 and 11 o'clock or at 1 and 7 o'clock and the conjunctiva is tagged with 5–0 silk or Mersilene suture. This procedure is useful in identifying the conjunctival edges at the time of closure.

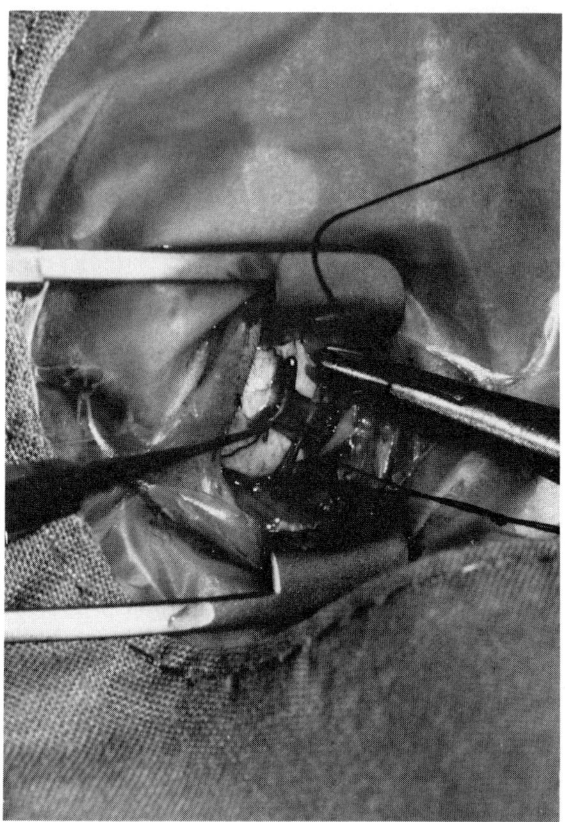

Figure 18–21 Isolation and tagging of muscles is done with a 2–0 silk suture, which is passed in a reversed manner under the belly of the muscle to prevent the needle's damaging the globe.

These silicone bands are soaked for approximately ten minutes in gentamicin sulfate solution. The implant is passed beneath the muscles, and a 5–0 Mersilene suture is placed around the two ends of the band in one quadrant, usually the inferior temporal (Fig. 18–22). The tightness (height of the buckle) should be conceptualized as an external purse string, counterbalancing the internal traction that results from myofibroblast contraction. The buckle should be only moderately high; if it is too high, the central retinal artery will pulsate or be occluded.

The buckle is placed at the arteriovenous shunt line or slightly posterior. Using a pediatric needle holder, an Ethicon 7–0 nylon suture on a tapered needle is passed through the sclera to secure the band (Fig. 18–23). The mattress suture should be slightly wider than the encircling band (Fig. 18–24). The scleral sutures should be superficial to avoid perforation of the globe, but sufficiently deep to avoid slippage.

Once the band is in place, drainage must be considered. If the detachment is shallow and concave with only slight residual fluid, the fluid usually resolves spon-

taneously. Should the child not require drainage, if the intraocular pressure is too high, Diamox (acetazolamide) 5 mg per kilogram can be administered intravenously. At the end of this procedure, the globe should not be left with a higher than normal intraocular pressure.

When the retina has detached 80 degrees, and the macula is involved, drainage is recommended. To prevent too high a buckle and to counteract hypotony, an intraocular injection of BSS with a 30-gauge needle is often given, via the pars plana, in the superior, temporal quadrant. This area of injection is determined by transillumination prior to drainage, but is usually 2 to 2.5 mm from the limbus. By first marking the pars plana with transillumination prior to drainage, it is possible to eliminate the complications arising from touching the lens or perforating the retina with the 30-gauge injection needle. The tip of the needle should remain visible at all times through the pupillary opening. It is especially important to do this when the retina is bullous.

A cut-down sclerotomy is performed posterior to the buckle in the quadrant having the highest retinal elevation. A double-armed mattress suture of Ethicon 6–0

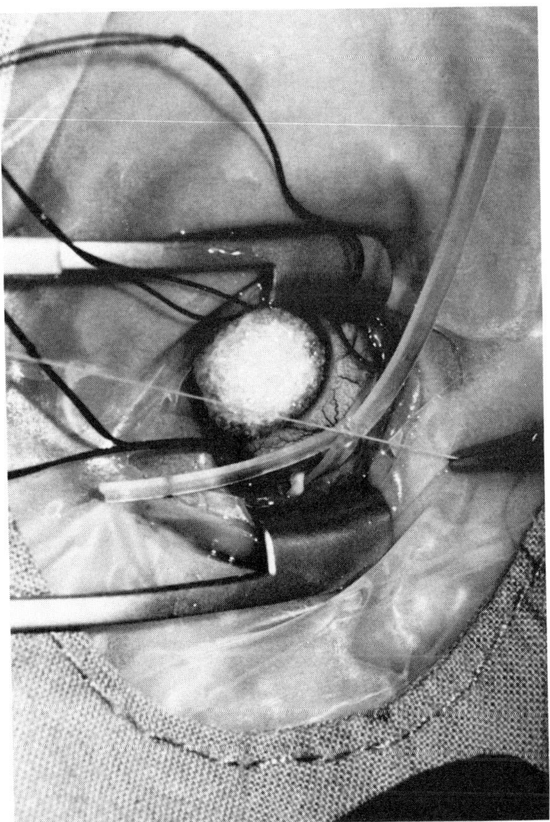

Figure 18–22 After cryotherapy, a number 240 or 40 band is passed underneath the muscles and tied in one quadrant with a 5–0 Mersilene suture.

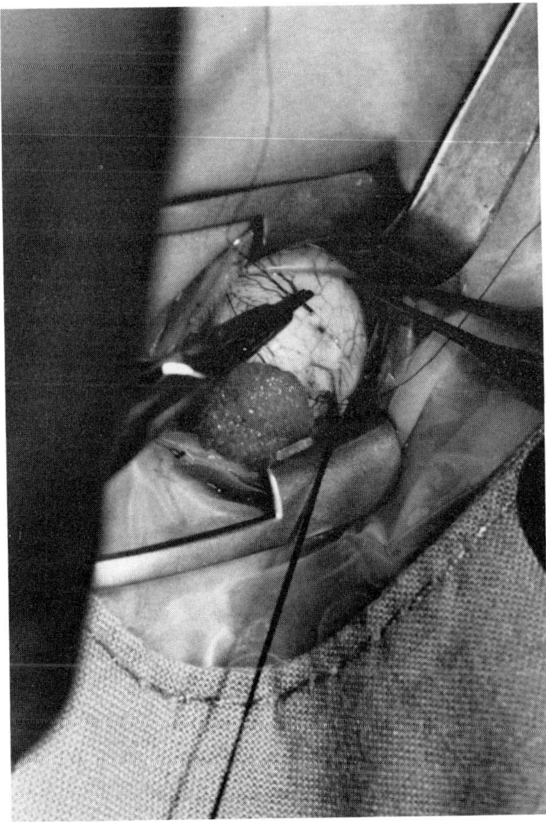

Figure 18–23 A 7–0 nylon suture is passed through the thin sclera to secure the band. The scleral sutures should be superficial to avoid perforation of the globe, but sufficiently deep to avoid slippage.

Mersilene is placed using a tapercut RV$_2$ needle. The suture loops are spread to expose the knuckle of choroid, and the needle is placed through the choroid into the pocket of subretinal fluid to be drained. Drainage should be slow. The mattress sutures are drawn up to close the sclerotomy site. The intraocular pressure is checked and should be high normal but not excessive.

Indirect ophthalmoscopy confirms that the buckle was placed correctly, that none of the sutures went too deep, and that no tears developed at the drainage site. As the retina settles and subretinal fluid is absorbed, a buckle that may have appeared low at the time of surgery becomes adequately high (Fig. 18–25). The optic nerve head is observed to determine whether its color is satisfactory and whether the central retinal artery is patent.

A culture of the band and sutures is taken, followed by gentle lavage of the globe area with Neosporin (polymyxin B - neomycin - bacitracin) and gentamicin sulfate solutions. The silk sutures are removed from under the muscles, and the conjunctiva is closed with a 6–0 plain suture. The previously placed conjunctival tagging sutures help identify the conjunctival edges, which reduces

the possibility of conjunctival cysts (Fig. 18–26). At this time, topical antibiotic and steroids are instilled. The vitreous should be relatively clear and without hemorrhage.

Postoperative care includes Garamycin (gentamicin), Econopred (prednisolone acetate), Mydriacyl 1 percent, and Neo-Synephrine 2.5 percent four times a day for two weeks. Systemic medications include Diamox

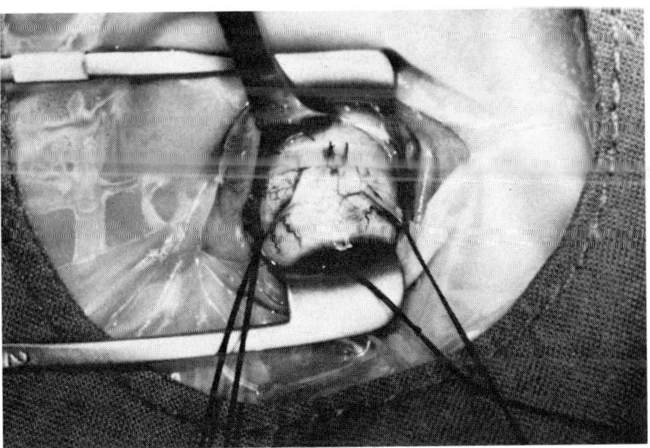

Figure 18–24 The posterior bite of the 7–0 nylon mattress suture is approximately 4 mm behind the anterior bite.

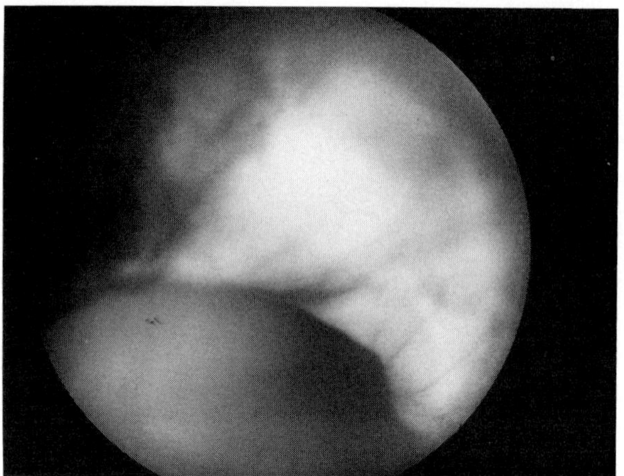

Figure 18–25 Fundus photograph demonstrating a high buckle following a successful scleral buckling procedure. To prevent erosion, the scleral buckle is transsected later (Color plate 13C).

(acetazolamide) 5 mg per kilogram per day, Ancef (cephazolin sodium) 25 mg per kilogram per day, and Decadron (dexamethasone) 0.5 mg per kilogram per day for one week. Lid edema is minimized with cold compresses.

RESULTS

The data base consists of 101 eyes of 75 infants with acute ROP (Table 1). Thirty-five of the eyes had prophylactic cryotherapy that was not successful in bringing about remission of the disease, because it was improperly placed or timed. The infants were from 7- to 38-weeks postnatal age at the time of scleral buckling. Thirty-eight eyes underwent revision(s) of the scleral buckle, 12 eyes have subsequently undergone open-sky vitrectomy. The average length of follow-up was 29 months. Thirty-one eyes were lost to follow-up, 16 of

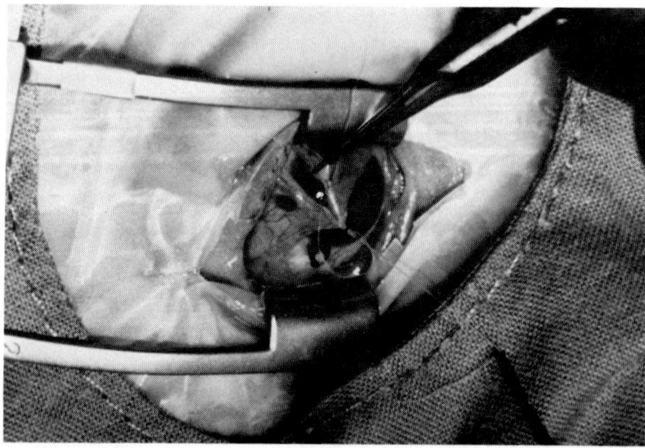

Figure 18–26 The conjunctiva is repaired with a 6–0 plain suture. Accurate apposition of the conjunctival edges reduces the likelihood of conjunctival cysts occurring.

these because of infant death. Success is defined as anatomic retinal attachment despite macular dragging. The overall success rate following scleral buckling was 54 percent. Success rate is not substantially different when analyzed according to birth weight, postnatal age of scleral buckling, or previous cryotherapy. The scleral-buckling technique evolved over a decade, and the population is not homogeneous with respect to vitamin E supplementation, duration of detachment, types of the detachment (tractional versus exudative versus rhegmatogenous), previous extent and placement of cryotherapy, and the increasing number of very-low-birth-weight survivors. Snellen visual acuities have been recorded for 11 eyes, and six eyes have "count fingers" vision.

COMPLICATIONS

Early Postoperative Complications

Vitreoretinal traction can persist when cryotherapy is not adequate to destroy all viable myofibroblasts, or when the external buckle is too low to compensate for internal, tractional forces. A buckle revision may be done to drain the recurrent, subretinal fluid or to move and tighten the buckle. If traction and membrane formation continue, further cicatricial RLF will develop.

Late Postoperative Complications

Despite successful reattachment, the band may cause constriction of the globe with growth of the infant's eye. The band must be transsected, ideally between three and six months, but always before one year postoperatively. Under general anesthesia, the conjunctiva and Tenon's capsule are incised in one quadrant. The band is identified through this small incision and transsected in one quadrant; complete removal usually is not necessary. The conjunctiva is closed with a 6–0 plain suture.

MORPHOLOGICAL INTERPRETATION OF SCLERAL BUCKLING

The morphological data base consisted of two eyes from two infants (patients 40 and 70) who underwent

TABLE 18-1 Scleral Buckling Cases

Patient Number	Case Number	Birth Weight (g)	Preop Cryo	Postnatal Age at Surgery (wks)	Number of Revisions	Success/ Failure	Visual Acuity	Follow-up (mos)	Figures
1	1	490	Y	17	0	S	UN	12‡‡	
2	2	520	Y	15	0	S	UN	6	
	3		N	14	0	S	UN	6	
3	4*	560	N	20	1	F	UN	6	
4	5*	600	Y	15	2	F	UN	16	
5	6	600	N	15	1	F	UN	3‡	
	7		N	16	1	S	UN	3‡	
6	8*	610	Y	16	2	F	HM	11	
7	9	610	Y	19	1	S	HM	12	
	10		Y	16	3	F	NLP	13	
8	11	625	N	14	0	S	NLP	39	
	12		N	18	0	F	NLP	38	
9	13	630	N	13	0	F	NLP	12‡	
	14		N	12	1	F	NLP	12‡	
10	15	650	N	21	1	F	LP	24	
11	16	660	Y	17	2	S	UN	3‡‡	18-1,2,3
12	17	670	N	21	0	F	UN	0‡‡	
13	18	680	Y	15	0	S	UN	2‡‡	
	19		Y	16	0	S	UN	2‡‡	
14	20	680	Y	13	0	F	UN	0‡	
15	21	700	N	11	2	F	UN	2‡	
16	22	700	N	12	0	S	CF	22	
17	23*	710	N	16	0	F	LP	21	
18	24	720	N	30	0	F	LP	14	
19	25	740	N	19	1	S	UN	22	18-10,11
20	26	740	Y	19	0	S	UN	18	18-4,5,6
21	27	750	Y	15	2	F	UN	6	
22	28	750	Y	8	0	S	CF	38	
23	29	750	Y	11	0	F	LP	8	
24	30	760	Y	17	0	F	LP	81	
	31		Y	18	0	S	LP	81	
25	32	790	N	17	1	S	20/400	50	
	33		N	16	2	S	20/400	50	
26	34*	800	Y	16	2	F	UN	7	
27	35	800	Y	13	3	S	LP	19	
28	36	810	Y	10	0	S	20/30	64	
29	37	840	N	14	1	F	LP	45	
	38		N	14	2	S	HM	45	
30	39	840	N	16	1	S	HM	24	18-7,8,9
31	40	850	N	19	1	F	UN	11	
32	41*	860	N	21	0	F	UN	10	
33	42	870	Y	38	0	S	HM	15	
34	43	880	N	14	0	F	UN	72‡	
35	44	880	Y	19	0	S	UN	8‡‡	
	45		Y	20	0	S	UN	8‡‡	
36	46	880	Y	19	0	S	HM	70	
37	47	890	N	14	1	F	LP	24	
38	48	890	Y	13	0	S	UN	6‡	
39	49*	900	N	14	1	F	LP	33	
	50		N	15	0	S	HM	32	
40	51	900	N	9	0	S	UN	1‡‡	18-27
41	52	920	N	27	0	S	CF	108	
42	53	920	Y	17	0	S	20/60	62	
	54		Y	17	0	S	20/80	62	
43	55	920	N	19	0	S	20/200	70	
44	56	920	N	17	0	S	UN	4‡‡	
	57		N	16	0	S	UN	4‡‡	
45	58	925	N	37	0	S	CF	92	
	59		N	36	0	S	20/200	92	
46	60	940	N	16	0	S	20/100	52	
47	61	960	N	17	0	S	CF	47	
48	62	960	N	15	1	S	HM	25	
	63		N	15	1	S	HM	25	
49	64*	960	Y	15	0	F	LP	17	
50	65	965	N	26	2	S	HM	67‡	
51	66	980	N	27	0	S	UN	13‡‡	

TABLE 18-1   Scleral Buckling Cases (Continued)

Patient Number	Case Number	Birth Weight (g)	Preop Cryo	Postnatal Age at Surgery (wks)	Number of Revisions	Success/ Failure	Visual Acuity	Follow-up (mos)	Figures
52	67	1,000	Y	11	1	F	UN	2‡‡	
	68		Y	11	0	F	UN	2‡‡	
53	69	1,010	N	14	0	S	HM	8‡	
54	70	1,015	Y	17	0	S	20/200	69	
55	71	1,040	N	23	1	S	LP	22	
	72*		N	24	0	F	LP	22	
56	73	1,060	N	15	0	F	LP	132	
	74		N	13	0	S	20/400	132	
57	75	1,065	N	14	0	F	LP	26	
	76		N	13	1	F	LP	26	
58	77	1,090	Y	13	0	S	UN	4	
	78*		Y	12	1	F	UN	4	
59	79	1,110	N	7	0	F	UN	0‡	
	80		Y	9	0	F	UN	0‡	
60	81	1,120	N	19	0	F	LP	10‡‡	
61	82	1,130	N	13	0	S	HM	19	
	83		N	14	2	F	NLP	19	
62	84	1,175	N	30	0	F	LP	55‡	
63	85	1,195	Y	13	2	S	HM	59	
	86		Y	27	0	F	LP	56	
64	87	1,260	N	22	0	F	NLP	6‡‡	
65	88	1,270	N	15	0	F	UN	9‡	
	89		N	16	1	F	NLP	9‡	
66	90	1,280	N	15	0	S	LP	70	
	91*		N	8	2	F	LP	72	
67	92	1,300	N	21	0	F	UN	11	
68	93	1,310	Y	20	0	S	CF	95	
69	94	1,320	N	20	1	S	HM	21	18-12,13
70	95	1,350	Y	16	0	F	UN	2‡‡	18-28
71	96	1,350	N	25	1	F	NLP	44	
72	97	1,350	N	9	1	S	NLP	8	
	98		N	8	0	F	NLP	8	
73	99*	1,400	N	22	1	F	UN	3	
74	100	1,420	N	14	0	S	20/200	50	
75	101	1,475	N	8	3	S	LP	70	

* = underwent open-sky vitrectomy; ‡ = lost to follow-up; ‡‡ = deceased

scleral buckling at the postnatal ages of 9 and 16 weeks, respectively. Both infants received interrupted, prophylactic vitamin E therapy; therefore, the spindle cell kinetics of unsupplemented infants should apply. That is, spindle cell activation should occur as early as 4-days postnatally; maturation, as early as 8-weeks postnatally.

The three light micrographs shown in Figure 18–27 demonstrate the retinal integrity of an infant of 900-grams birth weight who survived for 12 weeks and who underwent, at nine weeks, a successful scleral buckling procedure to correct a peripheral retinal detachment. The central (Fig. 18–27A), shunt (Fig. 18–27B), and peripheral (Fig. 18–27C) retinas have normal stratification of retinal neurons, minimal nuclear pyknosis, and extensive attachment between the retinal pigment epithelium and retina. There is an accumulation of debris in the subretinal space that might be a manifestation of high-light intensity damage to photoreceptors within the central retina. The debris may be accentuated by the previous retinal detachment in the peripheral regions.

The inner retinal vessels are intact centrally, are represented by the arteriovenous shunt at the demarcation line, and are absent among the peripheral, stacked spindle cells.

The three light micrographs shown in Figure 18–28 demonstrate the retinal deterioration of an infant of 1,350-grams birth weight who survived for 24 weeks and had an unsuccessful scleral buckling procedure performed at age 16 weeks. The central (Fig. 18–28C), mid peripheral (Fig. 18–28B), and peripheral (Fig. 18–28A) retinas are totally detached and dysplastic, with death of photoreceptors, formation of retinal rosettes, altered synaptology within the inner and outer plexiform layers, and degeneration of the ganglion cell layer. Preretinal membranes have developed on the vitreous surface, while a viscous fluid has accumulated in the subretinal space.

These two examples indicate that early scleral buckling can result in retinal morphology with no pyknosis of retinal neurons, while delayed procedures cannot

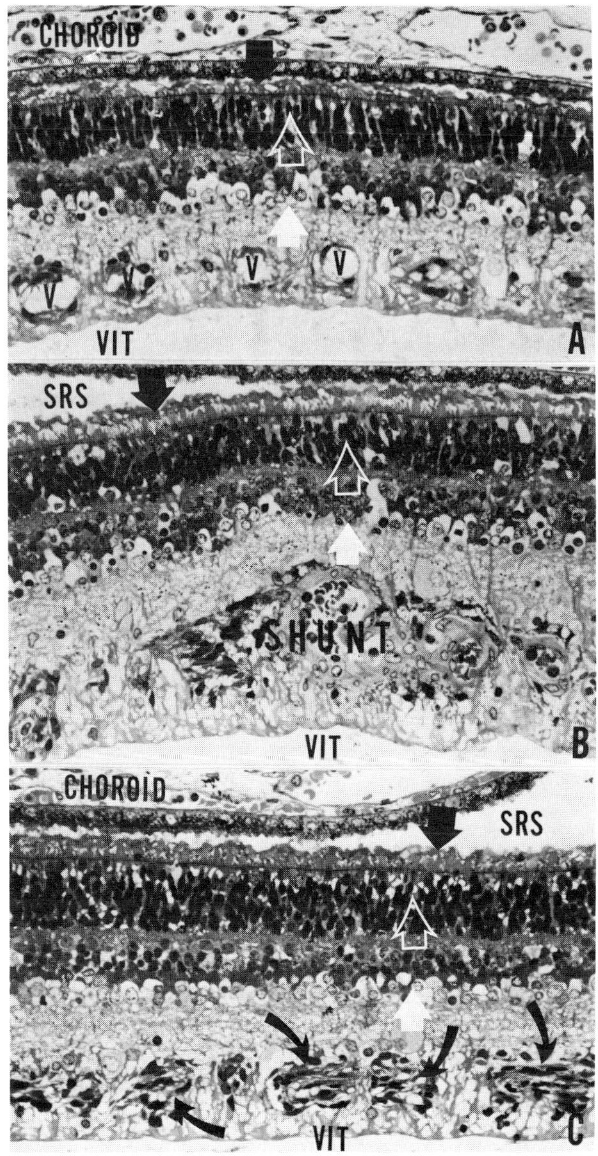

Figure 18–27 Light micrographs of the right eye of patient 40, who weighed 900 grams at birth. This eye underwent a scleral buckling procedure for a peripheral detachment when the infant was 9-weeks postnatal age. The infant died at 12-weeks postnatal age. Whole-eye donations were obtained at four hours postmortem. A, central retina; B, shunt; C, peripheral retina. The retina is attached with debris (   ) and fluid in the subretinal space (SRS). Because of the early, successful, scleral buckling procedure, the outer (open white arrow) and inner (solid white arrow) nuclear layers are morphologically intact, with the potential for restoration of good vision. V, inner retinal vessels; (   ), stacked spindle cells; VIT, vitreous. A-C=115×.

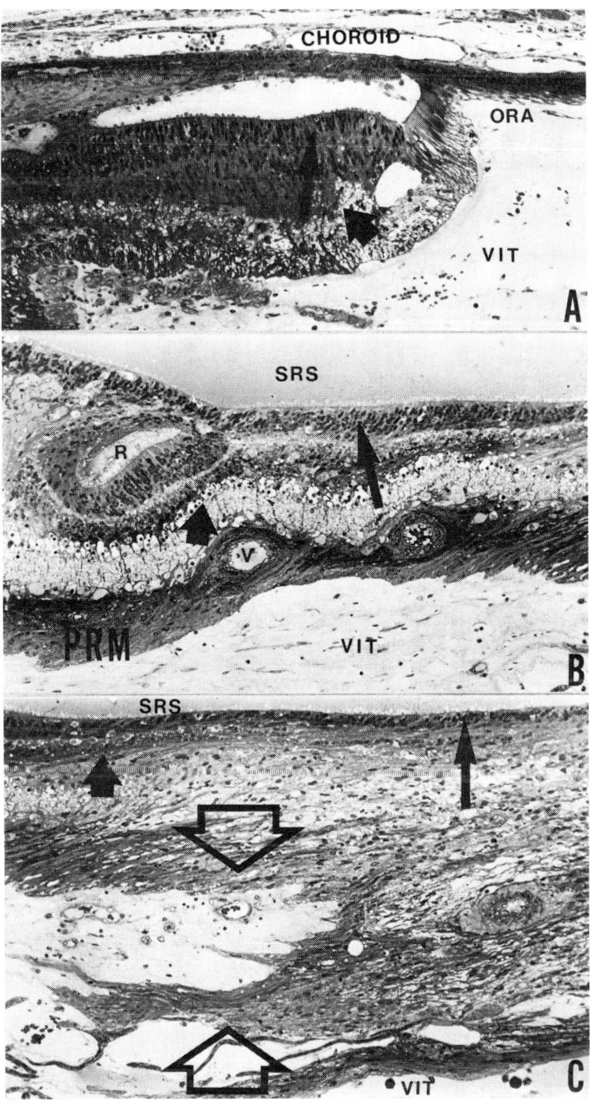

Figure 18–28 Light micrographs of the left eye of patient 70, who weighed 1,350 grams at birth. This eye underwent unsuccessful cryotherapy at 14 weeks-postnatal age and scleral buckling procedure at 16-weeks postnatal age. The infant died at 24-weeks postnatal age. Whole-eye donations were obtained at two hours postmortem. A, far peripheral retina attached at the ora serrata (ORA); B, mid peripheral retina; C, central retina. The retina is totally detached except at the ora serrata, with a viscous fluid in the subretinal space (SRS). Because of the late, unsuccessful, scleral buckling procedure, the outer (   ) and inner (   ) nuclear layers are morphologically atrophic with no potential for restoration of useful vision even if the retina were anatomically reattached by open-sky vitrectomy. R, retinal rosettes; V, inner retinal vessels; PRM, preretinal membrane (between two large arrow heads), preretinal mass with spindle cells, vessels, and cellular infiltrates; VIT, vitreous. A-C=65×.

reverse the death of nonregenerating, postmitotic, highly differentiated retinal neurons. Therefore, to minimize the possibility of such retinal death induced by prolonged retinal separation from the retinal pigment epithelium and choroid, in the acute stages of ROP one should attempt to reattach the retina as soon as possible.

REFERENCES

1. Tasman W, Annesley W. Retinal detachment in the retinopathy of prematurity. Arch Ophthalmol 1966; 75:608–614.
2. Faris BM, Brockhurst RJ. Retrolental fibroplasia in the cicatricial stage. The complication of rhegmatogenous retinal detachment. Arch Ophthalmol 1969; 82:60–65.
3. Tasman W. Vitreoretinal changes in cicatricial retrolental fibroplasia. Trans Am Ophthalmol Soc 1970; 68:548–594.
4. Tasman W. Retinal detachment in retrolental fibroplasia. Albrecht v Graefes Arch Klin Ophthalmol 1975; 195:130–139.
5. Harris GS. Retinopathy of prematurity and retinal detachment. Can J Ophthalmol 1976; 11:21–25.
6. Starzycka M, Ciechanowska A, Gergovich A. Retinal detachment in retrolental fibroplasia. Ophthalmologica 1980; 181:261–265.
7. Koerner FH. Retinopathy of prematurity: natural course and management. Met Ophthalmol 1978; 2:325–329.
8. Yassur Y, Grunwald E, Ben-Sira I. Surgical treatment of retrolental fibroplasia in infants. Met Ophthalmol 1978; 2:333–334.
9. McPherson AR, Hittner HM. Scleral buckling in 2½ to 11 month old premature infants with retinal detachment associated with acute retrolental fibroplasia. Ophthalmology 1979; 86:819–835.
10. Grunwald E, Yassur Y, Ben-Sira I. Buckling procedures for retinal detachment caused by retrolental fibroplasia in premature babies. Br J Ophthalmol 1980; 64:98–101.
11. Bert MD, Friedman MW, Ballard R. Combined cryosurgery and scleral buckling in acute proliferative retrolental fibroplasia. J Pediatr Ophthalmol Strab 1981; 18:841–844.
12. Baruch E, Bracha R, Godel V, Lazar M. Buckling procedure in infant retrolental fibroplasia. J Ocular Ther Surg 1981; 1:65–66.
13. McPherson AR, Hittner HM, Lemos R. Retinal detachment in young premature infants with acute retrolental fibroplasia, thirty-two new cases. Ophthalmology 1982; 89:1160–1169.
14. Topilow HW, Acherman AL, Want FM. The treatment of advanced retinopathy of prematurity by cryotherapy and scleral buckling surgery. Opthalmology 1985; 92:379–387.
15. Tasman W. Management of retinopathy of prematurity. Ophthalmology 1985; 92:995–999.
16. Kretzer FL, McPherson AR, Rudolph AJ, Hittner HM. Pathogenic mechanism of retinopathy of prematurity: a controversial explanation for the efficacy of oral and intramuscular vitamin E supplementation and cryotherapy. Bull NY Acad Med 1985; 61:883–900.
17. Soong HK, Eller AW, Hirose T, Hanninen L, Kenyon KR. In situ actin distribution in excised retrolental membranes in retinopathy of prematurity. Arch Ophthalmol 1985; 103:1553–1556.
18. Kretzer FL, Mehta RS, Johnson AT, Hunter DG, Brown ES, Hittner HM. Vitamin E protects against retinopathy of prematurity through action on spindle cells. Nature 1984; 309:793–795.

Treatment of Retrolental Fibroplasia with Open-Sky Vitrectomy 19

Alice R. *McPherson*, M.D.
Helen M. *Hittner*, M.D.
Robert A. *Moura*, M.D.
Frank L. *Kretzer*, Ph.D.

HISTORICAL DATA BASE

As active retinopathy of prematurity (ROP) resolves, cicatricial retrolental fibroplasia (RLF) ensues. Tasman[1] has classified the specific fundus changes seen in Grades I through V cicatricial RLF. Pathophysiologically, membrane formation occurs; these membranes exert intravitreal, tractional forces and have a sheetlike appearance. With membrane contraction, a tractional retinal detachment may be created, which may progress to various degrees of open and closed funnels. The hazy-white, avascular retrolental membrane creates a frontal opacity that masks the underlying, gray, vascularized retina.

Two surgical procedures have been developed to manage Grades IV and V cicatricial RLF. Controversy exists as to the advantages and disadvantages of closed vitrectomy versus open-sky vitrectomy. Tasman[2] reported the results of closed vitrectomy on four eyes (infant age between 2 and 22 months) with one (25%) anatomic success. Merritt, et al[3] reported the results of 12 closed vitrectomy cases (infant age between 4 and 18 months) with no anatomic successes. Lightfoot and Irvine[4] have reported anatomic reattachment in three of five eyes (60%, infant age between 4 months and 4 years) treated by closed vitrectomy. Machemer[5] has reported the results of both open (3) and closed (12) vitrectomy cases (infants between 4 and 24 months), with no successes with the open approach, but seven successes with the closed approach (58%). Trese[6] has reported anatomic reattachment in 45 percent of 40 consecutive cases (infants between 3 and 8 months) of closed vitrectomy. Charles[7] has reported anatomic reattachment in 50 percent of 416 consecutive cases (infants of at least 6 months of age, weighing 10 pounds and with Grades IV and V cicatricial RLF).

Schepens[8] has developed two types of open-sky procedures. The anterior, open-sky method includes surgery on the anterior segment in combination with a vitreous procedure limited to the area anterior to the equator. The subtotal, open-sky procedure includes surgery on all of the vitreous except the vitreous base. The vitreous base is not removed, since this would cause a detachment of the ora serrata, resulting in a giant retinal break. The open-sky technique offers the advantage of easier instrument access and interchange and promotes enhanced exposure of the far peripheral fields. The major disadvantage of open-sky vitrectomy is that the eye is exposed to atmospheric pressure. Consequently, the intraocular tissues can become edematous.

Hirose and Schepens[9] have reported anatomic reattachment in 38 percent of 184 consecutive cases of open-sky vitrectomy, but results differed depending on the configuration of the detachment. Open funnels responded better (83% success rate) than tightly closed funnels (22% success rate). Hirose and Schepens obtained ambulatory vision in 46 percent of the successes, and one patient showed 20/300 visual acuity six years after surgery.

SURGICAL TECHNIQUE

Subtotal, open-sky vitrectomy can be used to treat selected cases of advanced Grades IV and V cicatricial RLF (Fig. 19–1); it is inappropriate during Stages 1 to 4 active ROP or for Grades I to III cicatricial RLF (Fig. 19–2). Infants with organized retrolental membranes, with or without cataracts, are candidates for this procedure. Ideally, the eyes that will benefit most are found in infants between the ages of 5 and 12 months who have total, nonrhegmatogenous retinal detachment and who do not have glaucoma secondary to a flat cham-

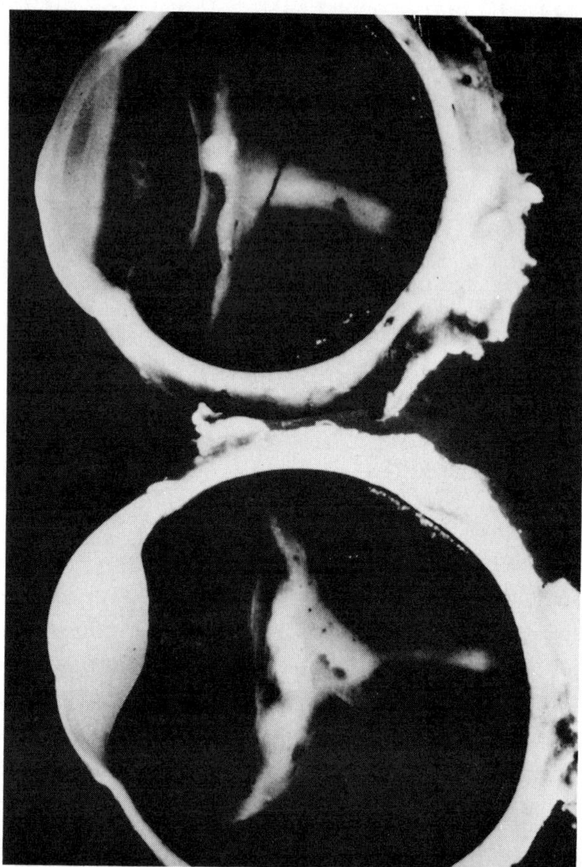

Figure 19–1 Cross-sections of two eyes with Grade V cicatricial RLF. There is complete retinal detachment with a closed funnel behind the retrolental membrane.

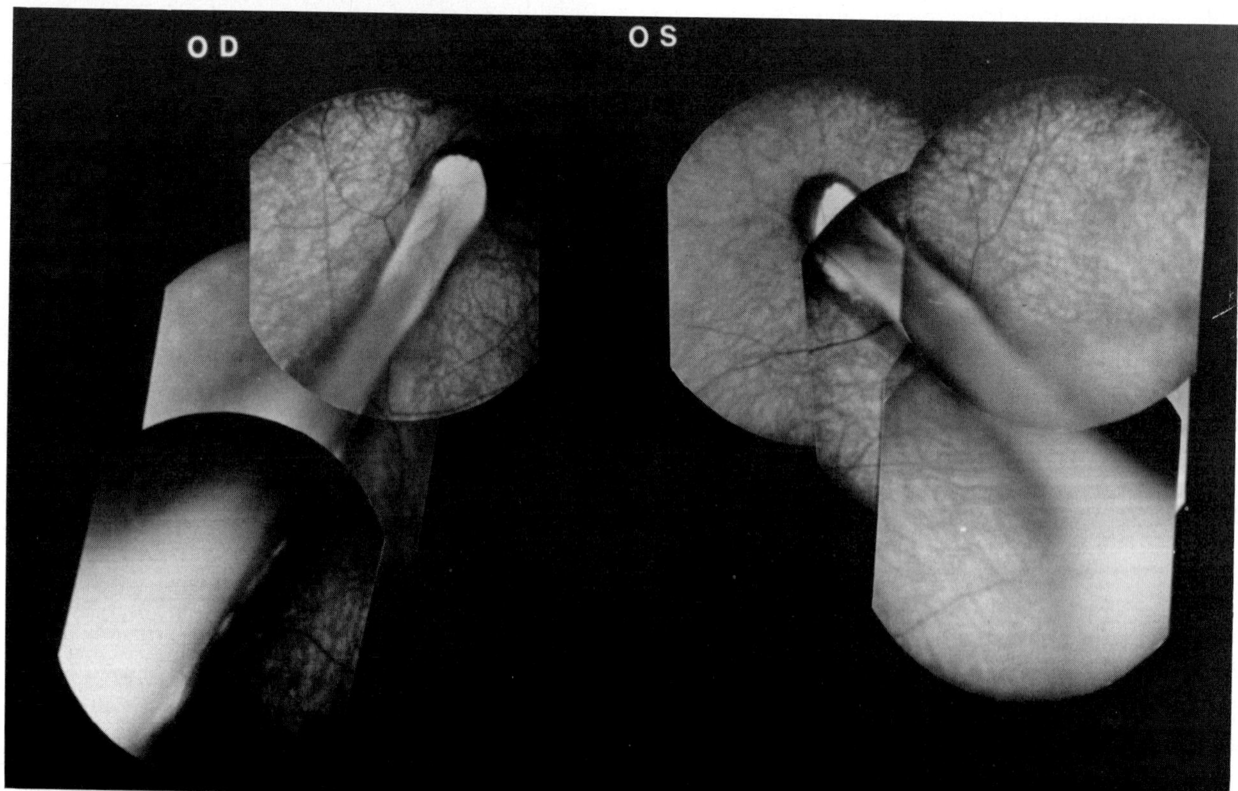

Figure 19–2 Retinal montages of two eyes with Grade III cicatricial RLF. The falciform folds are comprised of pleated retina and aggregated vessels. An open-sky vitrectomy is inappropriate for Grades I to III cicatricial RLF.

ber. Older infants can also undergo the procedure; however, the functional results do not appear to be as promising as those in children under 12 months of age.

Examination of the infant includes external and anterior-segment evaluation. The iris should be evaluated for neovascularization and extensive synechiae along the pupillary border (Fig. 19–3). Iris neovascularization, flat anterior chamber, and glaucoma are poor prognostic signs. The amount of neovascular activity in the retrolental region should be noted.

Ultrasonographic evaluation can be helpful. This technique may indicate whether a tightly closed detachment, an open-funnel detachment, or a retinal fold is present behind the retrolental mass (Figs. 19–4 and 19–5). In some instances, ultrasound might mislead the surgeon regarding the configuration of the detachment. This is especially true when dealing with closed-funnel detachments. Ultrasound might not demonstrate the closed funnel that will subsequently be found during surgery; therefore, ultrasonography is an ancillary test.

The instrumentation employed differs from the traditional, ocular microsurgery set. Special instruments that fit under a 125 mm focal-length surgical microscope have been devised (Figs. 19–6 and 19–7). The ends of these instruments are angled to fit inside the eye and allow the surgeon to keep his or her hands outside the surgical field. Modified Colibri or Castroviejo forceps, small de Wecker or Vannas scissors, aluminum spatulas, and a suction spatula to remove fluid close to the retina are the primary surgical instruments.

The surgical technique is summarized in Figure 19–8, Color plate 14.

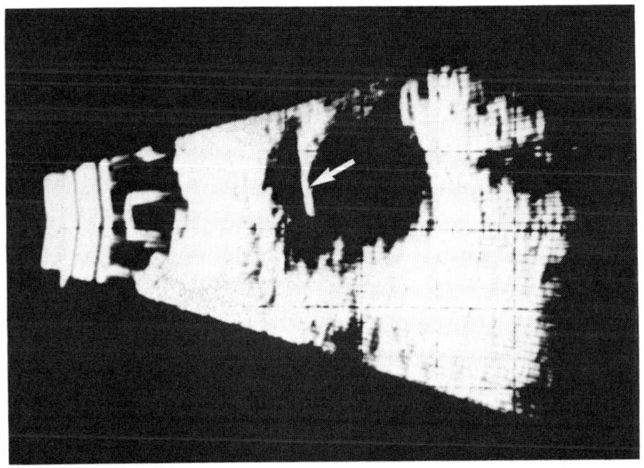

Figure 19–4   Ultrasonogram of Grade V cicatricial RLF in the vertical-nasal meridian. The echoes suggest an anteriorly placed membrane (　　　) without a funnel in this plane. This single ultrasonogram can be interpreted as an attached retina with peripheral membranes. Contrast this vertical-nasal plane with the horizontal-midline plane seen in the same eye in Figure 19–5.

A Flieringa ring or scleral supporter is sewn onto the sclera with an 8–0 Vicryl suture. This prevents collapse of the globe once the subretinal fluid is drained and the corneal button removed.

A sclerotomy is made anterior to the equator, and an Ethicon 6–0 Mersilene mattress suture is preplaced. This incision will permit lowering of the intraocular pressure through drainage. Since the exact configuration of the detachment is not always known, drainage should be done slowly to soften the globe, so that the anterior chamber can be deepened subsequently and maintained with Healon (hyaluronic acid). The drainage site is closed by pulling up the preplaced suture.

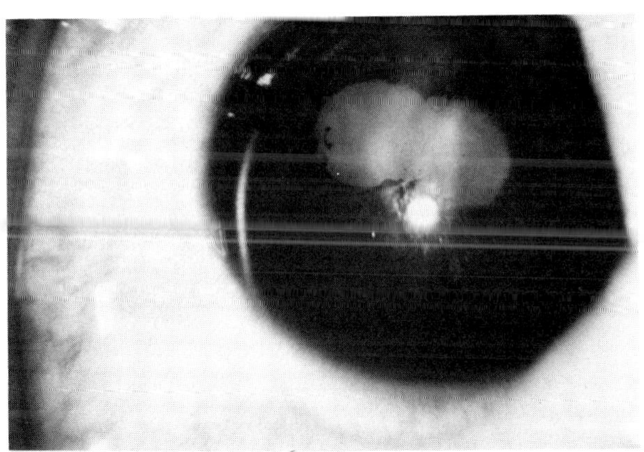

Figure 19–3   External photograph of the anterior segment, showing synechiae to the lens distorting the pupillary aperture. Often these are associated with narrow-angle glaucoma. The synechiae should be carefully noted preoperatively and released at surgery.

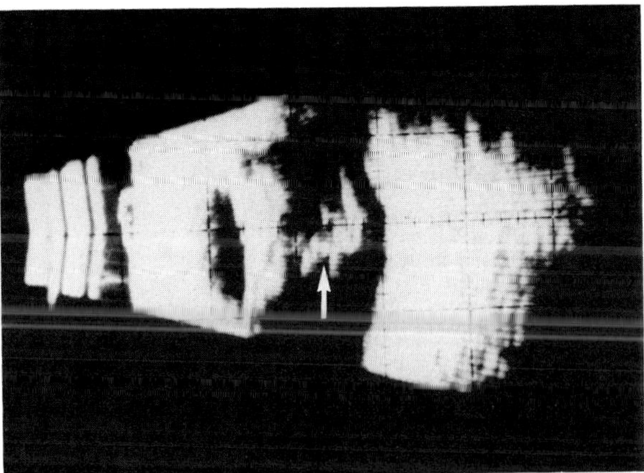

Figure 19–5   Ultrasonogram of Grade V cicatricial RLF in the horizontal-midline meridian of the same eye, as seen in Figure 19–4. The echoes show a retrolental membrane and the retina detached as a closed-funnel detachment (　↑　). This emphasizes the importance of examining many horizontal and vertical meridians.

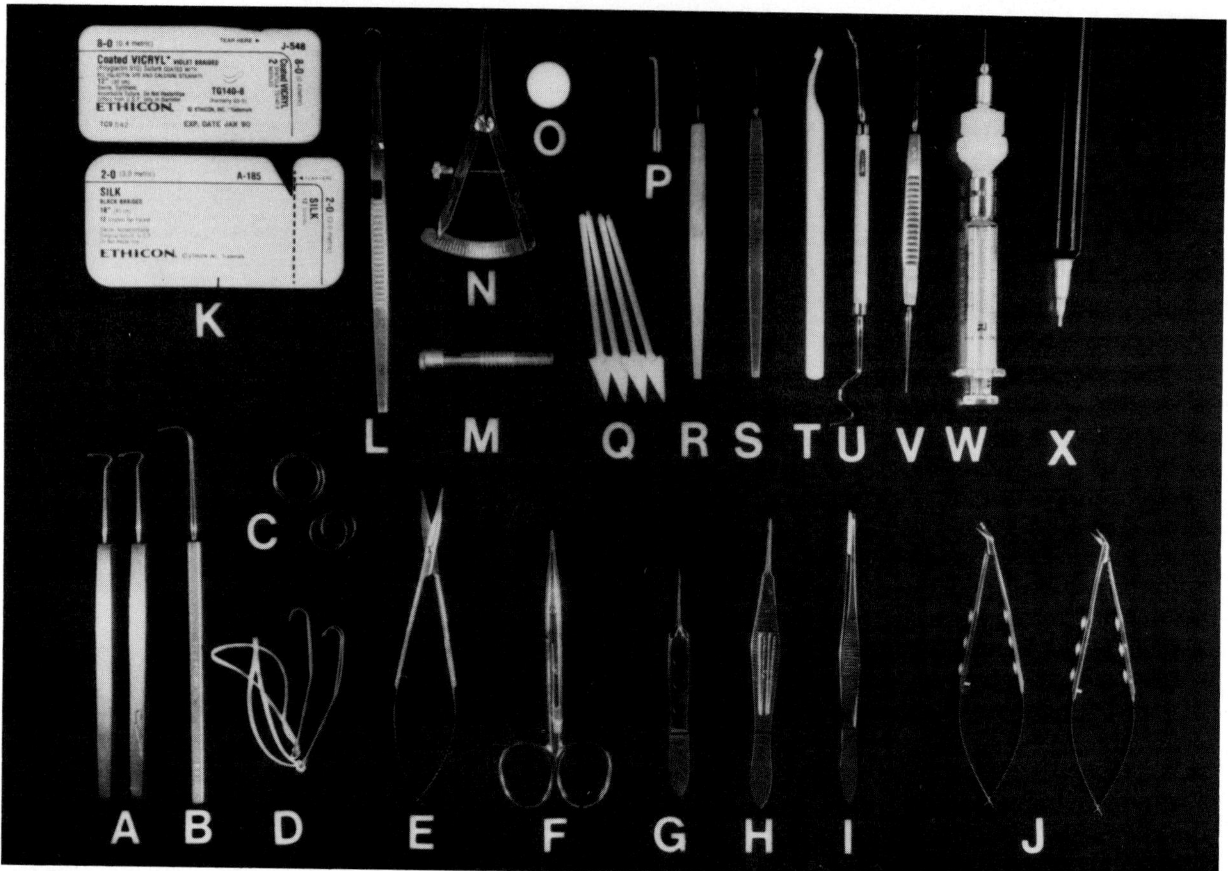

Figure 19–6 Instrument tray. A, Muscle hooks (Sparta 11–720); B, Cannulated muscle hook (Storz E-604 SP⁷/08862); C, Flieringa rings (Storz E-4034) size 12–16, special-order size 9, 10, and 11; D, Baby Jaffe lid speculum (Weck); E, Westcott tenotomy scissor (Sparta 12–451); F, Stevens tenotomy scissor (Storz E-3552); G, Fine Bishop Harmon forceps (Storz E-1502); H, 0.5 Castroviejo forceps (Storz E-1795); I, Bonaccolto utility forceps (Storz E-1906); J, Right and left corneal scissor (Katena L K4-1000, R K4-1010); K, Sutures-Sutupak-2.0 silk (muscle) 8–0 coated Vicryl; L, Baby orbit and scleral retractor; M, Paton see-through handle and blade (Storz E-3086); N, Castroviejo caliper (Storz E-2404); O, Teflon corneal base plug; P, Yellow perforating needle; Q, Weck-Cel sponges (Weck); R, Grieshaber baby scarifier knife (Grieshaber); S, Ziegler knife (Storz E-0153); T, Right and left Azar iris retractor, (L) Storz E-0773, (R) Storz E-0773; U, Rizzuti expressor and iris retractor (Storz E-0764); V, Double-ended spatula (Storz E-0474); W, 2-cc glass syringe with filter and 30-gauge ½-inch needle for fluid or air injection; X, Cataract straight probe.

The cornea is opened with a trephine, the size of which is determined by the diameter of the cornea, but the surgeon should usually leave 1 to 1.5 mm of clear cornea around the corneoscleral limbus. The trephine must be placed perpendicular to the surface and firmly rotated to produce a superficial groove. Topical fluorescein is placed in the groove to ensure that the button is properly centered. If it is centered, the corneal button is removed and stored in McCarey-Kaufman medium. This minimizes edema and swelling.

The iris-lens synechiae are released with a cyclodialysis spatula, and underwater diathermy is performed on the iris vessels. Intraoperative hemorrhage from the neovascular iris vessels may occur, obscuring visualization during surgery. Healon can be injected into the an-

terior chamber to deepen and maintain the depth of the chamber. Keyhole iridotomies are performed at 6 and 12 o'clock, and the lens is extracted with a cryoprobe (Fig. 19–8B, Color plate 14B). Alpha-chymotrypsin is not used. Tissue adherent to the lens should be separated. Often membranes will overlie the ciliary body, but blind dissection of these membranes under the iris is inadvisable. Traction on peripheral membranes can cause a tear in the retinal vessels, producing hemorrhage.

The retrolental membrane is then incised, dissected, and excised 360 degrees (Figs. 19–8C, 19–8D, and 19–8E; Color plates 14C, 14D, and 14E). These maneuvers are easier to perform through the open-sky technique than the closed-vitrectomy technique, because the exposure is better and bimanual manipulation is possible. Retrolental membranes in infants aged 7 months or less postpartum may have small vessels that will bleed should the membranes be pulled to a great extent; these vessels should be cauterized before excessive tension is placed on the membrane. This problem is not prevalent in older infants, whose membranes lack open vessels.

Vitreous remnants are removed from inside the funnel, and preretinal membranes are dissected. To minimize iatrogenic tears, the surgeon must pay particular attention to all vessels. It is preferable to let any hemorrhage stop spontaneously, because underwater diathermy can weaken the retina and produce tears (Fig. 19–9). It is important not to leave any blood on the retina or in the vitreous. Heparinized BSS Plus is used as the intraocular irrigating fluid to prevent fibrin clots. The viscosity of Healon is utilized to push back the retinal folds, visualize adhesions, and minimize tissue edema. The retina of a younger infant (7 months or less) is more

pliable than that of an older infant and so can sustain more expansion without breaking or tearing. To visualize the posterior pole for folds and membranes, the surgeon fills the eye with Healon, and a small round glass cover, made by Corning, is placed over the corneal opening.

After the intraocular portion is finished, it is important to check and cauterize any residual bleeding vessels, because blood acts as a chemoattractant for cell invasion into the vitreous. The iridotomies are then closed with 10–0 Prolene suture placed 1 mm from the pupillary border, ensuring an adequate pupillary aperture through which to view the fundus. Additional Healon is placed in the anterior chamber to prevent the development of irido-corneal synechiae. The corneal button is then resewn with interrupted or running 10–0 nylon sutures. Wound leakage would be disastrous, so the sutures should be tight. At the end of the procedure, 0.2 ml of 4 mg per cubic centimeter of dexamethasone are

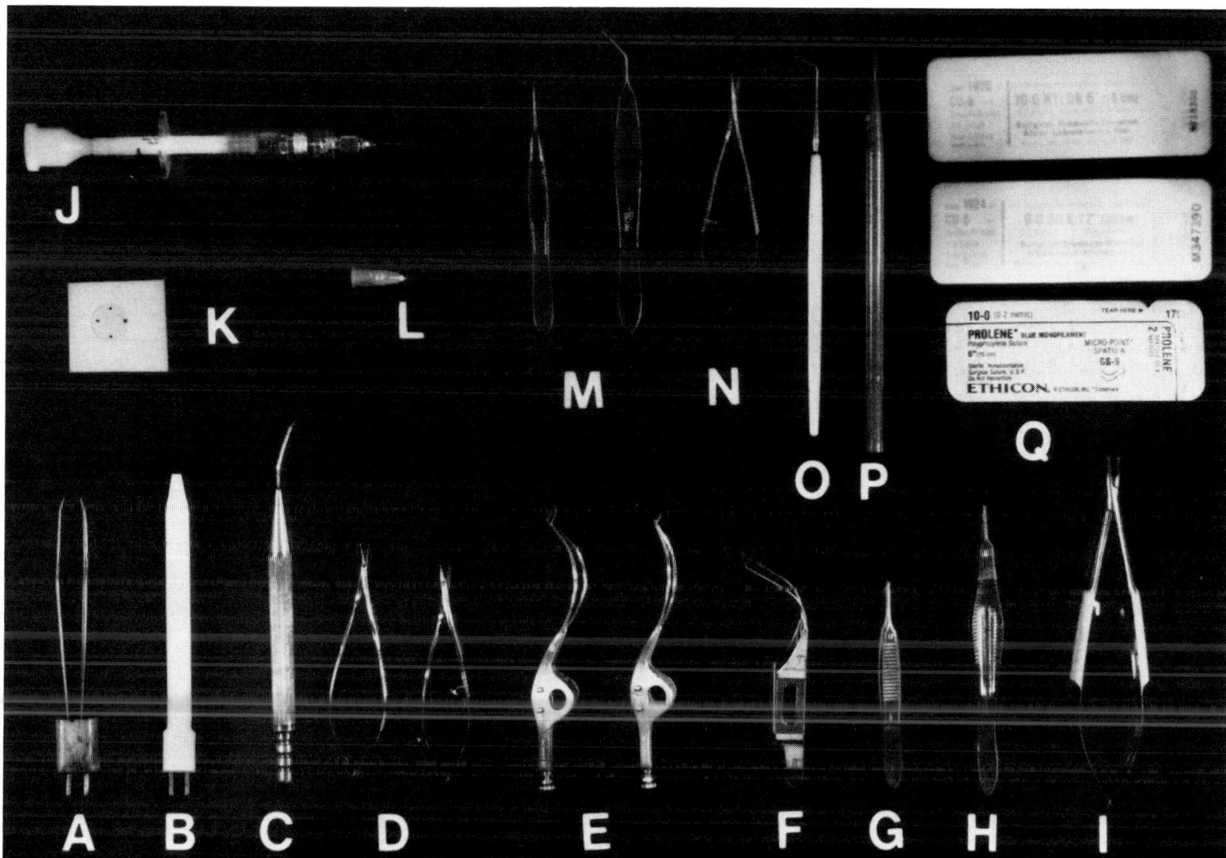

Figure 19–7   Instrument tray. A, Wetfield forceps (Mentor 22-1204); B, Wetfield hemostatic erasor, 20 gauge (Mentor 22-1260); C, Special irrigating dissector-spatula (AR McPherson Special); D, Vannas scissors; E, Open scissor (Grieshaber 614-10 and 614-20); F, Forceps (Grieshaber 615-20); G, 0.12 mm Bonn forceps (Weck 3100); H, 0.12 mm Castroviejo forceps (Weck 3441); I, Barraquer needle holder (Weck 4170); J, Healon with zolyse needle tip; K, Glass cover slip; L, Ashey needle; M, McPherson typing forceps (Weck 3548); N, Gaskin fragment forceps (Weck 3542); O, Cyclodialysis spatula (Storz); P, Superblade; Q, Sutures (1) 10–0 Prolene (Ethicon), (1) 9–0 silk (Alcon), (1) 10–0 nylon (Alcon).

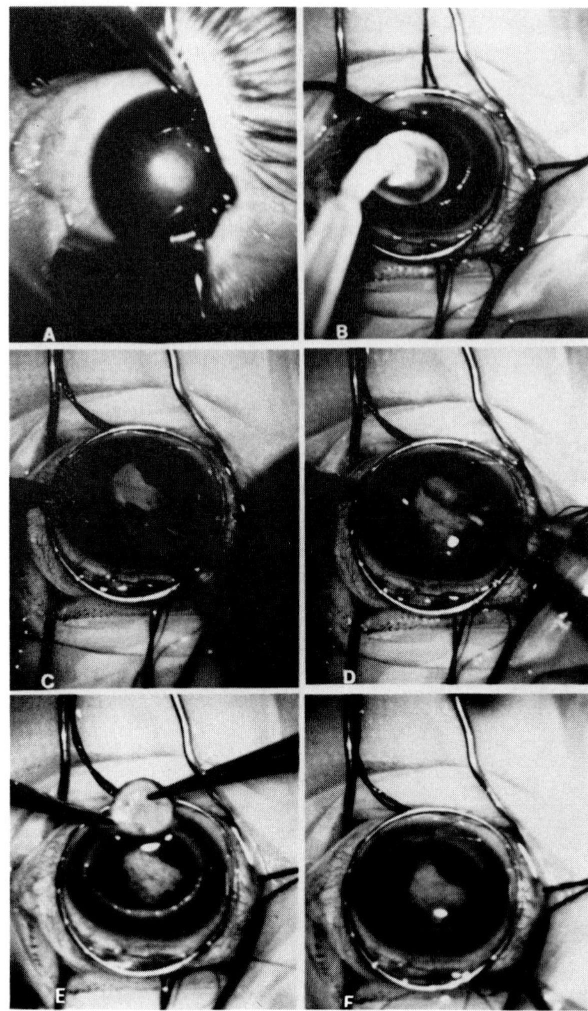

Figure 19–8 Summary of open-sky vitrectomy surgical technique. A External view of eye with closed-funnel retinal detachment; B The lens is extracted with a cryoprobe after iridotomies have been performed. Alpha-chymotrypsin is not used; C Incision of retrolental membrane; D Dissection of retrolental membrane; E 360-degree excision of retrolental membrane; F Detached retina seen through the pupil that has been opened by iridotomies. (Color plate 14)

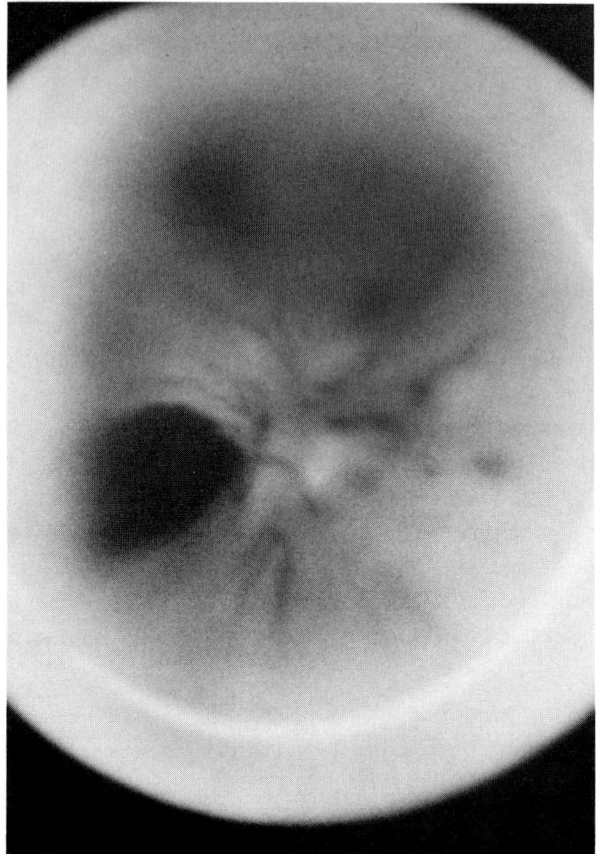

Figure 19–9 Fundus photograph showing an iatrogenic tear. This can be produced when underwater diathermy is utilized to control intraoperative hemorrhage.

injected into the anterior chamber. If additional Healon is needed, it is injected into the anterior chamber, and the intraocular pressure is checked.

One week after open-sky vitrectomy, the child is sedated for a postoperative examination. The cornea is checked to make sure sutures are intact. Any ruptured or loose sutures are repaired, since sutures rubbing against the cornea can produce corneal erosion. This can be treated with topical antibiotics and bandage lenses. The intraocular pressure is evaluated, since glaucoma can occur (Fig. 19–10), which can be managed with oral Diamox (acetazolamide) in a dosage of 5 mg per kilogram per day in three divided doses. Lowered intraocular pressure may also occur, and phthisis bulbi may ensue if membrane traction results in ciliary body

detachment. The anterior segment is scrutinized and large fundus drawings are made.

Usually, the infant is returned to the operating room at anywhere from several weeks up to three months for further evaluation, at which time additional membranes may be removed. The retina probably will not be com-

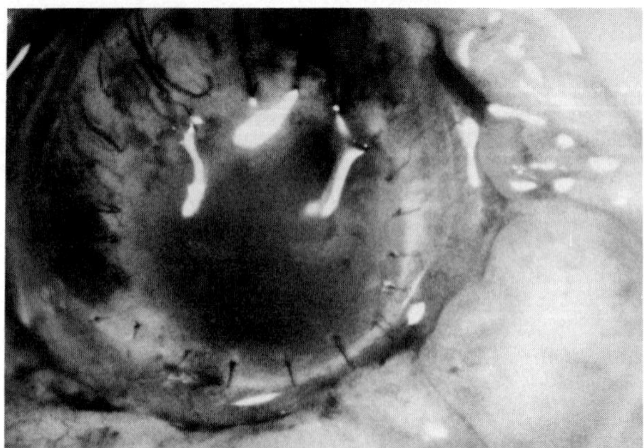

Figure 19–10 Photograph of the anterior segment showing ectatic thinning of the cornea when severe glaucoma occurs following open-sky vitrectomy.

pletely flat following the first open-sky procedure. Additional vitrectomy, Healon injections, and subretinal fluid drainage might be required to complete the process of flattening the retina.

RESULTS

The data base consists of 47 eyes of 32 infants ranging from 560- to 1,400-grams birth weight. The average follow-up was 9.7 months. All eyes treated were Grade IV or V cicatricial RLF. Thirty-eight eyes had closed funnels, while 9 had partially open funnels (Table 19–1). Success is defined as the ability to open the funnel with or without anatomic reattachment of the retina, along with maintenance of a clear cornea. Twenty-one eyes required additional vitrectomy, scleral buckling, and/or Healon injection. Twelve eyes required donor corneas. Successful reattachment was achieved in 6 eyes (13%), and two additional eyes had low residual detachments. Of the nine eyes with partially open funnels, two wwere anatomically reattached (22%; Figs. 19–11, 19–12, and 19–13; Color plate 15), and one additional eye had low residual detachment. Of the 38 eyes presenting with closed funnels, four were anatomically reattached (11%; Figs. 19–14, 19–15, and 19–16; Color plate 16) and one additional eye had low residual detachment. Two of the 47 eyes were anatomically attached and are able to fix and follow.

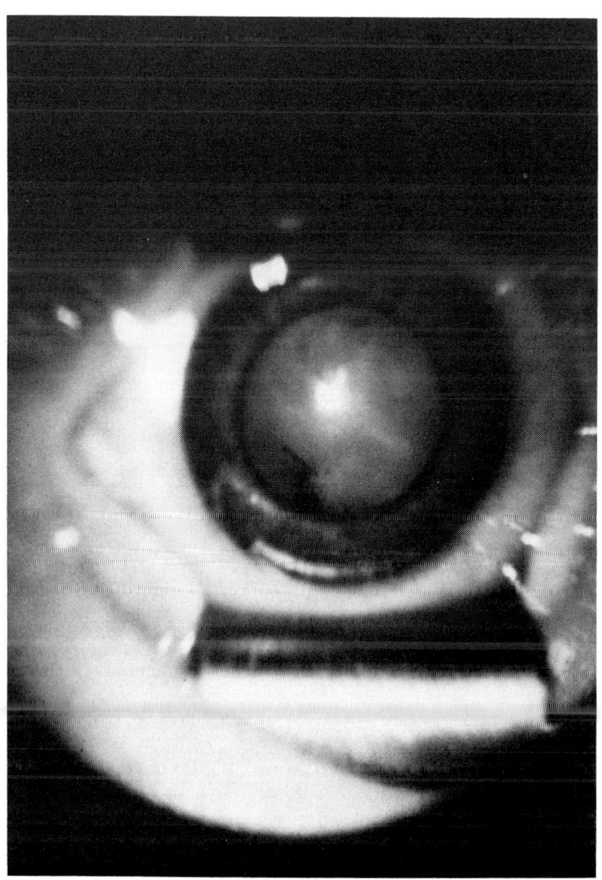

Figure 19–11 Preoperative appearance of retrolental membrane of patient 21, case 33 (Table 19–1). This infant weighed 860 grams at birth and developed a partially open funnel retinal detachment. Open-sky vitrectomy was performed at 5-months postnatal age. (Color plate 15A)

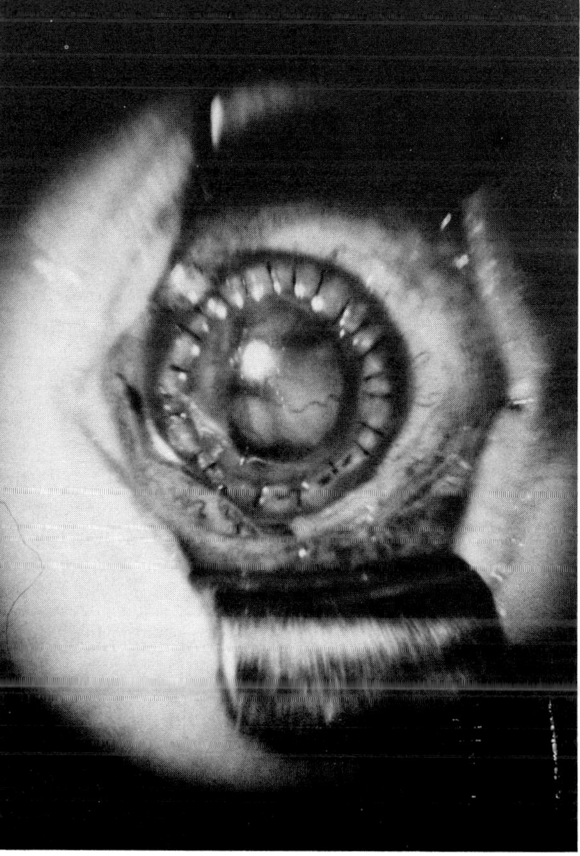

Figure 19–12 Postoperative appearance of anterior segment of patient 21, case 33 (Table 19–1). Through the clear cornea, the detached retina can be seen as anticipated following the first open-sky vitrectomy procedure. (Color plate 15B)

TABLE 19–1 Open-sky Vitrectomy Patients

Patient Number	Case Number	Birth Weight (g)	Previous Surgery	Postnatal Age at Surgery (mos)	Condition of Funnel	Number of Procedures	Additional Procedures	Donor Cornea	Success/Failure		Visual Acuity	Follow-up (mos)	Figures
									Open Funnel	Reattached			
1	1*	560		6	part open	1			S	F	UN	4	
	2*		bkl. rev ×1	6	closed	1			S	F	UN	4	
2	3*	600	cryo × 2 bkl rev × 2	11	closed	1			S	F	UN	14	
3	4*	610	cryo × 1 bkl rev × 2	7.5	part open	1			S	F*	UN	7	
4	5**	645		9.5	closed	1		X	F	F	NLP	7.5	
	6*			9	closed	2	Healon		F	F	NLP	7	
5	7*	680		12	closed	1			S	F	UN	14	
	8*			12	closed	1	Healon		S	F	UN	14	
6	9	700		11.5	closed	1	closed vit		S	S	UN	16	19–14,15,16
	10**			12.5	closed	2			F	F	UN	14	
7	11*	700		9.5	closed	2		X	F	F	UN	15	
8	12	700		6	closed	2			F	F	LP	14	
	13*			6.5	part open	1	Healon		S	F	LP	14	
9	14	710	cryo bkl	16.5	closed	1			F	F	LP	10	
	15*			12	closed	1		X	S	F	LP	13	
10	16*	720		14.5	closed	1			S	F	UN	3	
	17*			14	closed	1			S	F	UN	3	
11	18*	750	cryo ×2	7	closed	1	Healon	X	F	F	UN	3	
12	19*	750		9.5	closed	1			F	F	LP	14	
	20*			9.5	closed	1			F	F	LP	14	
13	21	780		7	closed	2		X	F	F	UN	11	
	22			8	closed	2	closed vit		S	F	LP	11	
14	23	800	cryo × 3 bkl rev × 2 drain Healon	6.5	part open	1	bkl		S	S	UN	6	
15	24	800	cryo × 2	12	closed	1		X	S	S	LP	11	
16	25*	820		24	closed	1	Healon		S	F	UN	7	
	26*			24	closed	1	Healon ×2		S	F	UN	7	

17	27*	820	ant vit	9.5	closed	2		X	S	F	UN	3	
18	28	840		7	part open	1	Healon, drain		S	F	UN	9	
	29*			6.5	closed	2		X	S	F	UN	9.5	
19	30	840	ant vit	17.5	closed	1			S	F	UN	12	
20	31*	840		13.5	closed	2		X	S	F*	UN	13	
21	32*	850	bkl	6	part open	1			S	F	UN	9	
	33*			5	part open	1			S	S	F+F	10	19—11,12,13
22	34*	900		4.5	part open	2	closed vit w/ Healon	X	F	F	LP	15	
	35**			5	closed	2	closed vit, Healon ×2	X	F	F	LP	14	
23	36	900	bkl, rev ×1	19	closed	1	closed vit, Healon		S	F	UN	17	
24	37*	910		11.5	closed	1			F	F	NLP	15	
25	38*	950		78	closed	1	iridectomy		S	F	UN	3	
	39*			78	closed	1	iridectomy		S	F	UN	3	
26	40*	950	cryo ×4	8	closed	1			S	S	F+F	13	
	41*		cryo ×3, ×1	7.5	closed	1			S	F	LP	17	
27	42*	1,010		8	closed	1			S	F	UN	4	
28	43*	1,040	bkl	16	part open	1			S	F	LP	11	
29	44	1,090	cryo ×1 bkl rev ×1	22	closed	1			S	F	UN	2	
30	45*	1,230	bkl rev ×2	69	closed	1		X	S	S	UN	6	
31	46	1,300		47	closed	1			S	F	UN	9	
32	47	1,400	bkl rev ×1 cryo	6	closed	1	Healon		S	F	UN	2	

F* = almost flat
  * = ultrastructural analysis of retrolental membrane ×1
 ** = ultrastructural analysis of retrolental membrane ×2

bkl = scleral buckle
rev bkl = revision of scleral buckle
part open = partially open

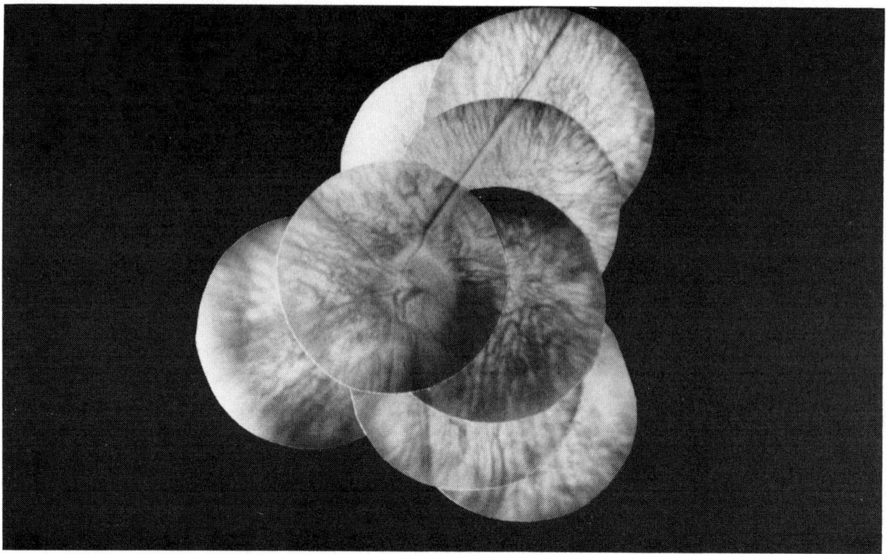

Figure 19–13 Postoperative appearance of attached retina of patient 21, case 33 (Table 19–1). This demonstrates a successful anatomical reattachment from a partially open-funnel retinal detachment. Visual acuity, 10 months postoperatively, is fixation and following. (Color plate 15C)

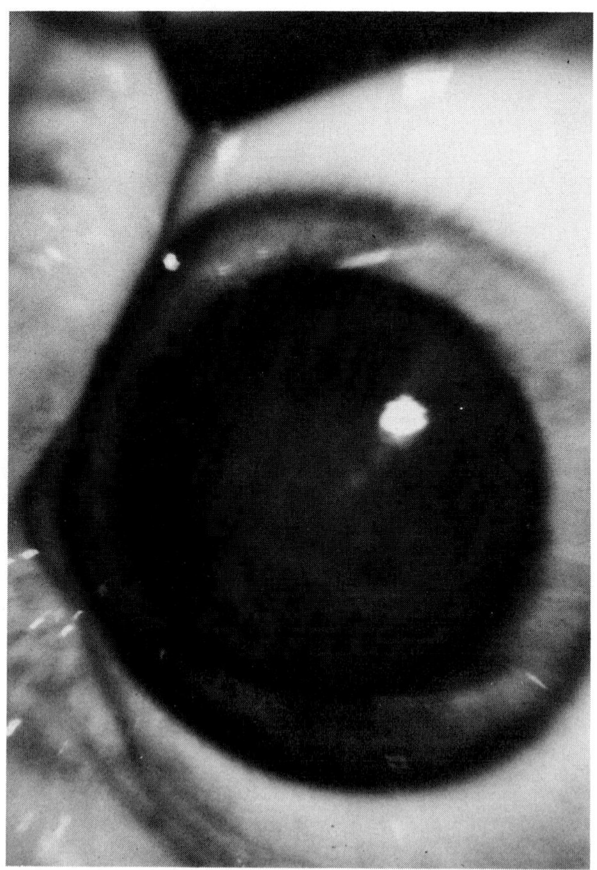

Figure 19–14 Preoperative appearance of retrolental membrane of patient 6, case 9 (Table 19–1). This infant weighed 700 grams at birth and developed a completely closed funnel retinal detachment. Open-sky vitrectomy was performed at 11.5-months postnatal age. (Color plate 16A)

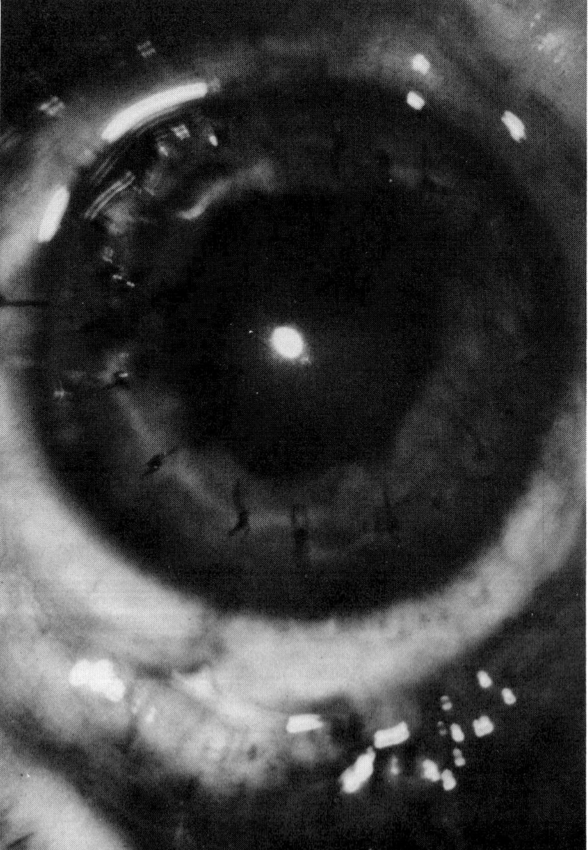

Figure 19–15 Postoperative appearance of anterior segment of patient 6, case 9 (Table 19–1). (Color plate 16B)

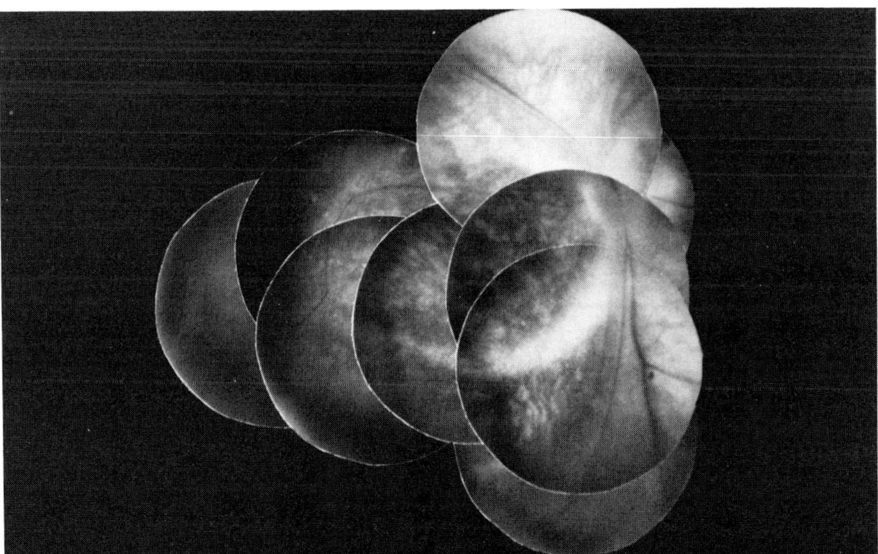

Figure 19–16   Postoperative appearance of attached retina of patient 6, case 9 (Table 19–1), which occurred following a closed vitrectomy. This demonstrates a successful anatomical reattachment from a completely closed-funnel retinal detachment. Visual acuity, 16-months postoperatively, is unknown. (Color plate 16C)

ULTRASTRUCTURAL INTERPRETATION OF OPEN-SKY VITRECTOMY

The natural history of the cellular (Figs. 19–17 to 19–19), fibrillary (Figs. 19–20 to 19–22), and vascular components of retrolental membranes have been studied through transmission and scanning electron microscopy. These membranes have been removed from open and closed funnels during open-sky vitrectomy that was performed between the postnatal ages of four months and six and a half years. The data base consists of 37 retrolental membranes from 33 eyes of 24 infants (Table 19–1). Ultrastructural analysis of all retrolental membranes was done without any knowledge of the clinical data. The membranes were fixed immediately in 2 percent glutaraldehyde and 2 percent paraformaldehyde in phosphate buffer.[10] The data are clustered into four groups, based on the cellular, fibrillary, and vascular changes as functions of postnatal age.

Group I

Ultrastructurally, from 4 to 5 months postnatal age (three retrolental membranes), the cellular components of these vascular, retrolental membranes are almost exclusively red blood cells and myofibroblasts arranged in sheets (Fig. 19–17A). Myofibroblasts are fusiform (Fig. 19–17B), have abundant, contractile, actin microfilaments streaming through the cytoplasm (Fig. 19–17C), and are the source of tractional retinal detachment.[11] The cells and vessels are interspersed in a honeycomb pattern of fibrillary material, as documented by scanning electron microscopy (Fig. 19–20).

Group I is, theoretically, the optimal time to perform open-sky vitrectomy, if cryotherapy obliterates the shunt to remove the anatomic site of continued myofibroblast invasion into the vitreous. The duration of retinal detachment correlates with the potential restoration of vision, since retinal neurons are postmitotic, nonregenerating cells that die when separated from their source of nutrition. These membranes still have patent vessels that may bleed during surgical dissection.

Group II

Ultrastructurally, during the sixth postnatal month (five retrolental membranes), the cellular components of the vascular, retrolental membranes are plasma cells (Fig. 19–18A), polymorphonuclear leukocytes (Fig. 19–18B), macrophages (Fig. 19–18C), and retinal pigment epithelium (Fig. 19–18D). With the invasion of these cells, myofibroblasts disappear from the vitreous. The ratio of these cell types varies; however, macrophages and retinal pigment epithelium are the dominant cells. In one infant (cases 32 and 33), the membrane removed at 5 months from the left eye was composed ex-

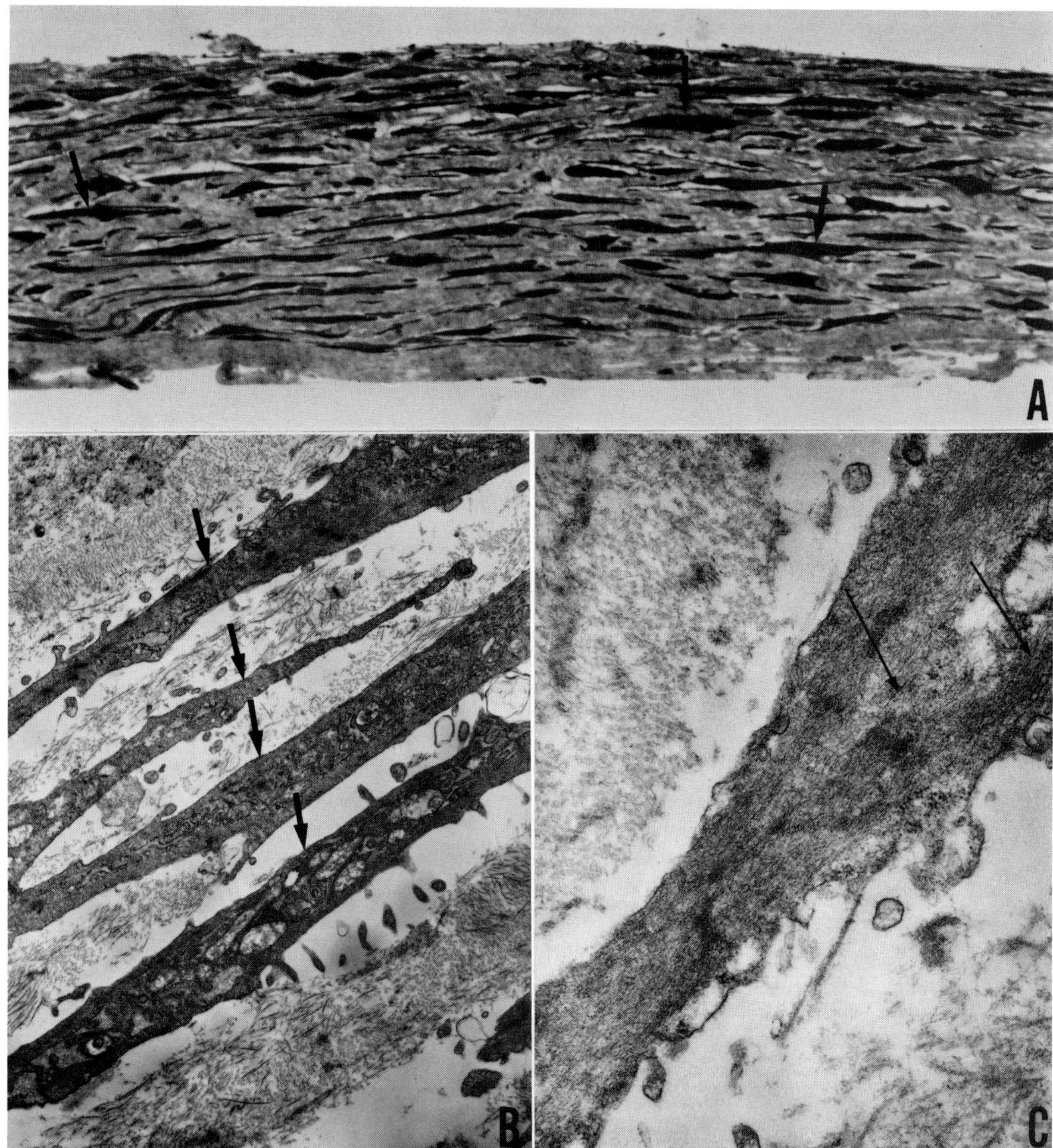

Figure 19–17   Light micrograph, A and transmission electron micrographs, B and C, demonstrating the myofibroblast vitreous invasion in Group I (4- to 5-months postnatal age). The myofibroblasts (➡) are arranged in sheets and fusiform in shape. The cytoplasm contains abundant contractile actin microfilaments (⟶). A = 470×. B = 8,700×. C = 26,000×.

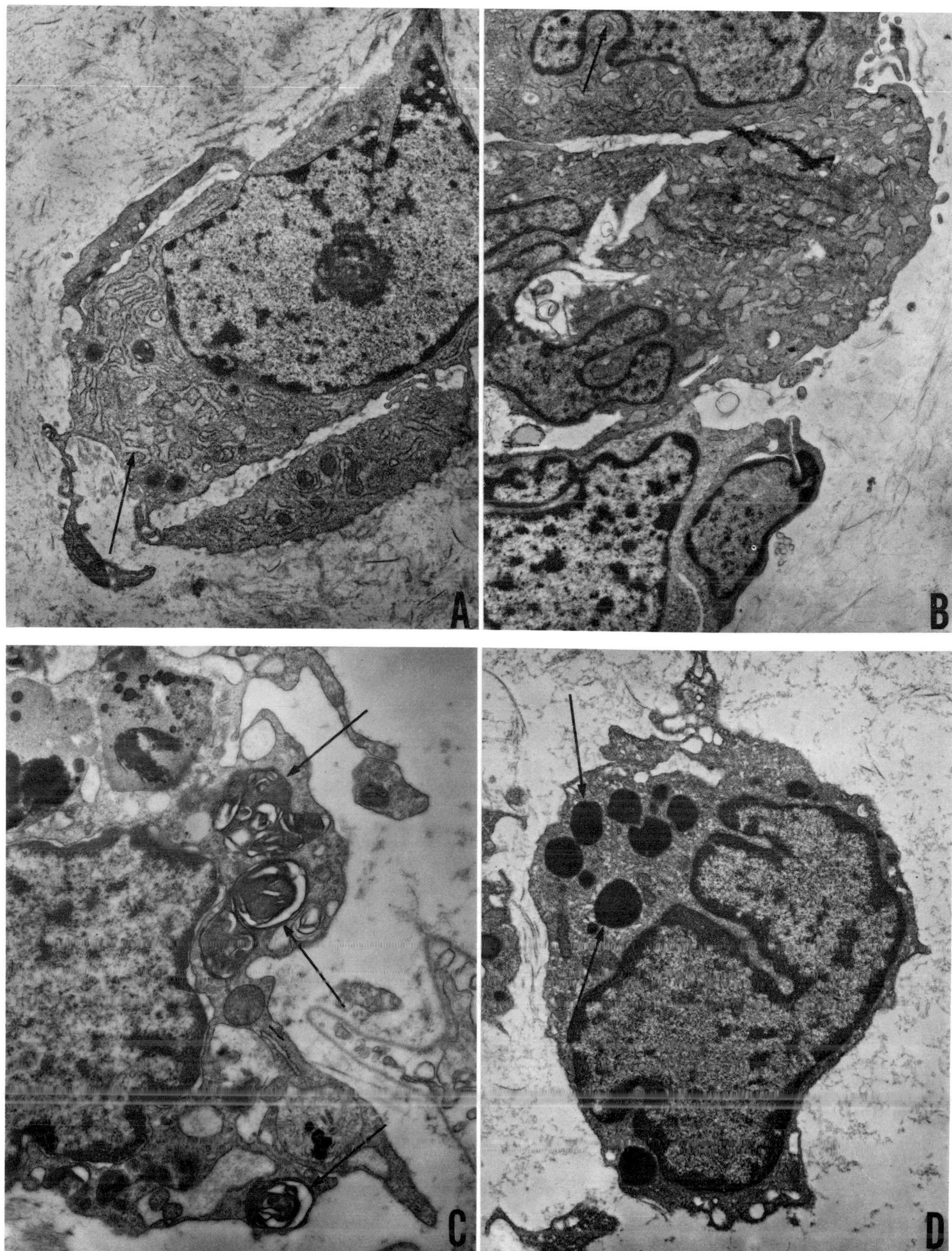

Figure 19–18 Transmission electron micrographs showing the four cellular components of the vascular retrolental membrane of Group II (6-months postnatal age). A Plasma cell with characteristic bloated rough endoplasmic reticulum (↗). B Polymorphonuclear leukocyte with characteristic multilobate nucleus (↗). C Macrophage with diagnostic phagosomes (↘). D Retinal pigment epithelium with diagnostic melanin granules (↘). A–D = 8,700×.

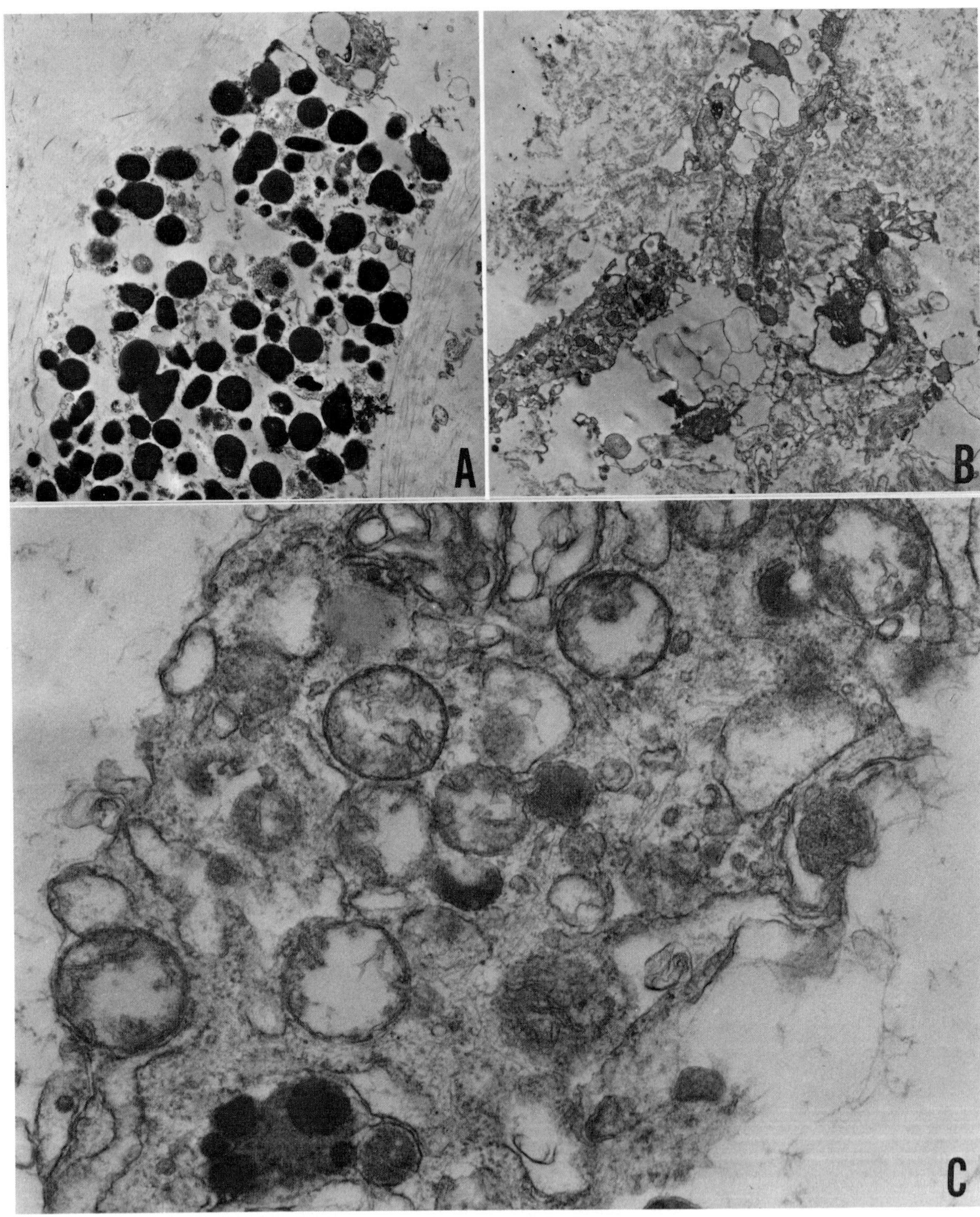

Figure 19–19 Transmission electron micrographs showing the components of cellular debris in the avascular retrolental membrane of Group III, (7- to 16-months postnatal age). A Free pigment. B Lysed cellular material. C Autolytic macrophages. These components indicate death of cells that invaded the vitreous during Group II. A = 6,900×. B = 5,400×. C = 34,000×.

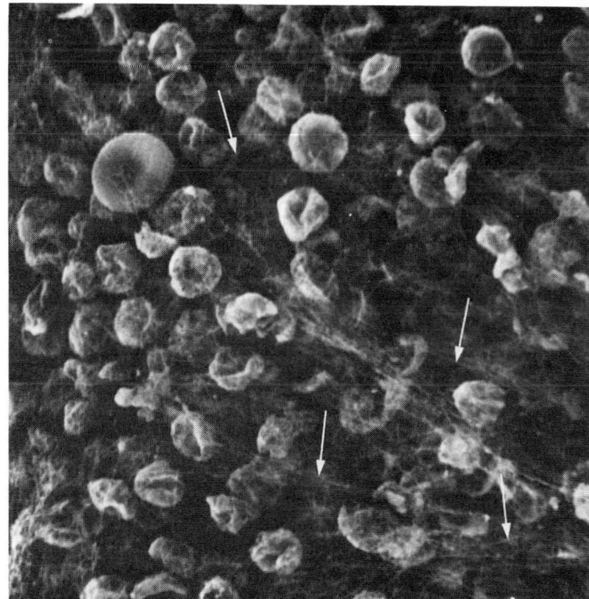

Figure 19–20 Scanning electron micrograph demonstrating the honeycomb pattern of fibrillary material (white arrow) of the vitreous in Groups I and II. Red blood cells are interspersed in the honeycomb pattern representing residual hemorrhage. 1,850×.

clusively of myofibroblasts, whereas the membrane removed at 6 months from the right eye was composed of macrophages, retinal pigment epithelium, plasma cells, polymorphonuclear leukocytes, and no myofibroblast sheets. In Group II, the cells are interspersed in a honeycomb pattern of fibrillary material, similar to that in Group I, as documented by scanning electron microscopy.

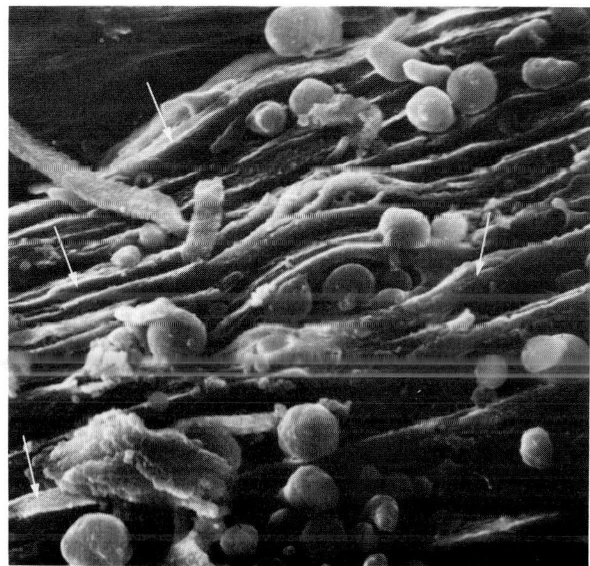

Figure 19–21 Scanning electron micrograph demonstrating the fibrillary material of the vitreous, which is condensed into sheets (white arrow) in Group III. Cell remnants are interspersed between the sheets. 690×.

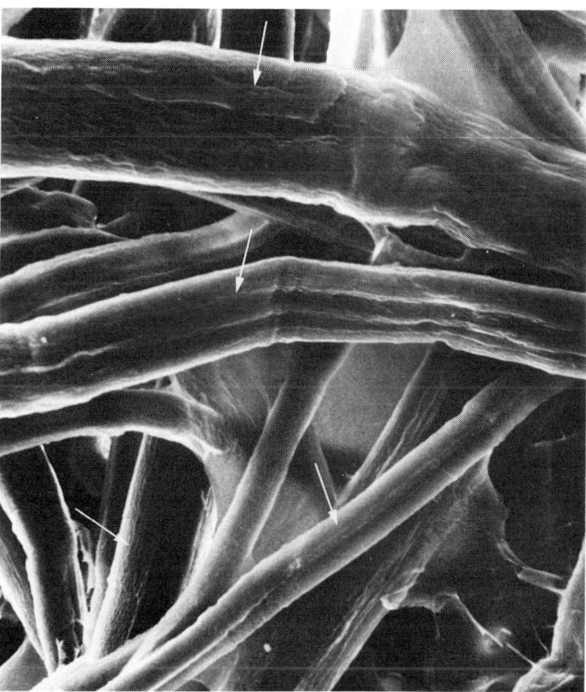

Figure 19–22 Scanning electron micrograph demonstrating the fibrillary material of the vitreous, which is condensed into cables (white arrow) in Group IV. No cellular or vascular components remain in this phase. 690×.

Clinically, Group II is still an appropriate time to anatomically open the funnel and press the pliable retina into apposition with the retinal pigment epithelium. Pliability probably correlates with the honeycomb pattern of the fibrillary material. These membranes still have patent vessels that can bleed during surgical dissection.

Group III

Ultrastructurally, from 7- to 16-months postnatal age (24 retrolental membranes), the cellular components of the retrolental membranes with ghost vessels become remnants of free pigment (Fig. 19–19A), lysed, cellular material (Fig. 19–19B), and autolytic macrophages (Fig. 19–19C). This indicates death of the cells that invaded the vitreous during Group II and that are not artifact because all samples were fixed immediately upon surgical removal and processed identically in a masked protocol. In one infant (case 35), the membrane removed at 5 months from the left eye was composed exclusively of myofibroblasts, while the membrane removed at 12½ months from the same eye and was composed of remnants of free pigment; lysed, cellular material and debris; and autolytic macrophages. In Group III, the cell remnants are interspersed between fibrillary material condensed into sheets, as documented by scanning electron microscopy (Fig. 19–21).

Clinically, in Group III the retina appears to be less pliable as it is maneuvered into apposition with the retinal pigment epithelium. This lack of pliability results from the condensation of the fibrillary material of the vitreous, and from extensive necrosis of the dead retinal neurons. These membranes do not bleed during surgical dissection, because the vessels are now ghosts.

Group IV

Ultrastructurally, between the second and sixth years of life (five retrolental membranes), the membranes are acellular and avascular. The fibrillary material is condensed into cables, as documented by scanning electron microscopy (Fig. 19–22).

Clinically, in Group IV the retina is difficult to maneuver into apposition with the retinal pigment epithelium, because it is extremely brittle owing to the cross meshwork of the firm vitreous cables, and owing to the extensive necrosis of the dead retinal neurons. These membranes do not bleed during surgical dissection, because the vessels have now atrophied.

REFERENCES

1. Tasman W. Vitreoretinal changes in cicatricial retrolental fibroplasia. Trans Am Ophthalmol Soc 1970; 68:548–564.
2. Tasman W. Late complications of retrolental fibroplasia. Ophthalmology 1979; 86:1724–1740.
3. Merritt JC, Lawson EE, Sprague DH, Eifrig DE. Lensectomy-vitrectomy for Stage 5 cicatricial retrolental fibroplasia. Ophthalmic Surg 1982; 13:300–306.
4. Lightfoot D, Irvine AR. Vitrectomy in infants and children with retinal detachments caused by cicatricial retrolental fibroplasia. Am J Ophthalmol 1982; 94:305–312.
5. Machemer R. Closed vitrectomy for severe retrolental fibroplasia in infants. Ophthalmology 1983; 90:436–441.
6. Trese MT. Surgical results of Stage V retrolental fibroplasia and timing of surgical repair. Ophthalmology 1984; 91:461–466.
7. Charles ST. Vitrectomy for retrolental fibroplasia. American Academy of Ophthalmology Annual Meeting, Atlanta, Georgia, November 12, 1984.
8. Schepens CL. Clinical and research aspects of subtotal open-sky vitrectomy. XXXVII Edward Jackson Memorial Lecture. Am J Ophthalmol 1981; 91:143–171.
9. Hirose T, Schepens CL. Open-sky vitrectomy in retrolental fibroplasia. American Academy of Ophthalmology Annual Meeting, Atlanta, Georgia, November 12, 1984.
10. Kretzer FL, Hittner HM, Mehta RS. Ocular manifestations of Smith-Lemli-Opitz syndrome. Arch Ophthalmol 1981; 99:2000–2006.
11. Soong HK, Eller AW, Hirose T, Hanninen L, Kenyon KR. In situ actin distribution in excised retrolental membranes in retinopathy of prematurity. Arch Ophthalmol 1985; 103:1553–1556.

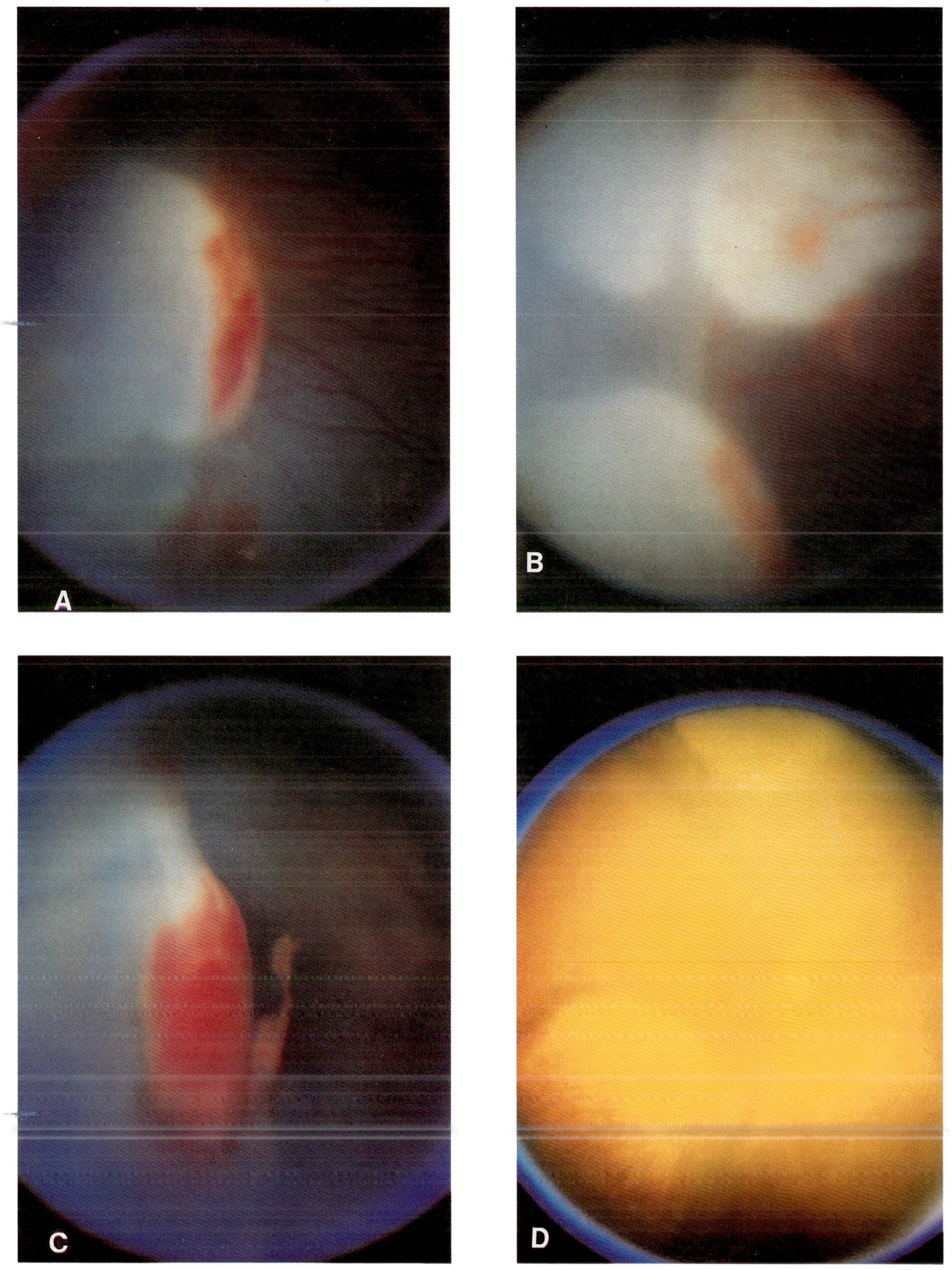

Color Plate 1

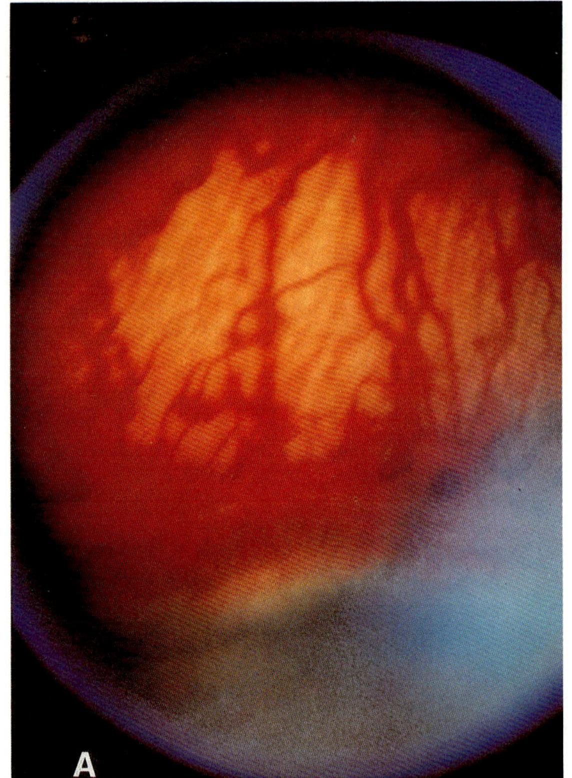

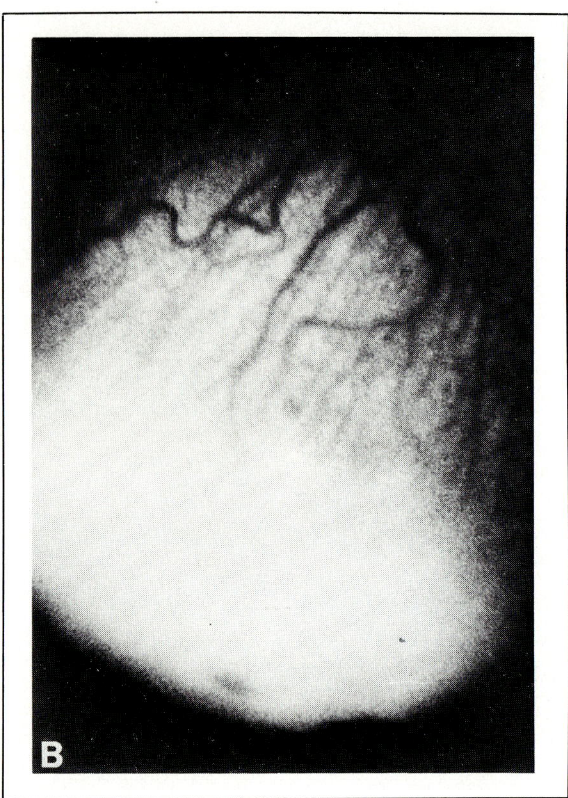

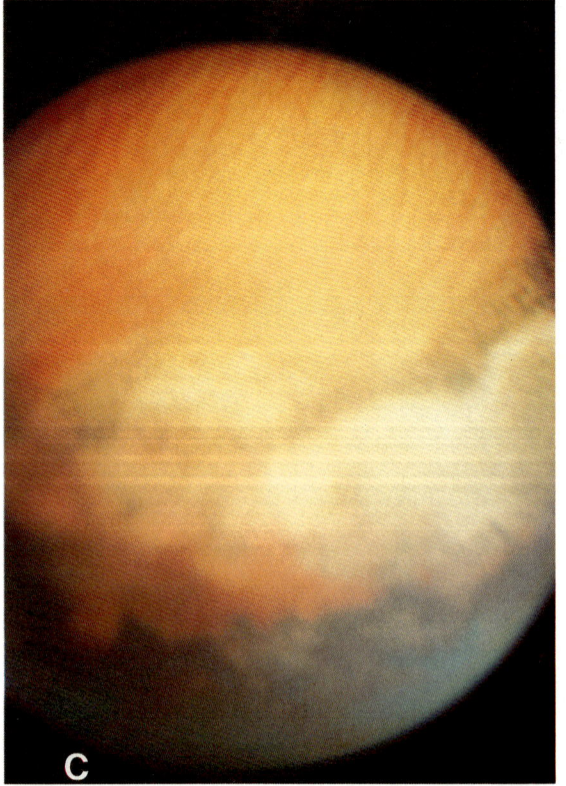

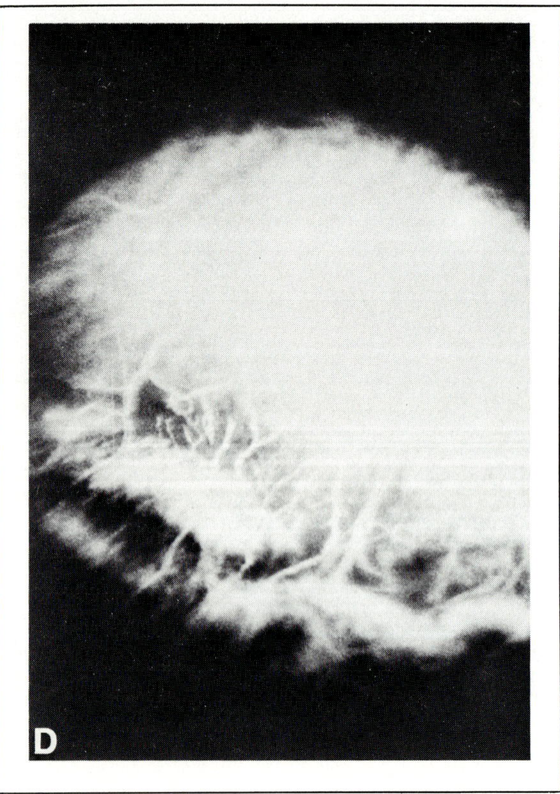

Color Plate 2

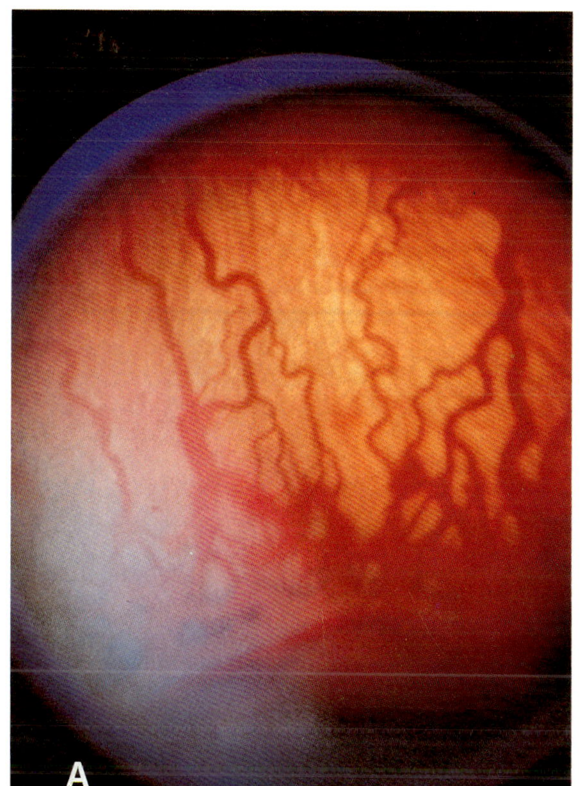

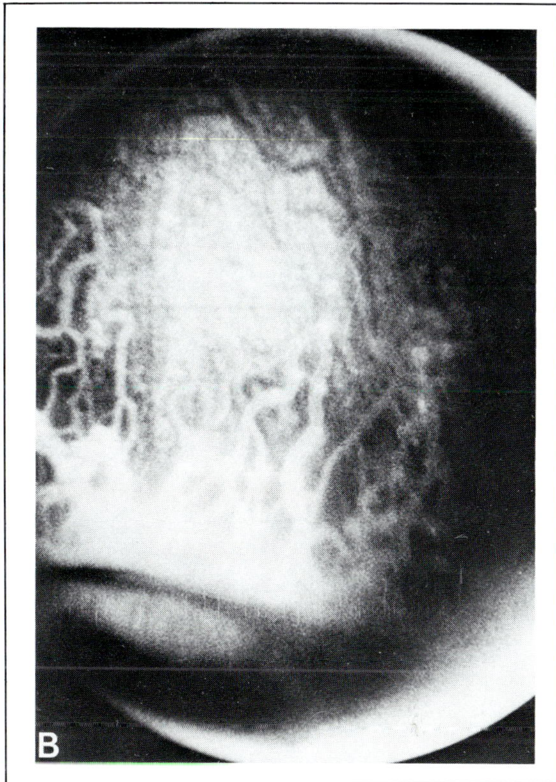

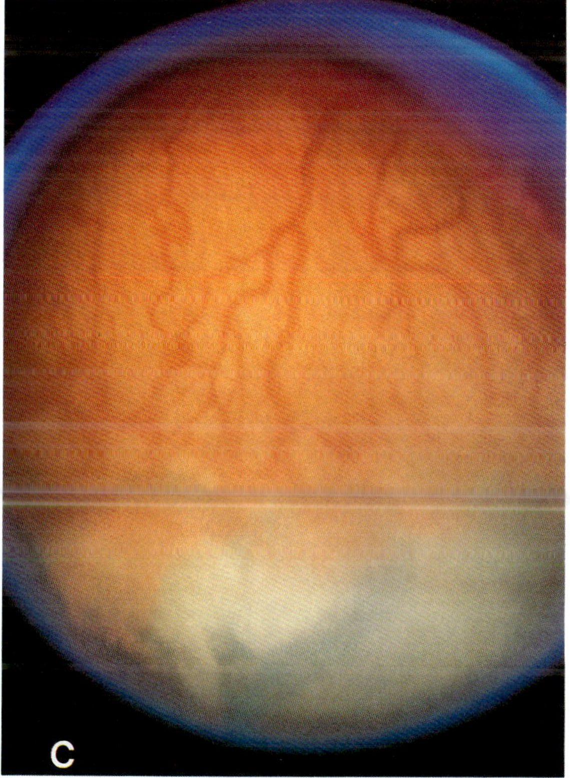

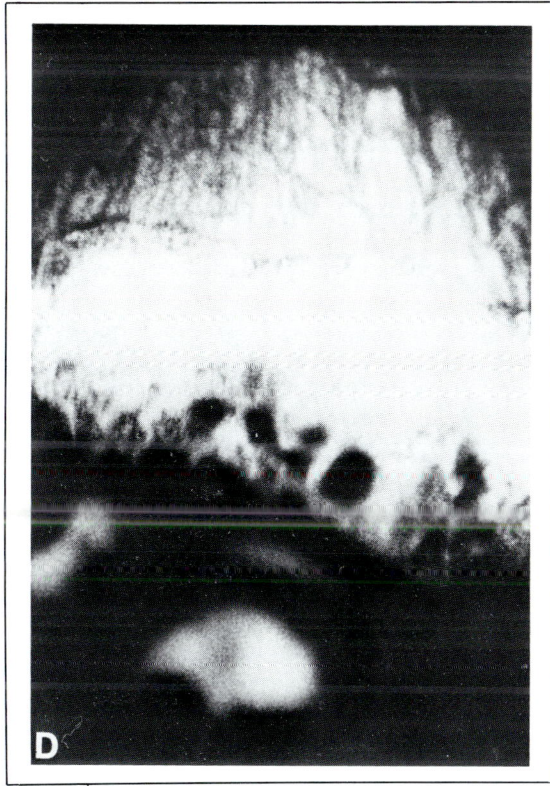

Color Plate 3

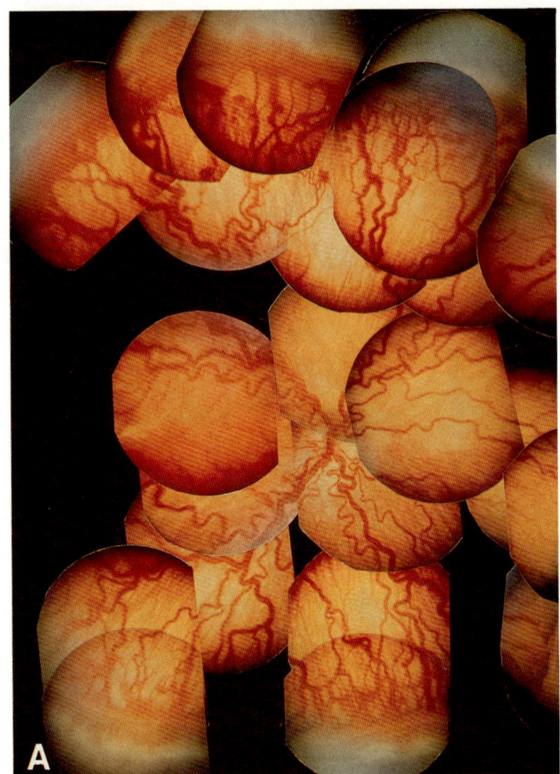
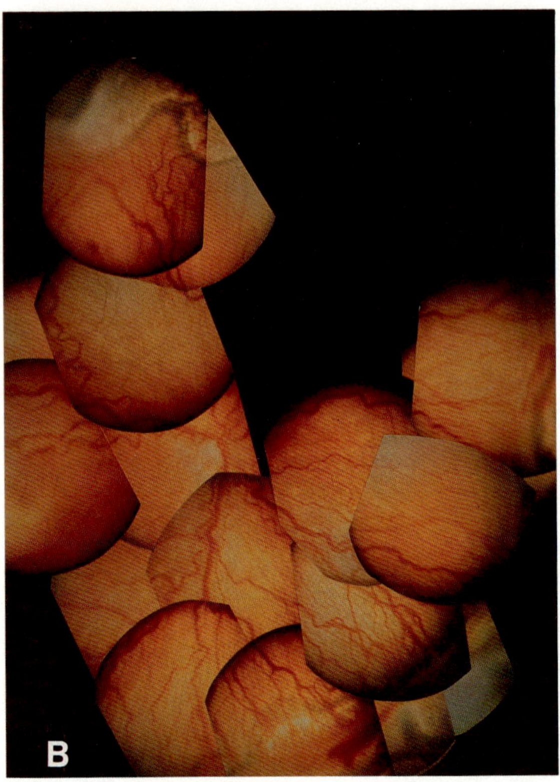
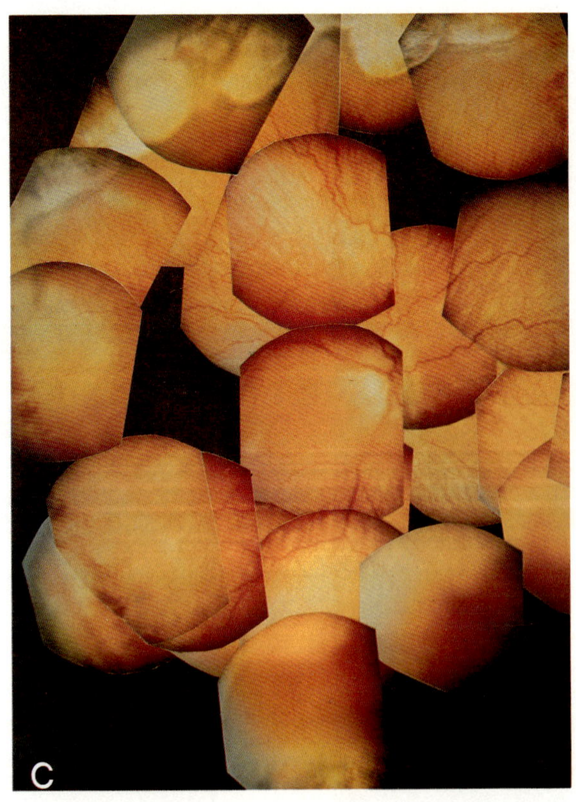

Color Plate 4

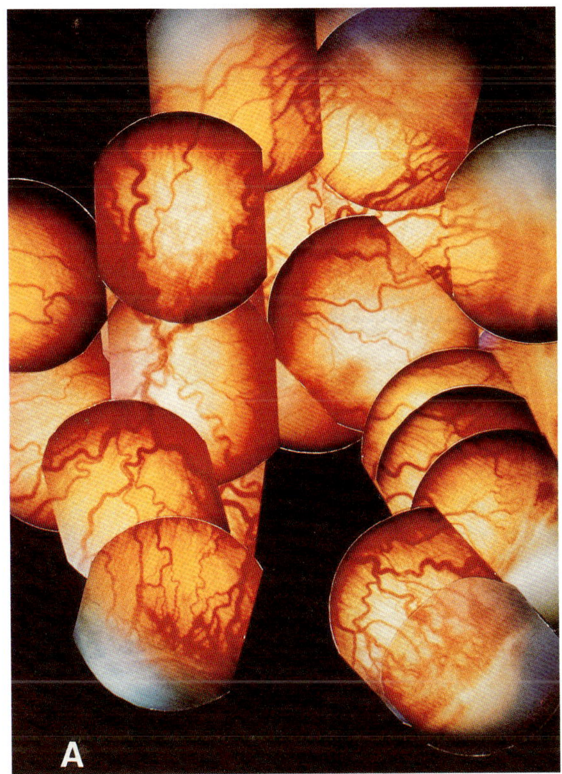

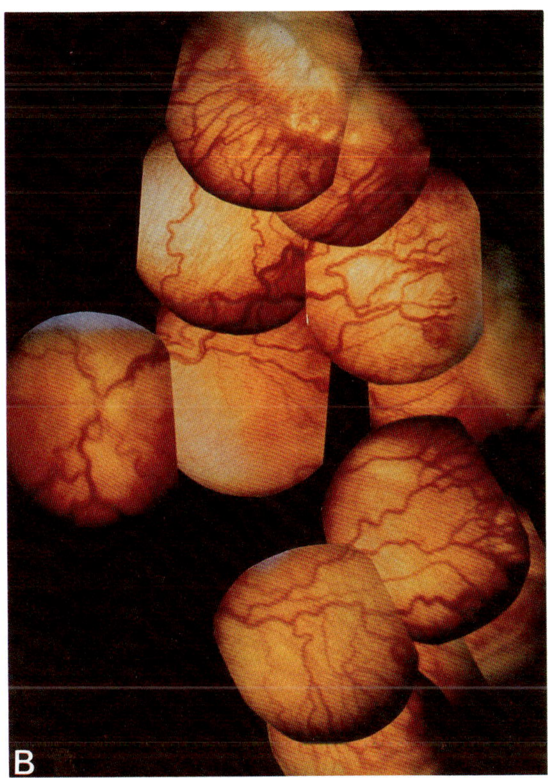

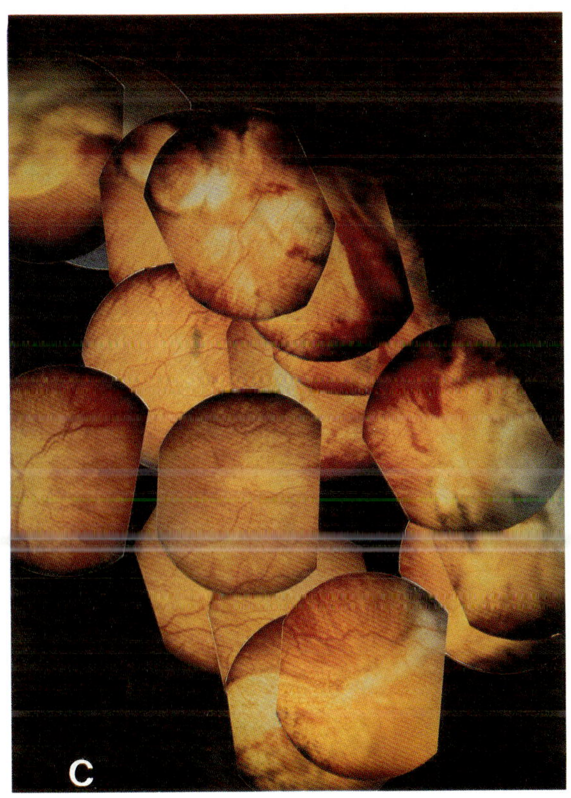

Color Plate 5

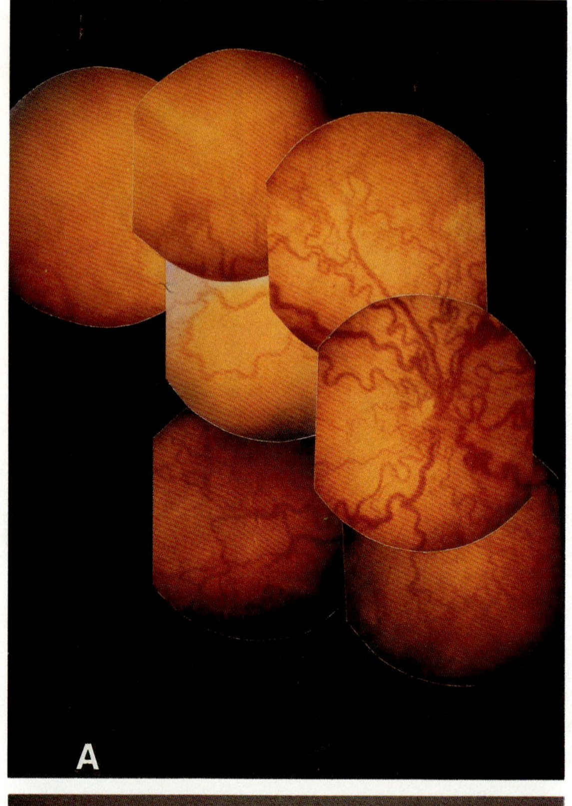

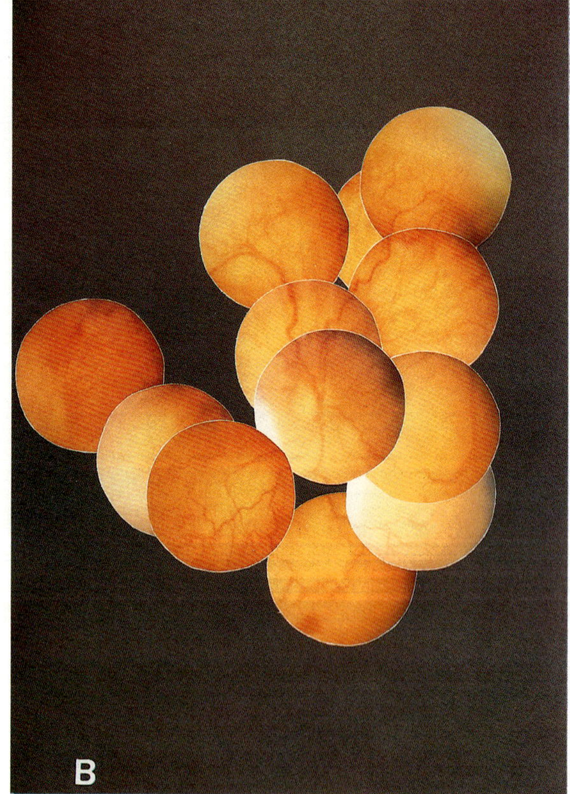

Color Plate 6

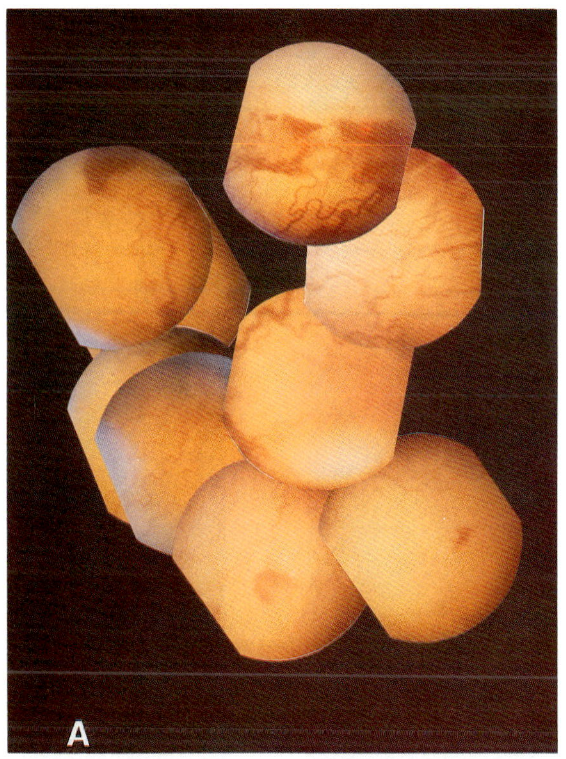

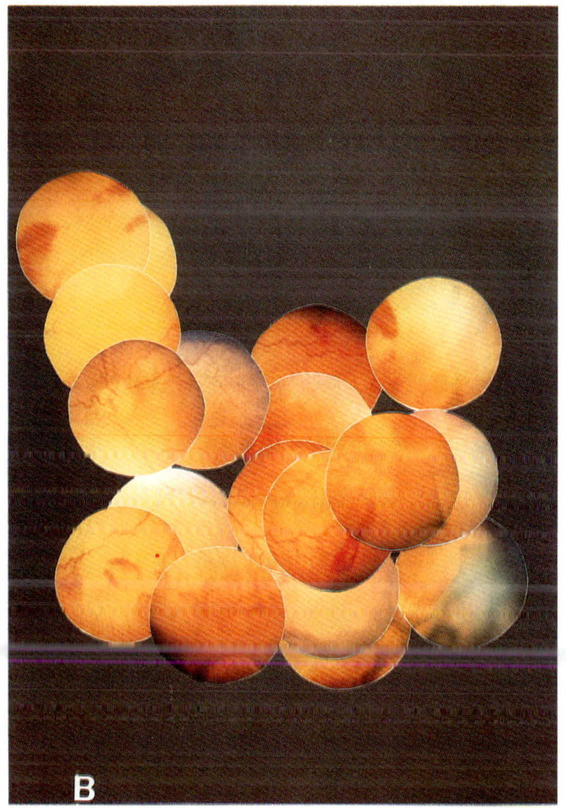

Color Plate 7

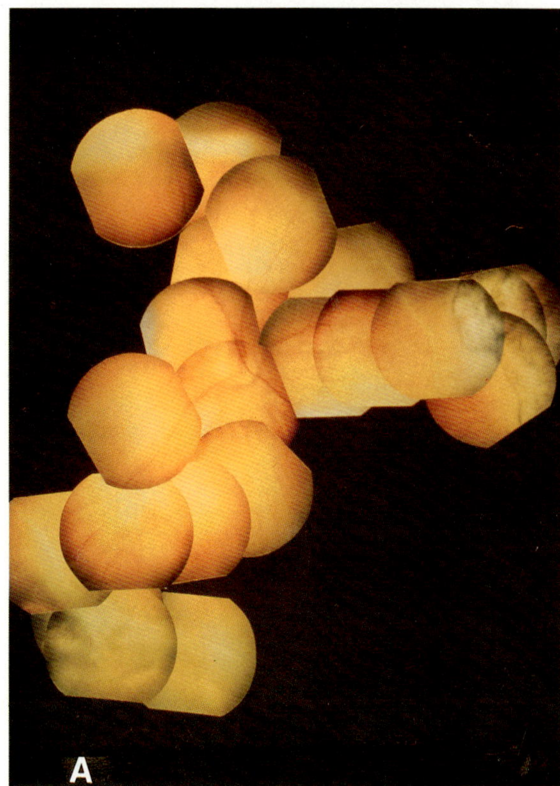

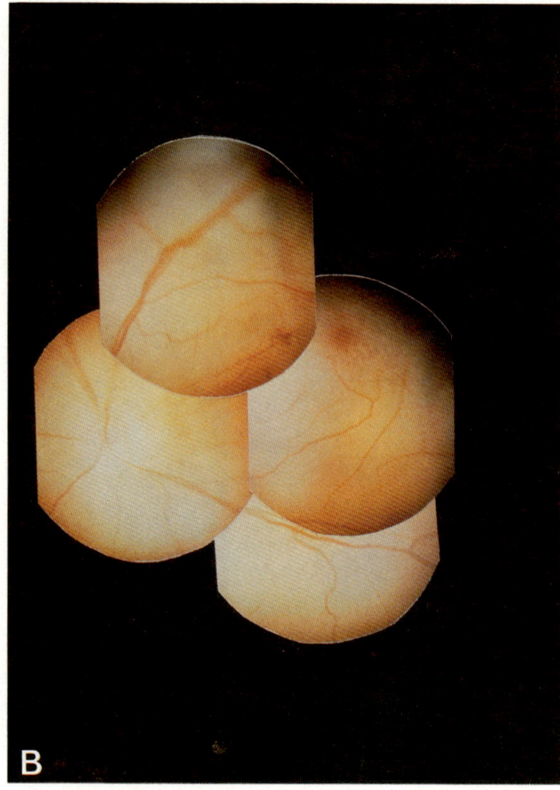

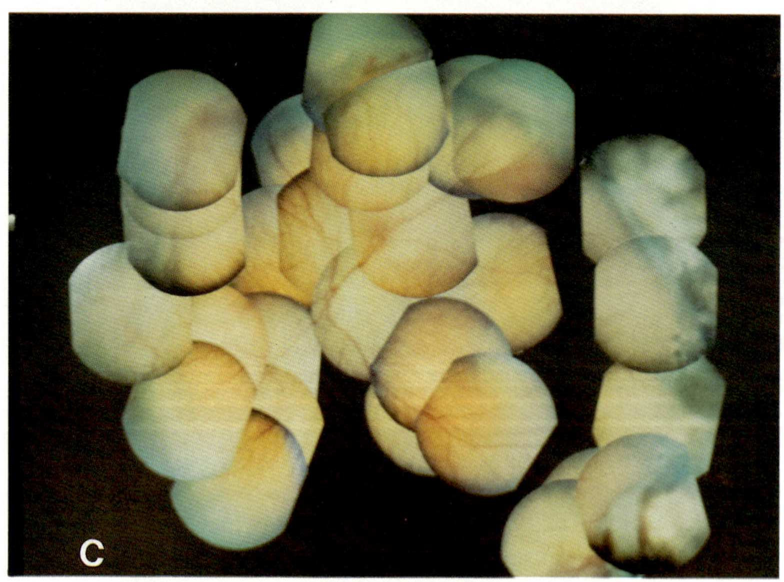

Color Plate 8

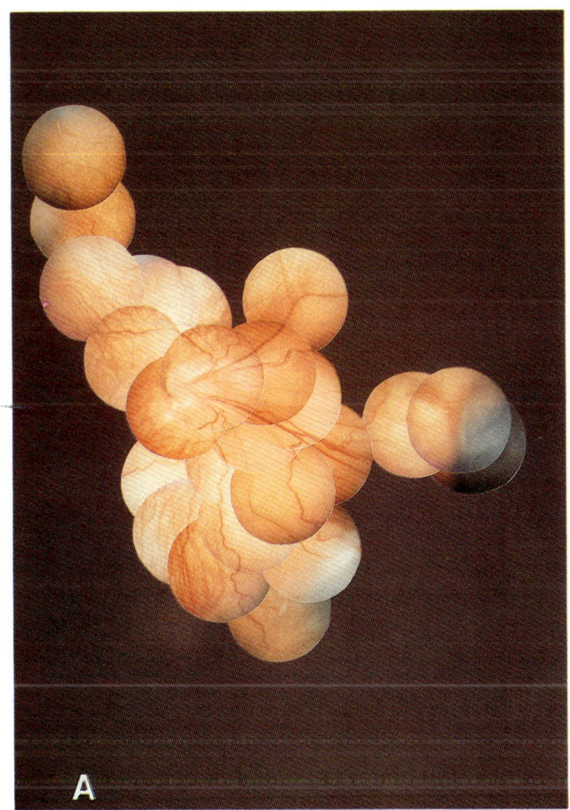
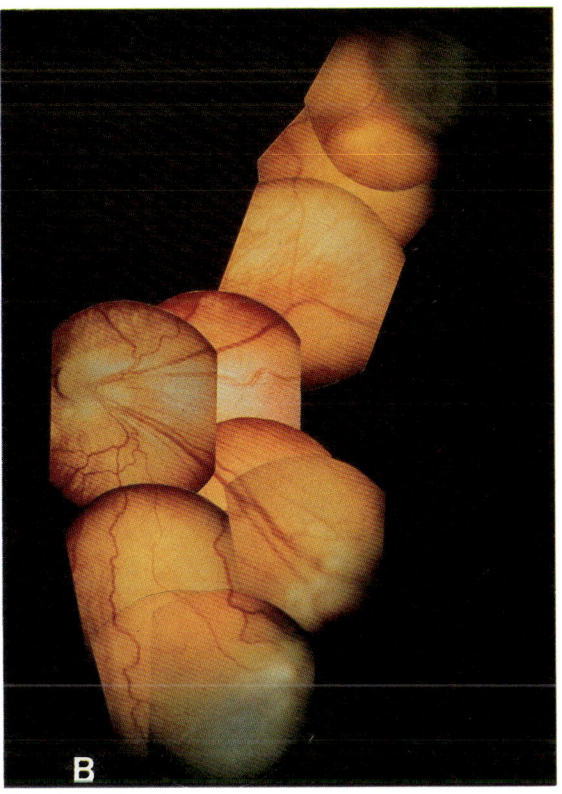
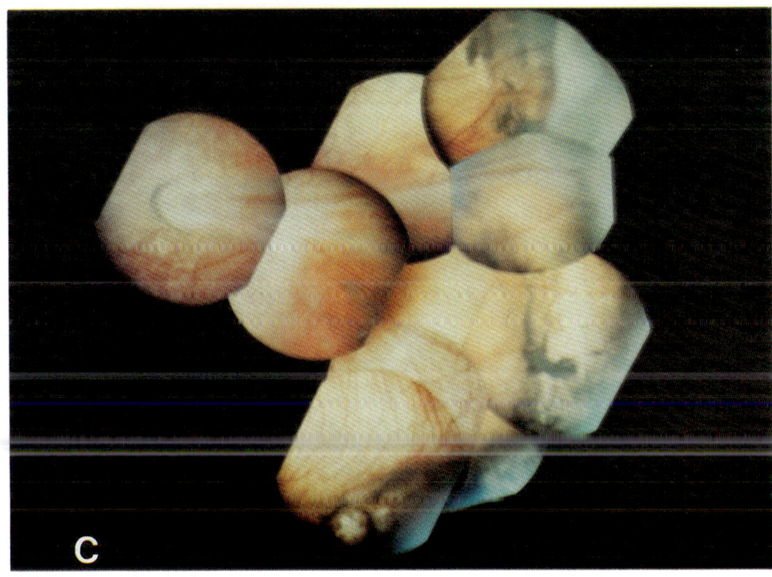

Color Plate 9

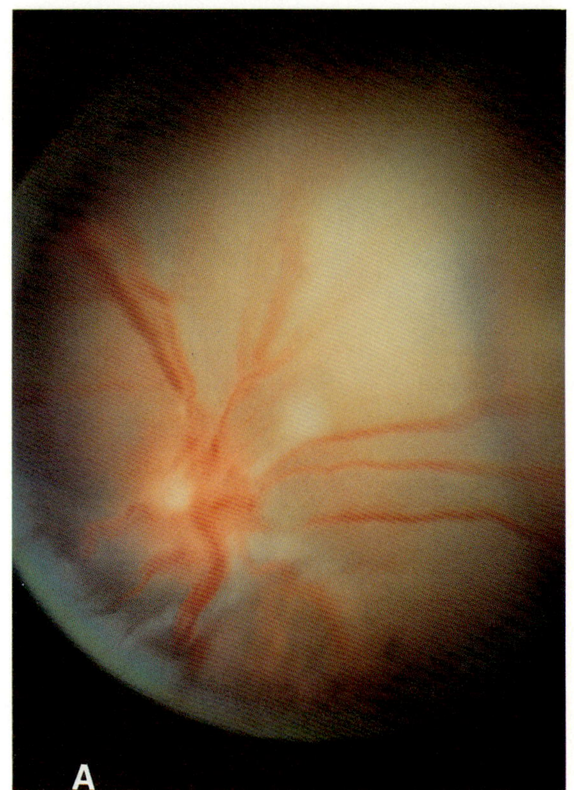

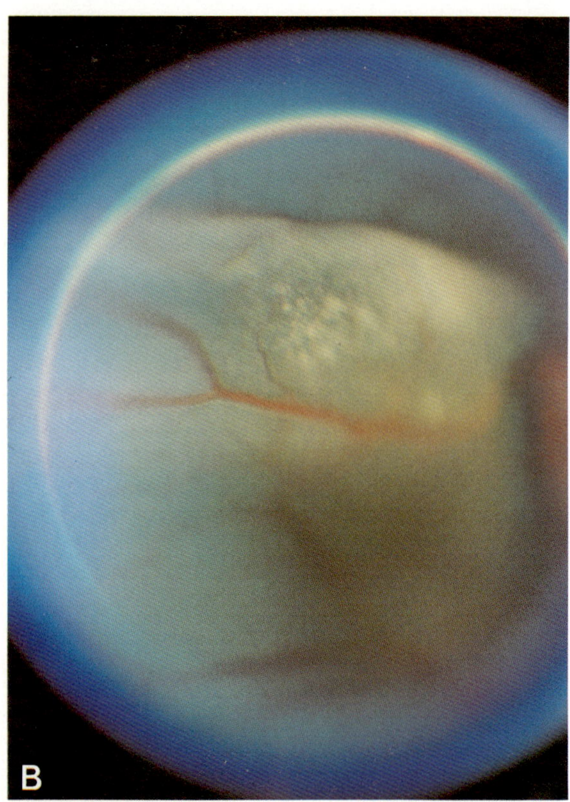

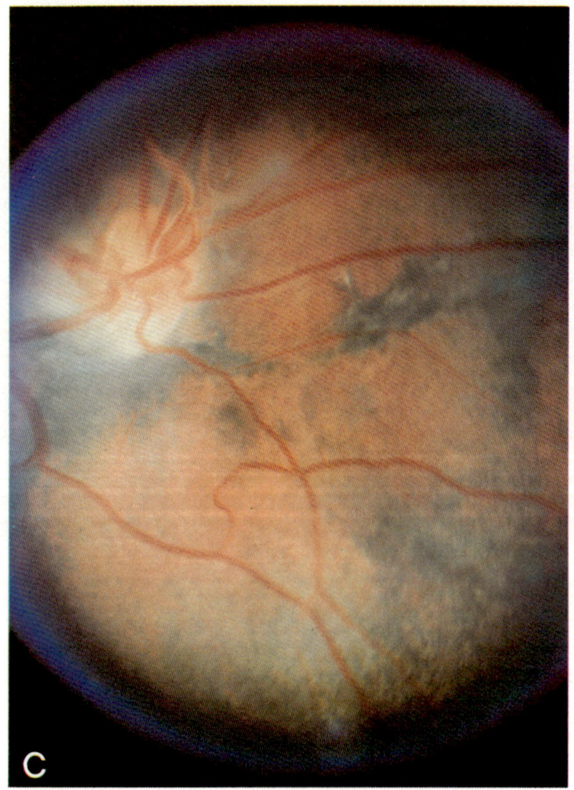

Color Plate 10

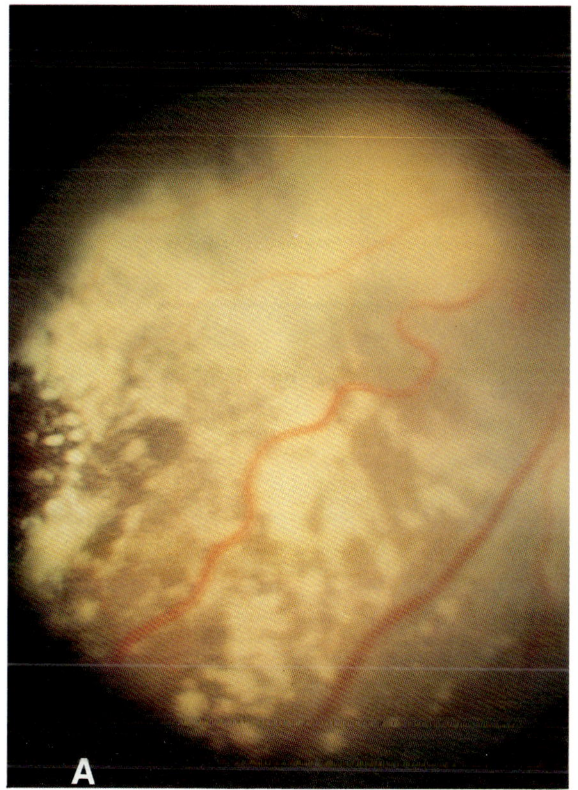

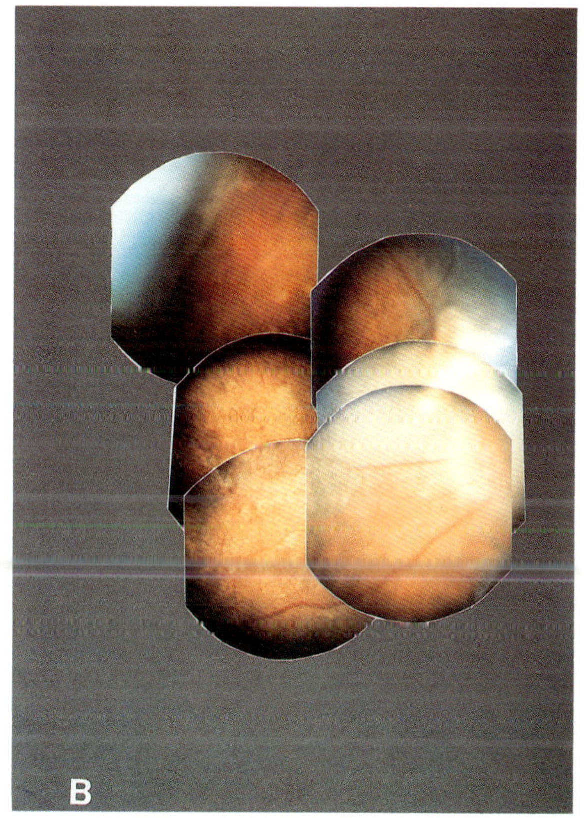

Color Plate 11

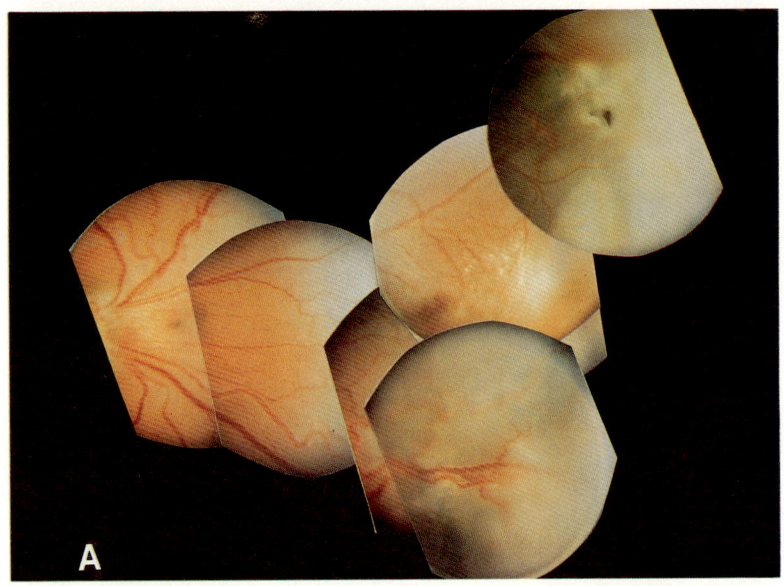

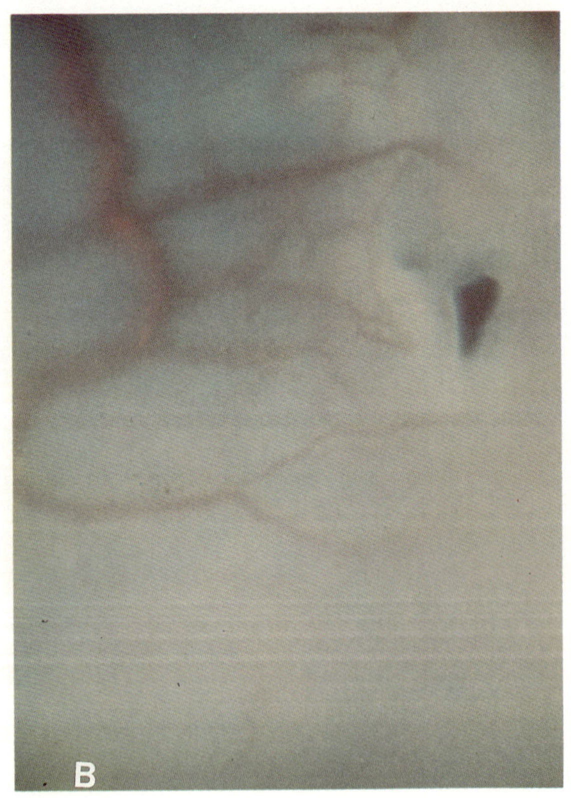

Color Plate 12

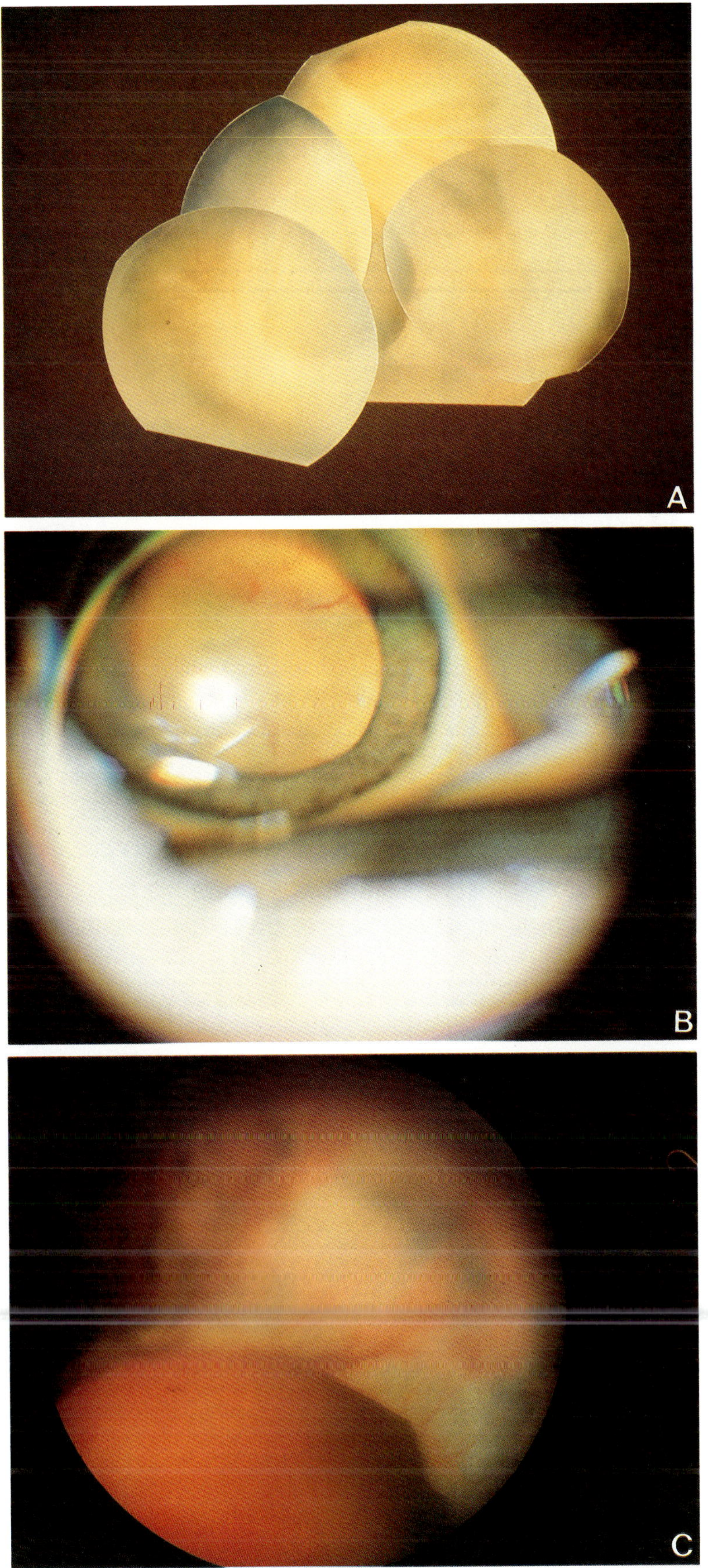

Color Plate 13

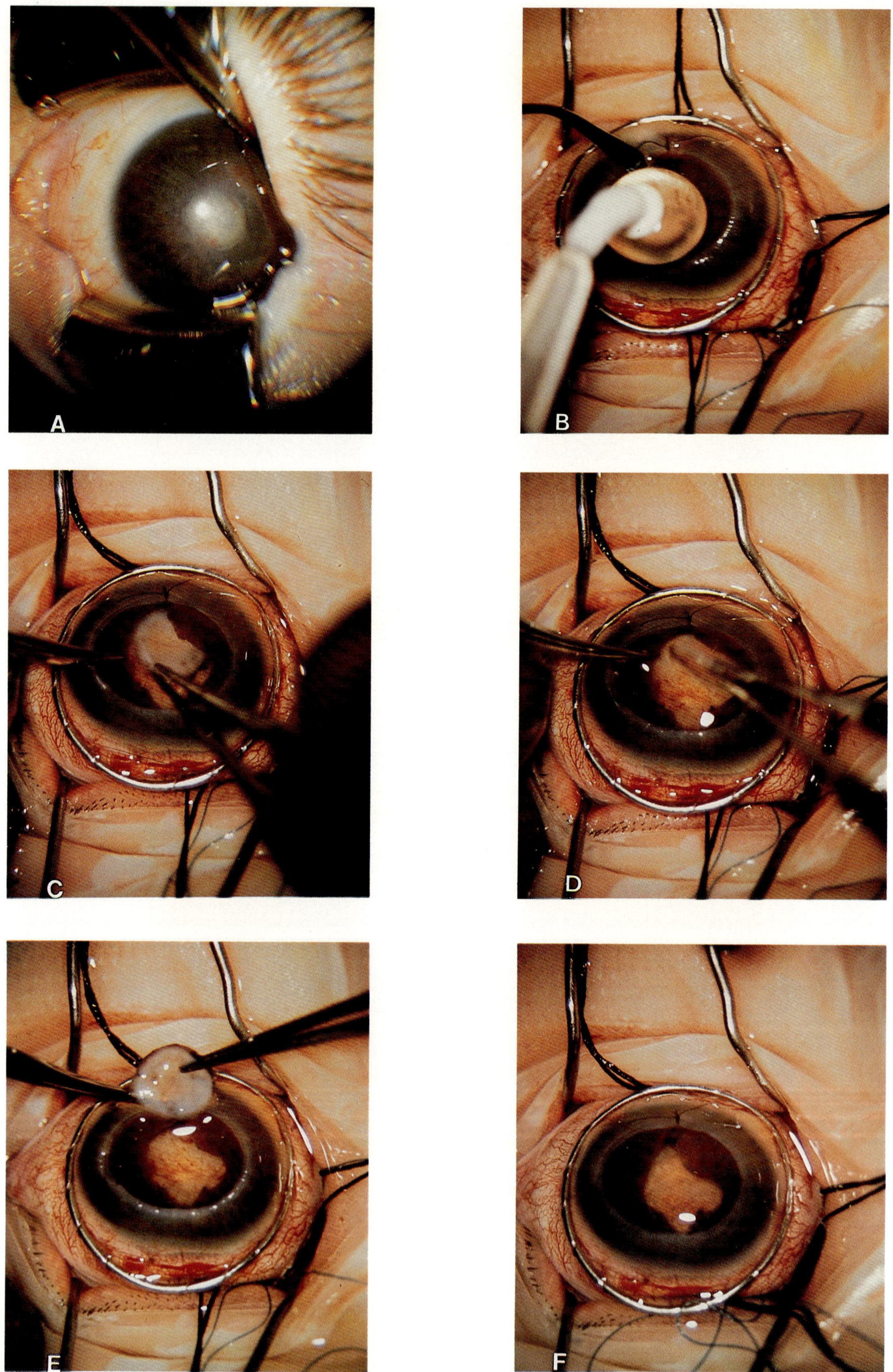

Color Plate 14

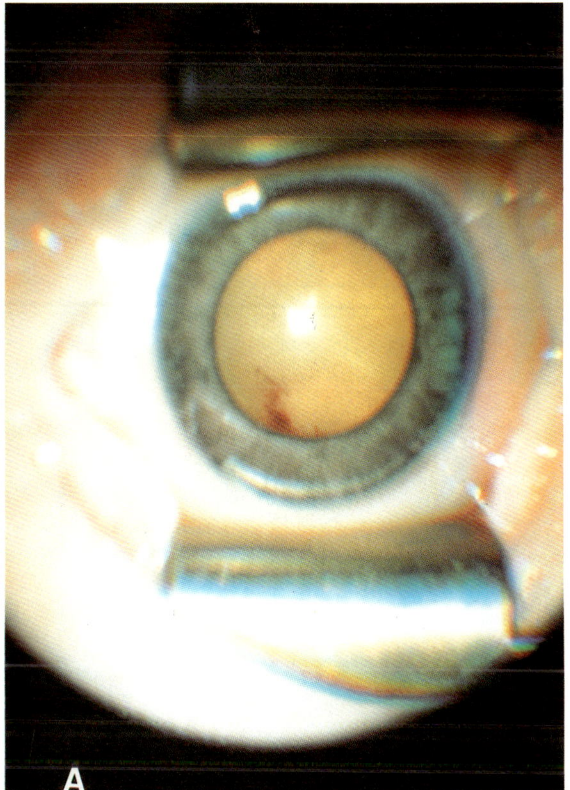
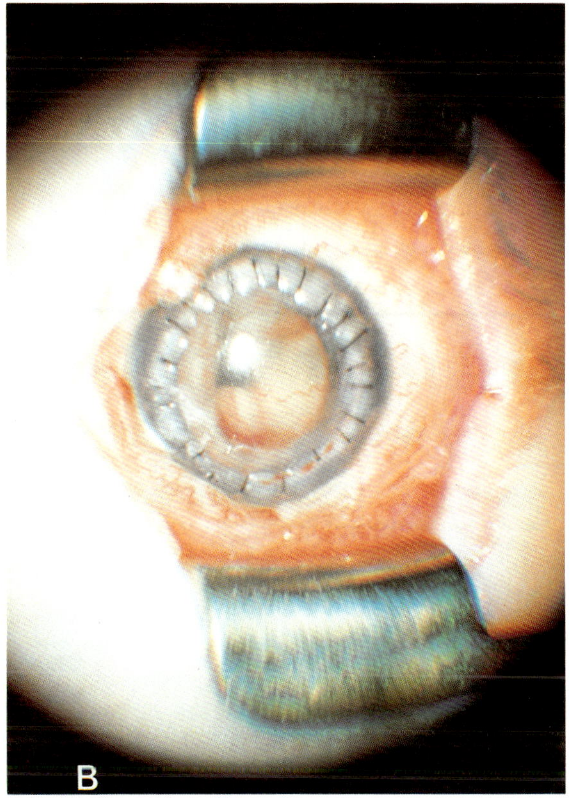
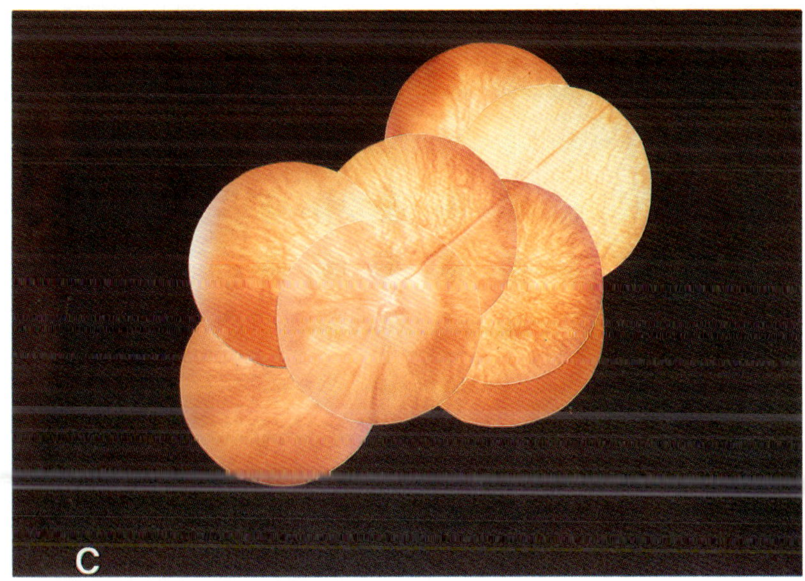

Color Plate 15

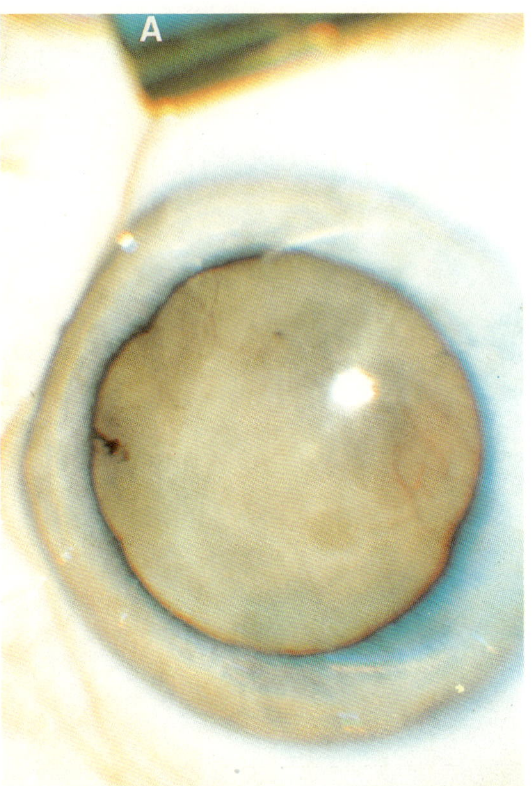

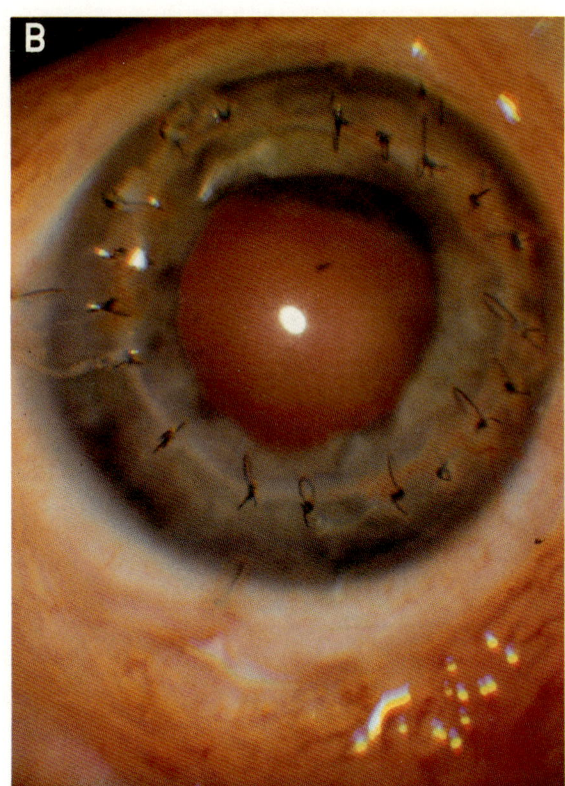

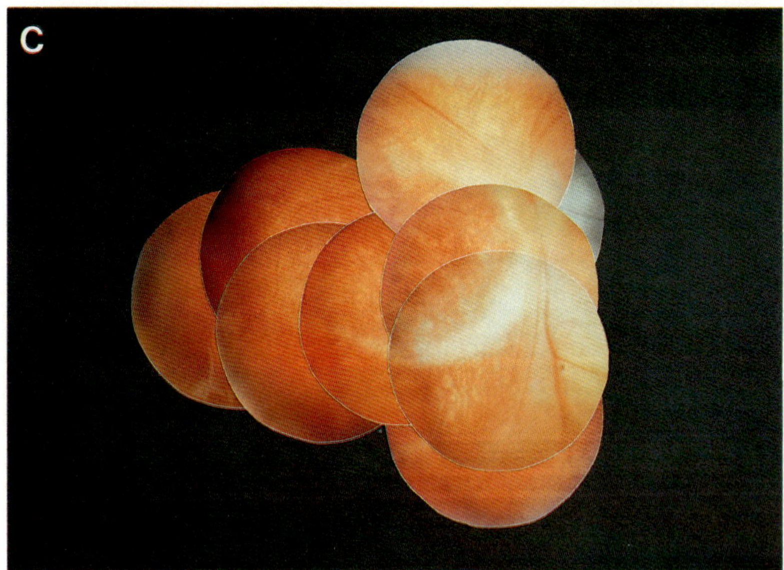

Color Plate 16

Vitrectomy with Ciliary Body Entry for Retrolental Fibroplasia   20

Steve Charles, M.D.

Despite medical therapy, cryotherapy, and scleral buckling, a considerable number of low-birth-weight infants develop end-stage retinopathy of prematurity (ROP). Surgery for the Stage 5 narrow- or closed-cone traction retinal detachment was not possible until I developed, in 1977, a transciliary body vitreous surgical approach with scissors delamination. In this chapter, I describe current indications, methods, and results.

SURGICAL ANATOMY

Current clinical practice frequently describes the typical anatomic picture with incorrect terms such as "disorganized retina," "retrolental mass," and "inoperable retinal detachment." A better understanding of the anatomic configuration permits more accurate preoperative evaluation and surgery. As in other disease entities, cellular migration and proliferation occur on retinal or vitreous surfaces. Cellular proliferation at the posterior hyaloid face (PHF) interface creates adherence between these layers and curved planar contraction (Fig. 20–1). As retinal detachment develops, this interface folds upon itself, creating apparent retinal-retinal adherence.

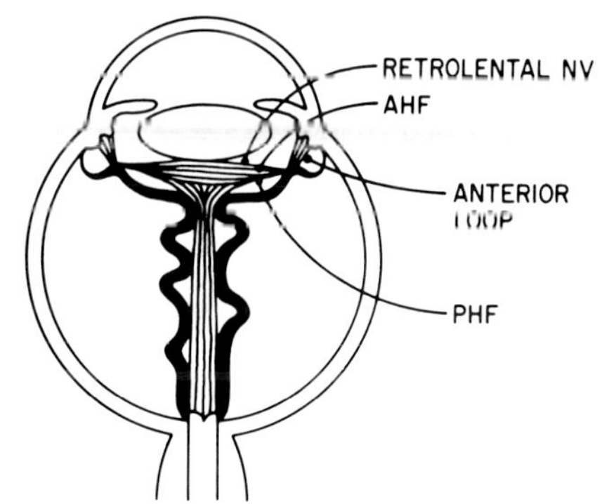

Figure 20–1   Proliferation life cycle

Marked adherence of PHF to equatorial retina pulls the equator anteriorly, creating a marked concavity of this preequatorial retina, often mistaken for a dialysis.

Anteriorly, proliferation occurs along the anterior hyaloid face (AHF)-lens interface, creating the well-known retrolental membrane (RLM). This is frequently incorrectly described as a retrolental mass when, in fact, it is a thin planar structure. The majority of vessels seen at this interface are actually retinal vessels translocated centrally because of the posterior interface contraction and resultant closed-cone traction retinal detachment. As the PHF-retinal interface moves anteriorly, it comes into contact with the AHF-lens interface, creating a four-layered complex known as the "retrolental membrane plate" or "complex."

PREOPERATIVE EVALUATION

Office Technique

Every attempt should be made to keep the infant cradled in a normal position in the parent's arms, rather than restrained. Eyelids should only be retracted manually if absolutely necessary. Because they have poor vision, these children usually squeeze their lids closed in response to physical stimulation of the lids, rather than to light. Under no circumstances should any form of sedation be utilized in the office environment because of the increased risk of cardiac and respiratory arrest. Frequently, quick looks as the child moves about without restraint or lid retraction is the best method.

Examination Under Anesthesia

Examination under anesthesia should only be undertaken if a form of therapy has a reasonable chance of being performed at the same time. Anesthesia risks are such that it should not be used for a work-up only because of protocol mentalities. The parents must have preexamination informed consent about surgical options, including none, lensectomy only, or lensectomy-vitrectomy, and in many instances either eye may be operated upon.

Electrophysiological Testing

The electroretinogram (ERG) is always nonrecordable in total retinal detachment. Almost all patients with an opaque retrolental plate have a total or near-total detachment. The ERG is useless in the evaluation of these children; anesthesia time should not be utilized for this purpose. There is no evidence that the visually-evoked potential (VEP) is of any predictive value with patients who have light perception. Light perception can be determined by children's blinking and head movements in response to light, without expensive inconclusive VEP testing. Sector scan, real-time contact ultrasonography, can be valuable primarily in evaluation of the opaque cornea and the rare, totally opaque retrolental-plate patient. The scan can be performed quite well in the office and does not require sedation or anesthesia. The closed-cone-traction retinal detachments are frequently misinterpreted as ''stalks'' or ''disorganized fibrotic tissue.'' Knowledge of the anatomy and surgical experience allow more accurate ultrasonographic diagnoses.

Many patients are said to have ''iris neovascularization,'' or rubeosis, when in fact they have persistent tunica vasculosa lentis. These patients can develop corneal edema secondary to corneal-iris contact from a pupillary-block mechanism. Persistence of tunica vasculosa lentis might play a role in the development of the retrolental plate, as well.

There is often thick yellow-brown material in the subretinal space. In late cases, it can be replaced by dense honeycomb-like plaques, dendritic configurations, and cholesterol crystals.

Timing

While emphasis has been on the early course of this disease, the period following six months needs greater attention. Dilated iris and retinal vessels indicate activity of the disease and are relative contraindications to surgery. Similarly, an exudative component to the retinal detachment, determined by retinal convexity and

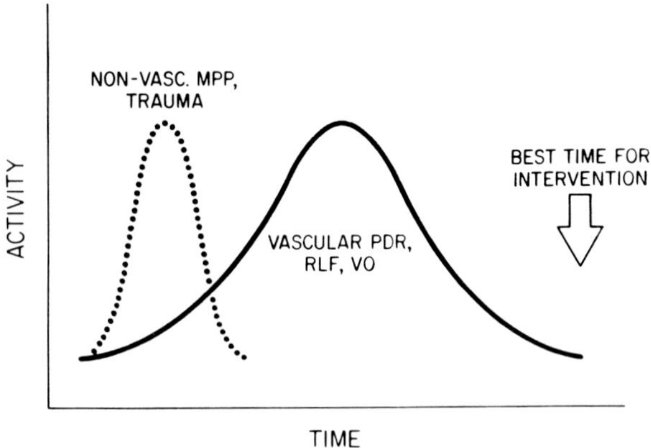

Figure 20–2 Basic anatomy of RLF

subretinal exudate, suggests delaying surgery. Surgery on active cases appears to have a higher reproliferation rate (Fig. 20–2).

Another advantage of delay is the reduction in anesthesia risk associated with greater body weight and better pulmonary function (Fig. 20-3). If there is any question about the medical situation, surgery should be delayed; there have been successful operations done on 18-month-old patients. There is an inherent compromise: early operations should result in better visual function and more straightforward surgical anatomy, but these are combined with greater medical risk and reproliferation.

Bilaterality

Because of the certainty of severe amblyopia, high anesthesia risk, and relatively poor prognosis, most unilateral cases should not be operated upon.

Risk Analysis

Because of the current 45 percent success rate, only ambulatory vision in successful cases, and high medical risk, care must be taken to secure informed consent. Competent anesthesiologists experienced in infant anesthesia must be included. Preoperative evaluation and postoperative medical management require an experienced neonatologist or pediatrician.

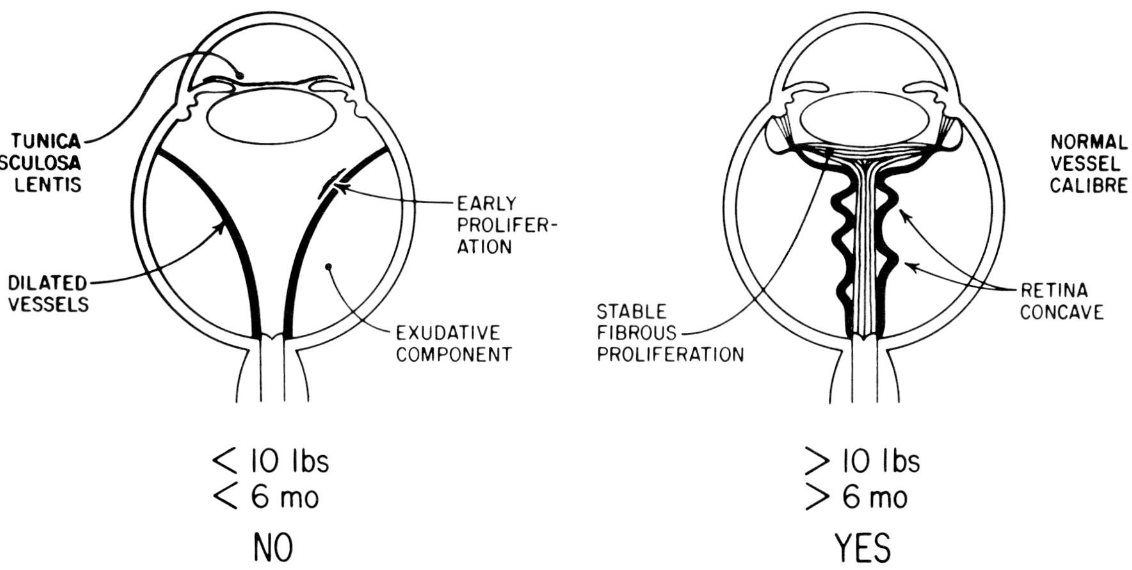

Figure 20–3 Indications in RLF

SURGICAL APPROACH

Combined Examination Under Anesthesia

If the office examination was inadequate to determine the need for surgery, mask insufflation anesthesia with quick, indirect ophthalmoscopy should confirm the need for surgery and indicate the best-prognosis eye. Because of the relationship between anesthesia and morbidity-mortality, there is no time for retinal drawings and prolonged photographic procedures. If the need for surgery is confirmed, the patient should be intubated, prepped, and draped.

Entry Site

Limbal entry creates striate keratopathy, regional corneal edema, wound leaks, and poor access to the preequatorial traction (Fig. 20-4). Pars plana entry brings the instruments into the subretinal space and creates an obligatory dialysis. Ciliary body entry approximately 0.5 to 1.0 mm posterior to the limbus is the safest. This entry into the iris root frequently requires sector iridotomy at this site or passage anterior to the iris. All incisions should be made with a single puncture with the 20-gauge shank, 1.4-mm blade lancet tip microvitreoretinal blade (MVR, from SSI). A 30-degree-bent, 20-gauge, blunt-

tipped infusion cannula (May) is utilized at a site slightly superior to the middle of the medial rectus. Bimanual technique allows small incisions, mobility of the globe, and interchangeability between nasal and temporal instruments. Coaxial illumination from the microscope without a fundus contact lens is used because of the anterior location of the retinal disease process. Standard sew-on infusion cannulas tend to strike the lid margins and rotate posteriorly into the subretinal space. Full-function probes with coaxial infusion are too large for these small eyes.

Lensectomy

An aspirating ultrasonic fragmenter (Mid Labs), combined with foot controlled delta (linear) suction, is

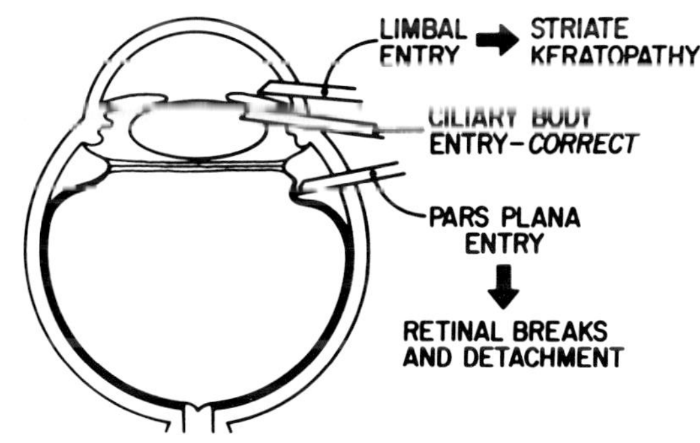

Figure 20–4 Entry in RLF

required in all cases. Even the best vitreous cutters (Microvit) are too slow for lensectomy. Care should be taken to remove all peripheral cortex, using scleral depression to visualize the periphery. Continuous and simultaneous aspiration and fragmentation should be used, because luminal fluid flow cools the sclera better than pulsed ultrasound (Fig. 20-5).

Anterior capsulotomy should be initiated with the MVR blade (Fig. 20-6). If any peripheral anterior synechiae or area of flat chamber are present, a micro iris spatula passed through the temporal incision can be used to press back the nasal iris diaphragm. The nasal infusion cannula can then be used to press down the temporal half of the iris. Anterior capsulectomy can then be performed with a 20-gauge, delta suction guillotine cutter (Microvit). If the retinal vessels are too active and the procedure performed only because of glaucoma and flat chamber, the wounds should be closed at this point.

Pupillary Dilation

Epinephrine is of little value here, because the iris is rigid and the drug can contribute to arrhythmias. Scissors should make multiple sphincterotomies rather than removing large amounts of iris with vitreous cutters. Scleral depression (Fig. 20–7) to visualize the periphery is preferable to extensive iridectomy. Care to avoid hypotony lessens pupillary constriction.

Retrolental Plate

Posterior capsule, AHF, PHF, and the internal limiting lamina (ILL) of the retina are usually in contact as a single

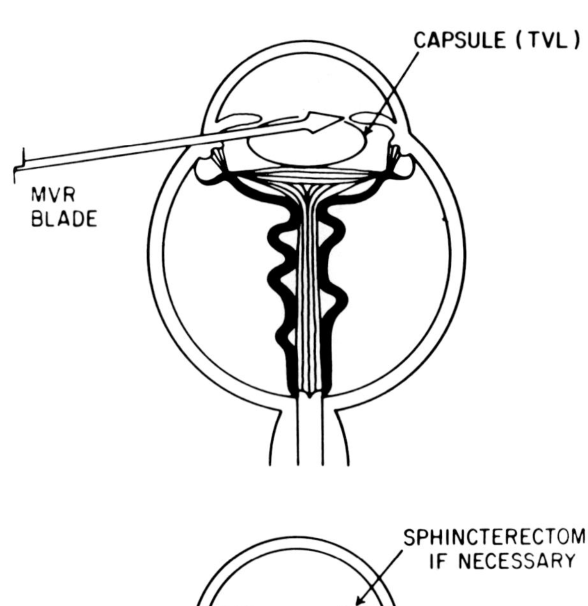

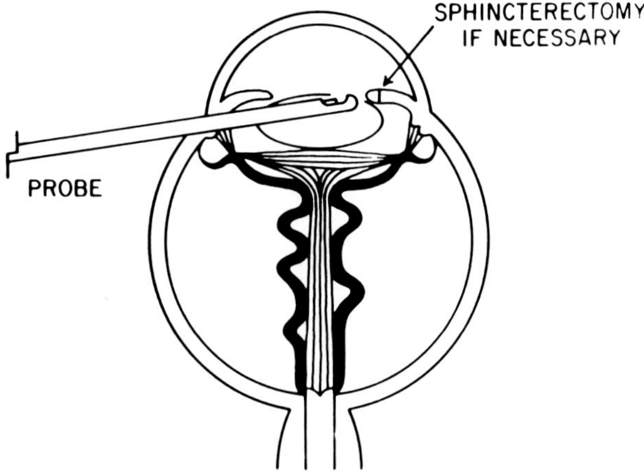

Figure 20–6 Anterior capsulotomy and capsulectomy, initiated with MVR blade

plate stretching from equator to equator. The retina is not in contact in a varying area centrally, depending on the narrowness of the conical detachment. At times, the peripheral edge of the plate can be seen, allowing the dissection to begin peripherally. The plate is of matte finish and white, while the retina is always shiny and pale

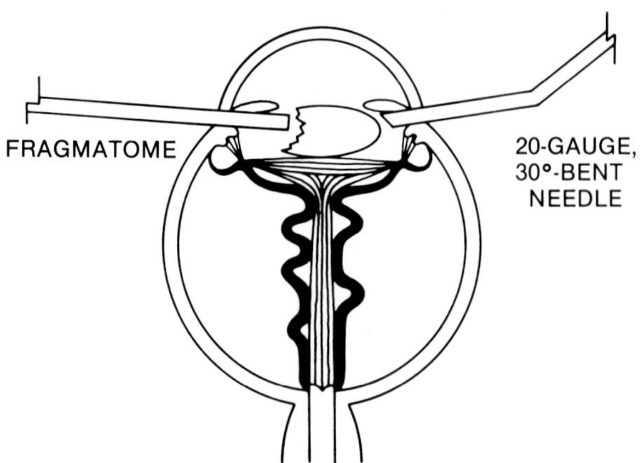

Figure 20–5 Aspirating ultrasonic fragmenter used in lensectomy

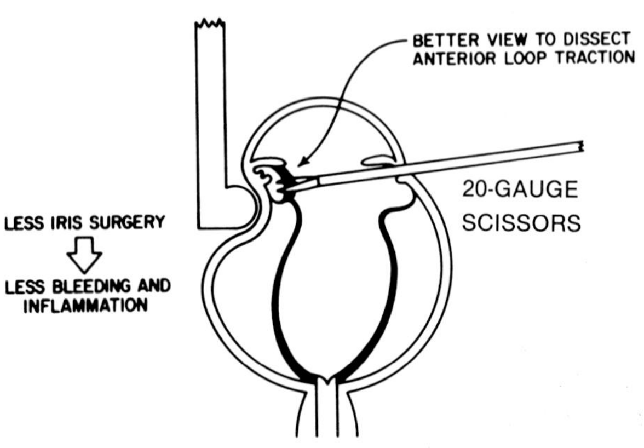

Figure 20–7 Scleral depression in RLF.

yellow. Recognition of this uniform finding in children and adults prevents anatomic confusion and disastrous results. Care must be taken not to displace the plate horizontally, as this will create large dialyses, frequently including the retinal pigment epithelium (RPE) and choroid.

The initial incision should be made, with the Charles modified Sutherland scissors (Fig. 20-8, Grieshaber) used for the entire dissection. The sharp tips are required for the initial incision in the plate, blunt tips and occasionally long 45-degree blades or vertical configurations to be used later. If the first incision is central, multiple radial cuts extending to the preequatorial area create a stellate appearance. These cuts should be full thickness, traversing posterior capsule, AHF, and PHF, allowing visualization of the pale yellow, shiny, retinal surface. If a preequatorial initial incision is used, circumferential cutting, 360 degrees (Fig. 20-9), should be done by alternating the scissors and infusion cannula from temporal to nasal. Following this circumferential cut, radial cuts through the plate, beginning peripherally, accomplish "segmentation" or "plate delamination."

Delamination

Because of marked adherence at the PHF-retinal interface, membrane peeling or stripping is *never* possible. Segmentation leaves too much epiretinal membrane (ERM) and structural rigidity. Small isolated areas of ERM can be left adherent to atrophic retina.

In all cases, delamination is the best method of removal of PHF/ERM. It is accomplished with the modified Sutherland scissors, the blades parallel to the retinal surface (Fig. 20-10). At times, 45-degree or vertical-modified Sutherland scissors are necessary to achieve this parallel orientation.

After the stellate cuts, multiple cuts, greater than 1,000, with the delamination scissors allow removal of

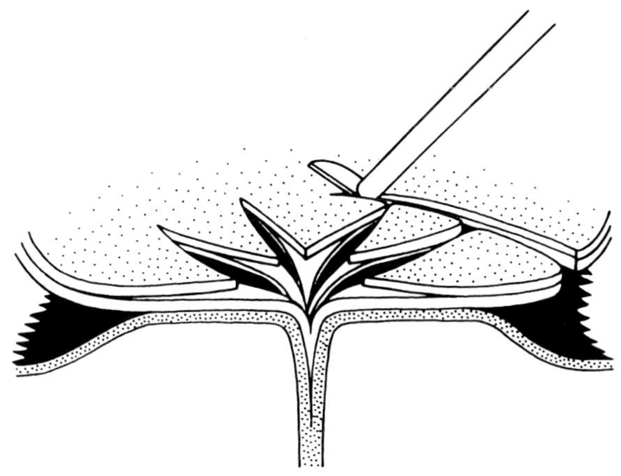

Figure 20–9 Anterior loop dissection

all PHF/ERM segments. After these are free-floating, they should be removed from the eye with the vitreous cutter. With experience, some PHF/ERM segments can be removed with the 20-gauge guillotine delta suction vitreous cutter (Microvit). At times the plate is calcified, requiring the Charles-modified long, thick-bladed Sutherland scissors, developed for the subretinal space.

Coagulation

In attempting to reduce retinal necrosis and reproliferation, bipolar diathermy to control bleeding should be avoided when possible. The infusion cannula can wash blood away from the dissection site; intermittent elevation of the infusion bottle can be used to control bleeding as well.

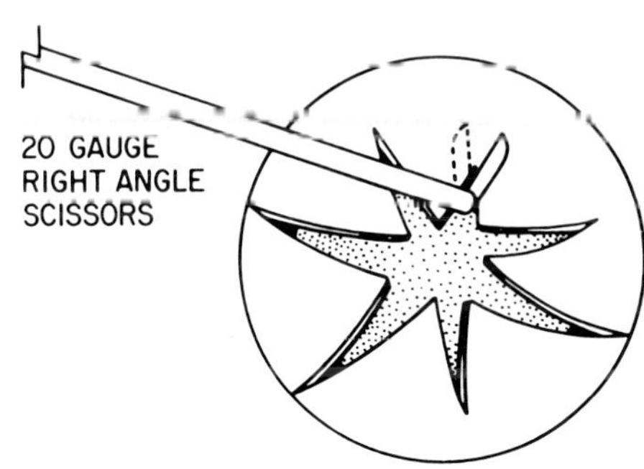

Figure 20–8 Stellate incisions in RLM

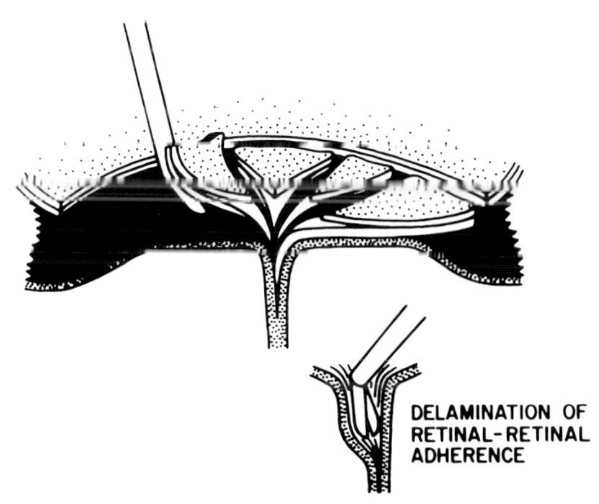

Figure 20–10 ERM delamination

Vitreous Substitutes

Infusion fluid (BSS Plus), hyaluronic acid, air, and 15 percent air perfluoropropane mixtures have been used with, at present, inconclusive differences.

Infusion fluid requires no positioning, does not enhance reproliferation, clears blood rapidly, and requires no FDA approval. But the lack of surface tension allows transretinal fluid flow through tiny retinal breaks-dialyses, causing rhegmatogenous detachment.

Hyaluronic acid is a pseudoplastic, non-Neutonian fluid having minimal surface tension. It easily reaches the subretinal space through small retinal breaks. Hyaluronic acid prolongs the presence of attractants, growth factors, blood, cells, and protein, all instrumental in reproliferation. Because of reproliferation, low surface tension and a high incidence of glaucoma, hyaluronic acid is no longer utilized.

Air-gas mixtures have a 50 percent higher surface tension than silicone but can cause iris-retinal contact with postoperative iris-retinal adherence. Air (gas) has some role in stimulating reproliferation, presumably because of prevention of aqueous contact with the intraocular surfaces. Air lasts only 3 to 4 days, while a nonexpansile 20 percent SF-6 mixture lasts 7 days, and 15 percent perfluoropropane lasts 30 days. Air (gases) are utilized when a retinal break is seen or subretinal fluid is seen internally or externally, as a result of communication of the subretinal space with the subnonpigmented epithelial space, at the entry wounds.

Silicone might be a good choice in these cases, but it can cause glaucoma and corneal changes and is not approved by the FDA. Many surgeons remove the silicone after the cases stabilize, in three to six months.

Fluid-Air (Gas) Exchange

Foot-controlled power injections should be used to infuse air (gas) through the infusion cannula (Fig. 20-11). Fluid egress should be through a tapered extrusion needle foot controlled by a delta linear suction system (Microvit).

Subretinal Fluid Drainage

Internal drainage of subretinal fluid (SRF) should be avoided, because structural rigidity of the retina often prevents complete reattachment, and subretinal air or gas will follow the needle into the subretinal space via surface tension. External drainage of subretinal fluid is done in all cases, except reoperations with minimal elevation. Foot-pedal control by the delta suction system, consisting of a 25-gauge ⅝-inch needle placed obliquely through the equatorial sclera, is the safest and most efficient method of drainage (Fig. 20–12). A marked transretinal pressure gradient should be avoided, as it can cause relief tears of the retina (Fig. 20–13). Frequently, subretinal fluid will be communicated from the subretinal space to the supranonpigmented epithelial space in the intraocular space (Fig. 20–14).

Scleral Buckling

Delamination of the equatorial PHF/ERM surface, combined with circumferential dissection of preequatorial plate, or anterior loop traction, eliminates the need for scleral buckling. The problem of scleral intrusion of the buckle is avoided (Fig. 20–15).

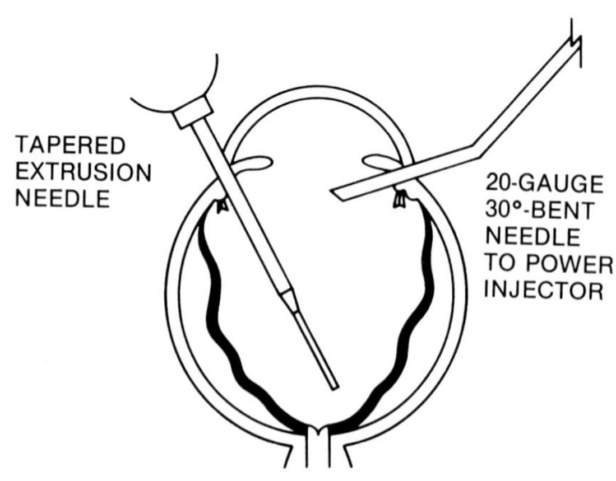

Figure 20–11   Internal fluid/gas exchange

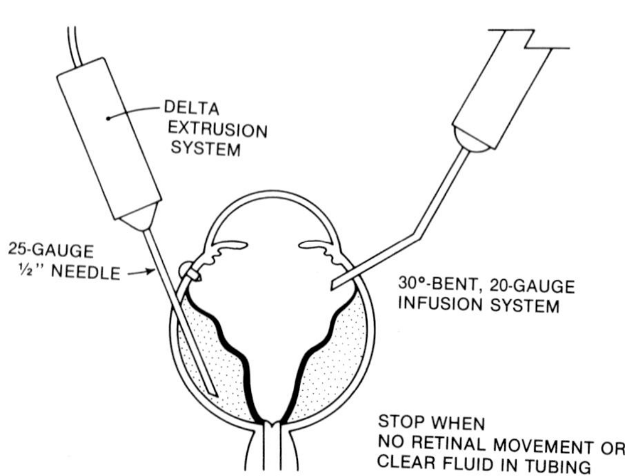

Figure 20–12   Subretinal fluid drainage

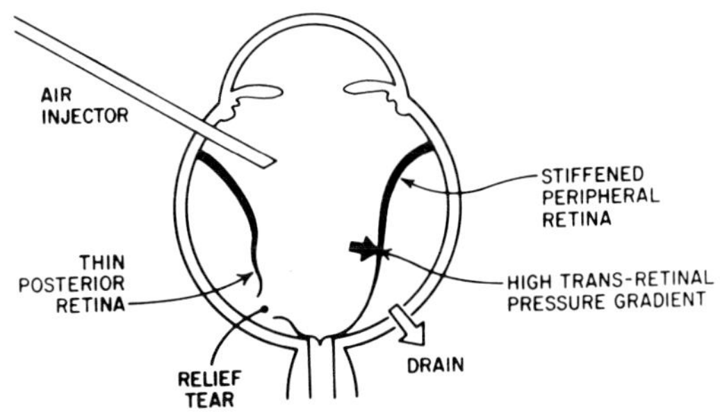

Figure 20–13 Subretinal fluid drainage-induced retinal break

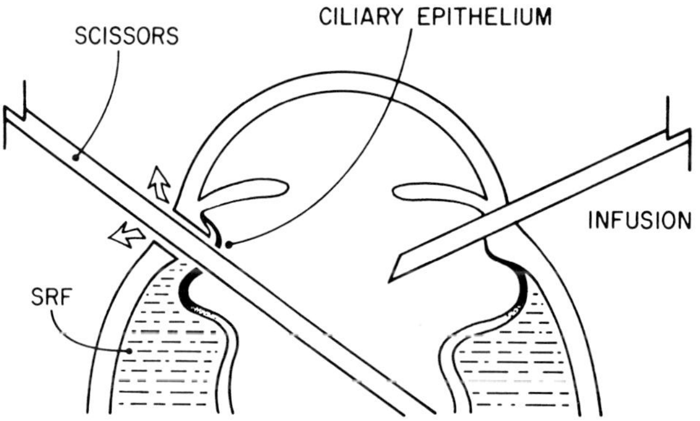

Figure 20–14 Drainage of subretinal fluid through sclerotomy

Scleral buckling increases iris-retinal adherence by translocating equatorial sclera-retina centrally and anteriorly toward the capsule remnants and posterior iris surface. Scleral buckling necessitates rectus muscle traction sutures and traction-induced bradycardia. Sufficient anticholinergic agents to block this reflex can cause tachycardia and postoperative pulmonary problems. Occasionally, circumferential segmental buckles are done for retinal breaks. In these instances, carved, hard silicone exoplants should be utilized because of flexibility, speed, and low extrusion rate.

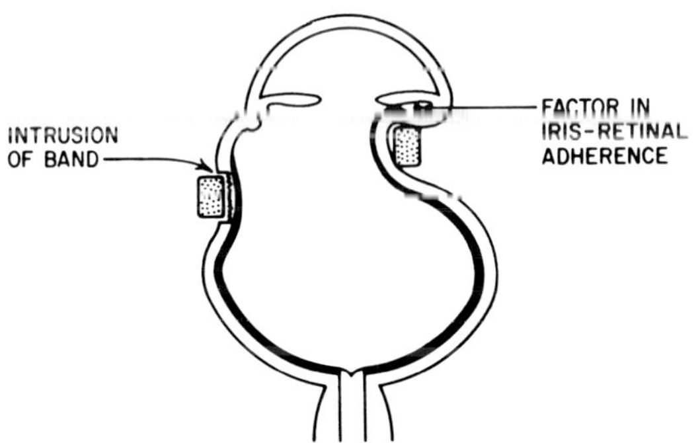

Figure 20–15 Scleral buckling problems in RLF

Retinal Suturing

Surface tension agents and buckles are usually insufficient for major retinal choroidal dialyses, so that retinal suturing is required. A simple method is to push the retina into position with the infusion cannula, with a scleral plug in the opposite opening. A 5–0 monofilament nylon suture with a long needle is then placed through the sclera, retina, and sclera again in a single looplike pass and tied externally (Fig. 20–16).

Retinal Glue

Cyanoacrylate, polymer glues have been utilized when scleral buckling was not practical, but it is thought that retinal structural rigidity would prevent retina-RPE contact at a retinal break. Cyanoacrylates are not approved by the FDA, and it is hoped that better, more flexible, less toxic glues will be developed. The glue is applied after fluid/gas exchange, followed by needle drainage of subretinal fluid and removal of the gas (Fig. 20–17).

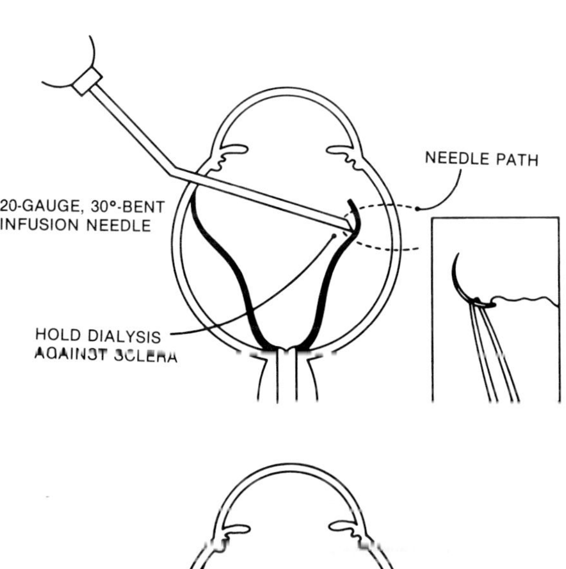

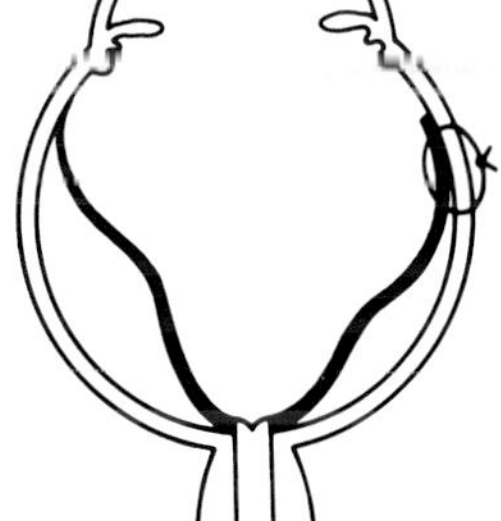

Figure 20–16 Retinal suturing for RLF

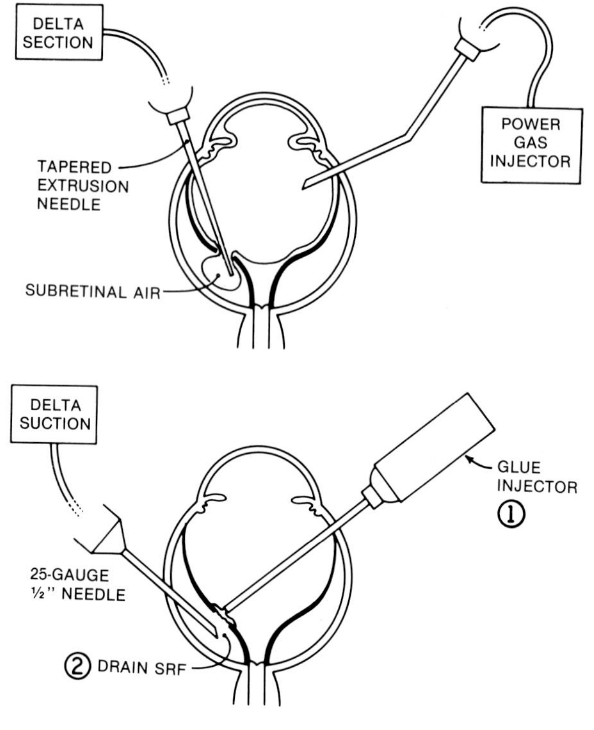

Figure 20–17 Retinal glue for RLF

Wound Closure

At the end of the dissection, after possible use of surface tension agents and subretinal fluid drainage, a 22-gauge tapered, flexible intravenous cannula (Jelco) is substituted for the infusion cannula (Fig. 20-18). Two

passes of an 8–0 monofilament nylon shoelace suture are then placed around the cannula, three loops made, and the knot pulled up as the assistant withdraws the cannula, retaining normal intraocular pressure.

Reproliferation

A significant number of cases that have had complete delamination of all PHF/ERM redetach as a result of recurrent proliferation. Factors in this reproliferation include lens material, blood, surgical disruption of ILL, diathermy, and surface tension agents. Iris-retinal adherence is a frequent configuration (Fig. 20–19), but many other localized or widespread reproliferations on the retinal surface are prevalent. It is hoped that glue will reduce reproliferation by elimination of surface tension agents.

Antiproliferative agents such as 5–fluorouracil have been utilized but have therapeutic ratio problems and pharmacokinetic problems of four to six hours duration. While hyaluronic acid can double the duration of 1 mg of intraocular 5–fluorouracil, this positive effect is counterbalanced by the stimulation of reproliferation. Ten mg of subconjunctival 5–fluorouracil are instilled, but this specific use of this approved drug has not been approved by the FDA. Subconjunctival triamcinolone acetate, 20 mg of Kenalog, is utilized in all cases to reduce inflammation.

The surgical approach to reproliferation utilizes the same delamination technique as in primary surgery.

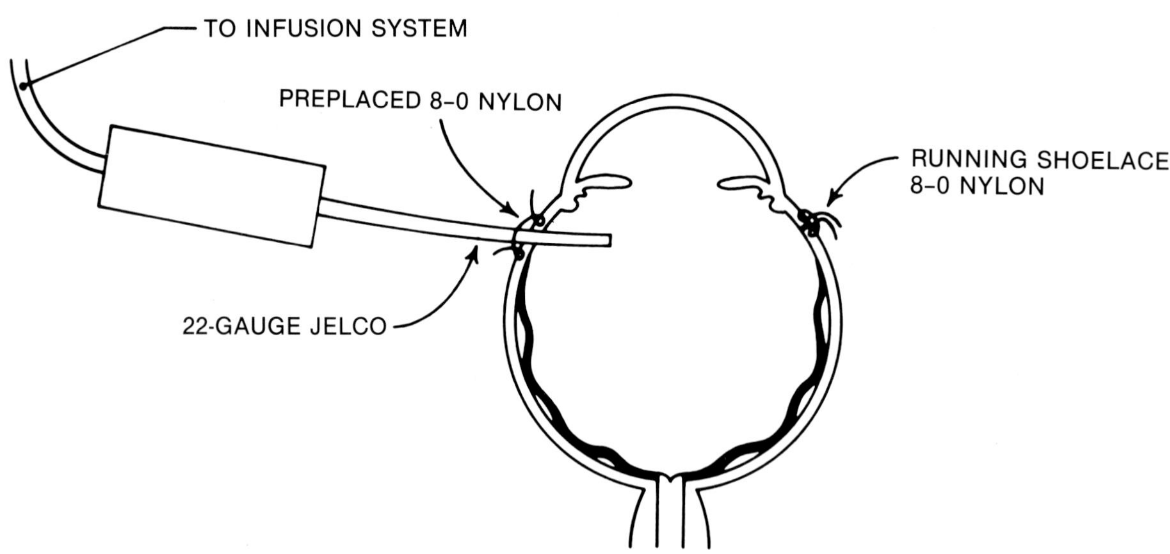

Figure 20–18 Wound closure

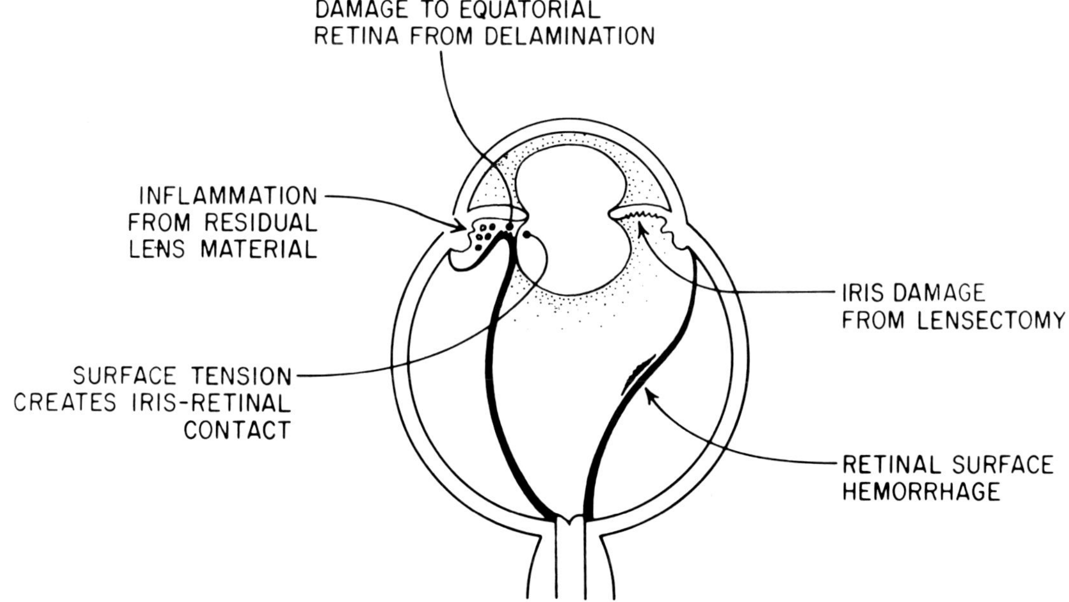

Figure 20–19 Pathogenesis of iris-retinal adherence

When this retinal adherence is present, infusion cannulas and instruments must be made very anterior by an MVR-blade puncture through the iris root or the potential space iris and equatorial retina (Fig. 20–20).

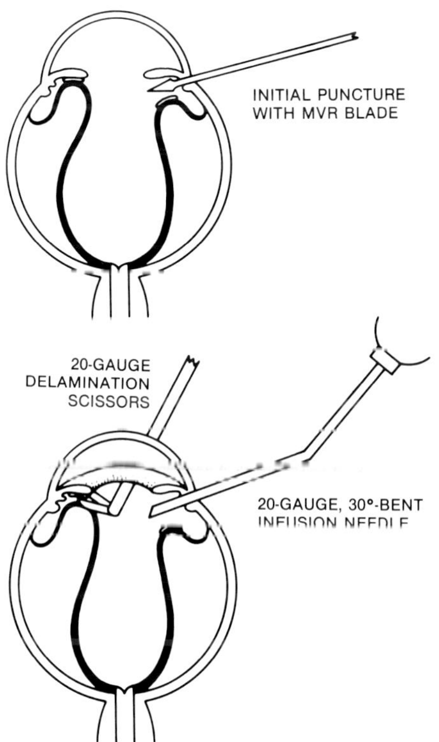

Figure 20–20 Reoperation for iris-retinal adherence

Visual Rehabilitation

Residual subretinal fluid is pumped out very slowly by the RPE, often requiring 2 to 6 months for maximal reattachment. Only when reattachment occurs can slow repair of rod and cone outer segments begin. Animal studies have shown a rough correlation between the durationof retinal detachment and recovery period. After reattachment occurs, full retinoscopic correction of 18 to 30 diopters should be worn full-time, even without evidence of visual behavior. Full visual recovery can take as much as 2 to 3 years postoperatively because of these factors and slow central nervous system development. The parents and consulting physician should be informed of this slow recovery so as to encourage full-time use of aphakic correction.

Slow visual recovery, the difficulty of visual testing in children, and recent progress in the management of these patients make statistical interpretation of results difficult.

A consecutive series of 580 eyes operated upon by the author (January 1977 to September 1985) demonstrated a 46 percent anatomic success rate. Another 31 percent had minimal or no return of epiretinal membrane, concave retina, but the retinas were not attached. Some will ultimately attach, but the remaining infants will be afflicted by rigidity of the retina or subretinal proliferation. Phthisis is very rare in the group, because of removal of cyclitic membrane. The ultimate anatomic success rate with current methodology is in excess of 50 percent and probably approaches 60 percent, depending on case selection.

Less than 3 percent were inoperable at the primary surgery, with an average of 1.3 operations per eye done. Essentially all anatomic failures were because of reproliferation. It is estimated that there will be a small, late failure rate because of glaucoma, although this has not been noted in the early series.

Visual success rates were about 10 percent less than anatomic success rates and depend on visual criteria. Hand motion perception is of little value to these patients and is not considered a visual success. Unequivocal ability to pick up small objects and ambulate in familiar surroundings without striking obstacles are minimum criteria for visual success. A few older children can now read large print, and one child sees 20/200. The families were informed that none of the children will attain reading or driving visual levels.

Irreversible photoreceptor degeneration, the effects of subretinal blood, the possible failure of development of photoreceptors, retinal hypoxia, and central nervous system changes result in attached retinas but no useful vision. Amblyopia is a certainty if one eye is functionally superior to the other.

The current method returns 35 to 45 percent of otherwise inoperable Stage 5 total traction retinal detachments to functional vision. It is anticipated that improvements in vitreous substitutes, glues and antimigration proliferation therapy will reduce reproliferation. Lasers or material science technology might improve cutting capability and facilitate delamination.

As in other proliferative retinopathies, prevention is the ultimate goal, with this methodology used in the interim.

These data were collected and analyzed statistically by Patrick Riddle, M.D.

The author acknowledges illustrations and photography by Ned Hockman, Professor of Cinema at the University of Oklahoma, and typing by Sabrina Early.

INDEX

Numerals in *italics* indicate a figure, page numbers followed by a "t" indicate tabular matter.